Iyengar

Iyengar

The Yoga Master

EDITED BY KOFI BUSIA

Shambhala
Boston and London
2007

SHAMBHALA PUBLICATIONS, INC.
Horticultural Hall
300 Massachusetts Avenue
Boston, Massachusetts 02115
www.shambhala.com

9 8 7 6 5 4 3 2 1

First Edition
Printed in the United States of America

⊛ This edition is printed on acid-free paper that meets the
American National Standards Institute z39.48 Standard.
Distributed in the United States by Random House, Inc.,
and in Canada by Random House of Canada Ltd

Designed by Jeff Baker

Library of Congress Cataloging-in-Publication Data
Iyengar, B. K. S., 1918–
Iyengar: the yoga master / B. K. S. Iyengar; edited by Kofi
Busia.—1st ed.
p. cm.
Includes index.
ISBN 978-1-59030-524-9 (alk. paper)
1. Iyengar, B. K. S., 1918– 2. Hatha yoga. I. Busia, Kofi
(Kofi A.), 1951–
II. Title.
RA781.7.L887 2007
613.7'046—dc22
2007001680

This book is dedicated to Yogacharya Sri B. K. S. Iyengar in honor and appreciation of his life and work.

Contents

Contents

EDITOR'S NOTE

The English alphabet has five vowels and twenty-one consonants, whereas Sanskrit, the language of India—and of yoga—has fifteen vowels and thirty-three consonants. There is obviously going to be a problem representing all those different sounds. English also has conventions for using capital letters that raise issues that do not arise in Sanskrit. Chögyam Trungpa Rinpoche, author of the classic book *Cutting Through Spiritual Materialism* and many other works, used to counsel his editors to spell words such as *christianity, buddhism, zen,* and *islam* in lowercase. The fact that many readers might take offense at this surely illustrates his point that the capitals put people into a state of reverence that might not always be helpful when they should be bringing the intellect to bear.

For example, if the phrase "the saintly Ramanuja would sometimes become merged with God" is an acceptable use of capitalization, then what about "the saintly Ramanuja would sometimes become merged with Brahman"? God (as understood in the West) is not the same as Brahman, although it (It?) can play the same role. But if we recognize that role and write *Brahman* rather than *brahman,* then should we not write *Purusha* rather than *purusha,* to represent the indivisible, ineffable Spirit of the universe—or should that be spirit? And shouldn't we be writing *Nature* and *Prakriti* to represent the complement to Spirit, instead of *nature* and *prakriti*?

This book follows the standard English convention for *God,* for words like *Buddhism* and *Newtonian,* and for the personal names of the various divinities such as *Krishna.* But as what some cognoscenti might consider a strange exception, everything "conceptual" is set in initial lowercase, except for Ishvara, which can be roughly translated as "lord." We did this to indicate its special iconic status in yoga philosophy. Ishvara is—roughly speaking—that part of purusha that is always pure. It is unembodied, indivisible spirit, even though parts of that same purusha do somehow seem to become embodied in each of us as our separate, infinite souls.

Since this book is dedicated to B. K. S. Iyengar, we have followed his example of openness, clarity, and simplicity. It is our hope that many people new to yoga will read this book and be inspired to take up yoga. Although the chapters range from the simple to the sophisticated, all Sanskrit terms have been transliterated as phonetically as possible. So you will mostly find *Shiva* rather than *Siva* and *Vishnu* rather than *Visnu*. Knowledgable Sanskrit scholars are asked to forgive this indulgence. There was once a time when they also were not sure how to pronounce things. An immediate exception is, of course, with Sri B. K. S. Iyengar himself, who always uses the *Sri* spelling with his name. In deference to him, and to any other people whose names demand it, we used *Sri* (instead of *Shri*). In general, however, the Sanskrit words you see in this book can be pronounced as they are written. So, it's *chakra* and *chitta,* to make it clear that the sound is *ch* as in *church,* rather than *cakra* and *citta,* because people might otherwise inadvertently pronounce these with a hard *c* as in *cat,* or with a soft *c* as in *citation.* But if *chakra* is written with *ch,* then what about the aspirated sound, which should then logically be represented by *chh?* Fortunately, that letter occurs so rarely that we have followed the general convention of ignoring it.

But to ignore Sanskrit aspirations completely would then ask the English letter *t* to do the work of four different Sanskrit letters, which seems rather onerous for one poor letter. It would be representing the two variants of *t* in the Sanskrit alphabet, along with the two aspirated or *th* variants of those. Since English simply does not have enough letters, some compromises are necessary. So, whenever you see a *th* it is to be pronounced like the *th* in *Thomas* rather than like that in *the.* As in many other books, we do not distinguish between the two different kinds of *t* or *th*. But in spite of these good intentions, the conventions for yoga poses are now so entrenched that we were loath to go against them. One or two of the contributors also had their personal foibles about how they preferred things to be spelled within their individual essays. You will therefore see the occasional anomaly such as the word for "west" being spelled *pashchima* when it is used outside a pose name, but becoming *paschimottanasana* when used inside one; or a word being transliterated one way in one chapter only to be spelled slightly differently in another. Please excuse these differences.

Another use of capitalization is as a way of distinguishing names or styles of yoga such as Bikram Yoga, Anusara Yoga, or Iyengar Yoga; from the more generalized philosophies, methodologies, or approaches such as karma yoga, jnana yoga, or bhakti yoga. So, Ashtanga Yoga would refer to the specific school or style of practice founded by Pattabhi Jois; whereas ashtanga yoga would refer to the philosophical classification and exposition of yoga proffered by Patanjali. Kundalini Yoga would refer to the school established by Yogi Bhajan; whereas kundalini yoga would refer to the energy-based approach to yoga associated with the chakras and with Tantra practices.

Introduction

It is hard to know when this book started, so I'll say that it was 1969 or 1970 while I was a student. I was standing in the University Gym. My friend Jeremy happened by, and I asked him, "What are *you* doing here?" He was not exactly the kind of person you expect to see in a gym. He said, "I've come for a yoga lesson." I chuckled—the knowing kind of chuckle you give when you've just been handed some good dinner-table gossip concerning someone else's absurdity. "Well," said Jeremy, "I really think *you* should have a lesson before you react like that." My father had tried to bring me up to be just, so I decided that my friend had a point. I picked up my badminton kit and followed him. *Anyway,* I thought to myself, *it's surely better to laugh knowingly, with lots of juicy details, than to laugh in ignorance.* But my life was about to change.

A lifetime before that, way back in 1952, Yehudi Menuhin was giving violin recitals in Mumbai (Bombay), India. A yoga master named Sri Bellur Krishnamachar Sundararaja Iyengar was summoned to give the maestro a private lesson. In 1954, Iyengar visited the United Kingdom for the first time as Yehudi Menuhin's guest, and the path that gradually led me to him was begun. While in London, Iyengar gave private lessons to Menuhin and a few other notable musicians. Slowly but steadily, word spread. In 1960, he gave one of his incomparable lecture-demonstrations in Highgate, London. It was attended by two hundred people, and the audience was agog. As president of the Asian Music Circle, Menuhin arranged for Iyengar to give another lecture-demonstration at the Institute of Recorded Sound. Interest in Iyengar continued to grow. In September, he gave a few more demonstrations around London, and a month later, he gave a private class at the home of Ayana Angadi, the director of the Asian Music Circle. He only had three students, but their enthusiasm knew no bounds, and they proved to be the most fertile soil. The bountiful seeds of interest in yoga he planted in them sprouted. Everyone else is descended from them, because they were his first three real students in the West. It was now up to them to tell others about him. I think it is fair to say that they did an excellent job. The conventional wisdom is that their names were Diana Clifton, Beatrice Harthan, and Angela Marris.

Iyengar came to London all through the sixties and seventies, usually at the invitation of the Menuhins. But he would also teach others. Things changed a little on June 20, 1961, when Ayana Angadi and Angela Marris, also a member of the Asian Music Circle, decided that regular classes would be a good idea and that they should be held in Ayana's home. Iyengar was quite willing. The morning class consisted primarily of musicians, as well as Beatrice Harthan, a lawyer. The evening class was attended by Patricia Angadi, Diana Clifton, Angela Marris, Silva Mehta, Eilean Moon, and Daphne Pick. Silva had already studied with Iyengar in India, so she became the unofficial leader of the group. Beginning on July 18, 1961, the group of six and Beatrice decided to practice together every week. Some say that this is when "Iyengar Yoga" was really born.

A year later, Iyengar returned to London and really began to be noticed. Of particular note was the BBC television broadcast "Yehudi Menuhin and his Guru." The Asian Music Circle again arranged a tour of lectures and classes in June and July, and Iyengar gave his first public classes in North London. The demand was such that before he left, he authorized his students from the previous year, who had been practicing diligently and consistently together, to begin teaching in his name—as long as they taught in pairs to support each other. The first "official" Iyengar teachers in the Western tradition were Diana Clifton, Beatrice Harthan, Angela Marris, Silva Mehta, and Eilean Moon. I had the good fortune to get to know them all except Eilean.

Angela Marris and Beatrice Harthan worked very hard and were rewarded when, the next year, Iyengar was able to come and spend six weeks. He taught seventy pupils in London and twenty in Brighton. Among his Brighton students were Aldous Huxley, Jacqueline du Pré, Clifford Curzon, Olivia de Havilland, Moira Shearer, and Sir Paul Duke. He also gave three lecture-demonstrations in London, including a particularly notable one at the Commonwealth Institute.

In 1964 and 1965, B. K. S. Iyengar was back in Britain teaching on his now yearly tours in London and Brighton. The year 1965 was particularly notable as the year his stunning book *Light on Yoga* was published.

In 1966, he gave classes to a hundred people in London, including another lecture-demonstration at the Commonwealth Institute. In 1967, he began training teachers for the London County Council, which would not accept any yoga teachers unless he had personally authorized them. In 1968, he gave a demonstration to five hundred people in Manchester, and by 1969, he had a regular presence in that city and northern England. Also in that year, yoga classes for the general public—taught specifically with Iyengar's method—were officially introduced into the adult education curriculum of the Inner London Education Authority (ILEA). These classes and the heady enthusiasm of those who taught them were the foundation on which Iyengar Yoga all around the globe was built. To this day, Sri Iyengar's gratitude to these students and teachers knows no limit.

It was around this time that, with a knowing little smile on my face, I trailed behind my friend Jeremy and walked into my first yoga class. It was taught by a truly wonderful woman called Penny Nield-Smith, to whom I owe a debt I can never repay. Regional and local authorities across the length and breadth of England were following the ILEA's lead, wanting to run public classes in yoga taught by people endorsed and validated by B. K. S. Iyengar. Teacher training commenced in the north of England in 1969 and was conducted yearly until 1976. But I knew very little of any of this as I lightly swung my badminton racquet and went to my first yoga class. I was just a perfectly ordinary and reasonably contented young man, trying to find a meaningful sense of direction for his life. It would take me decades to realize that what I was looking for was waiting for me behind that door.

In 1970, the first official Iyengar teacher-training program was established under the auspices of the ILEA at the College of Physical Education, Paddington. It was taught by Silva Mehta. Iyengar Yoga was now growing throughout the United Kingdom at phenomenal speed, and Iyengar Yoga teachers were being trained as fast as possible to feed the insatiable demand. I suppose I was lucky to be around, because I was about to join them, albeit reluctantly.

My friend Jeremy lasted a mere three weeks in yoga. I don't recall ever actually deciding that I wanted to "do" this yoga thing. Yet there I was, very soon a regular feature in Penny Nield-Smith's classes. Somehow, some mysterious force compelled me to go back week after week. Her classes grew bigger and bigger. She was a phenomenal teacher. She was soon doing three classes back-to-back. I attended the middle class, and we were regarded as the "most competent" group. In my case, it simply meant that I had gotten in on the ground floor because I had attended the very first class at the University Gym. I don't know why this should have counted for so much, given that it took me about four months to work out that this "yoga stuff" would be a lot easier to do if I stopped showing up every week in thick, tight jeans and refrained from spooning down my yogurt and my orange while walking to my class. I was that kind of student. Penny was heroically patient with me.

One day, I told Penny that from then on I would arrive early for my own class and stay on a little after mine had ended. By overlapping both of her other classes, I could take the class registers for her. I would mark everyone off, collect any money, give out change, field questions, and leave everything in the corner beside her bag. Then she could just scoop it all up and rush off to the railway station to catch her train back to London.

My offer to help Penny must have gotten lost in translation. She seems to have interpreted it as a declaration that I had a secret yearning to become a yoga teacher. I didn't. I just wanted to help her out a little. To this day, I really do not know where she got that idea.

After I'd been studying with Penny for about a year, she told me that her teacher, a man called B. K. S. Iyengar, was coming to London to teach. She wanted me to have some classes with him. By this time, she had been transformed into a minor divinity in my life. I would have done anything she asked. If she wanted me to take classes with some stranger, I was only too happy to go. So I said okay. By way of preparation, she encouraged me to have a look at *Light on Yoga*. I glanced at it. I really can't say it did anything for me—just some strange man doing some impossible contortions in a string of black-and-white photographs at the back of the book. Now *that* was the weird kind of stuff I thought Jeremy had been talking about when he first told me he was going to a yoga class. I didn't want anything to do with any of that. My life was normal, and I wanted to keep it that way. I couldn't even be bothered to look at the introduction. I put the book down again. Penny was another matter; for her, I would go. I had become devoted to her. Penny Nield-Smith has been dead for many years now, but my heart is still devoted to her and I salute her.

A week later, Penny told me that she'd tried to get me into some of B. K. S. Iyengar's beginning classes, but they'd all been full. She'd therefore signed me up for some intermediate classes and a couple of advanced ones for good measure. Apparently she'd gone to a lot of effort to put in a good word for me with the organizers who had okayed it. I shrugged my shoulders noncommittally and said that it was fine.

So I went for my first class with Sri B. K. S. Iyengar. He didn't seem to have a first name. Everyone called him Mr. Iyengar or else referred to him as B. K. S. Nothing particularly memorable or magical happened. After all, I didn't really care who or what he was. My only reason for being there was that Penny had asked me. She introduced me to the man whom I would eventually take as my guru. "This is my pupil Kofi," she said. "I would like him to become a teacher." At that, I lost all interest in him as my eyes snapped to attention and locked themselves on Penny in blank astonishment. Hey! This was the first I'd heard of any such thing. B. K. S. looked me up and down and smiled wryly. I guess I didn't look much like yoga teacher material. That was an assessment I agreed with.

As I waited, I looked around. Some of the people who have contributed to this volume were there. Unlike me, they all looked like the real business. A few other people, who had clearly paid to come and watch as if this were some kind of exhibition, sat on the sidelines.

The class started. I couldn't understand a word of this man's instructions, nor had I seen or done the majority of these poses before. At one point, the master looked at me and said, "So you want to be a yoga teacher?!"

Now it's true that my mind can be very slow sometimes, but even I could see where that particular question was going. A well-developed sense of self-preservation kicked in, and I spoke up immediately. This needed nipping in the bud. "No," I informed him clearly but firmly. I pointed straight at Penny. "*She* is the one who wants me to be a yoga teacher. Me? I know nothing about it. It has nothing to do with me. Go talk to her."

The people around me seemed surprised that I should speak this way. But it was not them around which danger hovered. So I did my nipping.

The next day, I was slated to play with the big kids. Wasn't *that* going to be fun? Not having yet troubled, in spite of Penny's advice, to look at *Light on Yoga,* I showed up for the advanced class in total ignorance. That was probably the best thing I could have done. I had absolutely no fears, no expectations, and no concerns. There's really not a lot anybody can do when someone wants one of your body parts to go somewhere it just won't go. Nothing you can do but smile. So I did a lot of smiling. That day, I relied a lot on the power of simply smiling. I left this Mr. B. K. S. Iyengar to it and let him haul any part of my body he wanted in any manner that struck his whim. He'd soon realize that God had made me from a particularly intractable sample of high-grade concrete, and that would be that. In the meantime, if he wanted to waste his energy, it was his energy, so why worry? It made no difference to me. Every time he came to me, it was the same. I thought, *My body is not going to cooperate with you, sir, and you will surely find out soon enough.* I had not the slightest concern.

At one point, I was supposed to put my forearms on the ground and kick up and balance—except that nothing moved. Indeed, my head went downward at high speed. A tall, willowy lady called Angela tried to help me out by showing me what to do. Her legs went flying up with elegance and grace. Then another one called Agnes joined in. Iyengar told me to go over by the door, except I still didn't understand a word. Somebody was kind enough to translate, so I put my forearms on the floor on either side of the door. He told me to try kicking up there. It didn't make the slightest bit of difference; I still had the world's heaviest torso. People called Dona, Maxine, Victor, Angela, Agnes, and a host of others would try to show me what to do from time to time. It was all very well for *them.* My legs were locked to the ground with high-grade glue. So I just chuckled and smiled. An awful lot of hauling about and smiling went on that day. He did the one; I did the other. The next day, I was none the worse for wear, and everything still worked as it should. But it could only have been some inner trait hell-bent on lunacy and suicide that propelled me to the next class. It certainly wasn't sanity. More probably, I still hadn't caught on to what was going on around me.

The next time I saw Penny, it was as if nothing had happened. She asked me how I had got on, and I shrugged my shoulders and said, "Fine." She had asked Mr. Iyengar what he thought about me becoming a yoga teacher. He had apparently grunted and said, "He'll do." It really meant nothing at all to me. She gave me a signed copy of *Light on Yoga* to mark the occasion. I still have it. So without knowing it and without really trying, I was now a bona fide Iyengar-approved yoga teacher with no classes of my own to speak of and absolutely no motivation in that direction, for I had no real intention of taking this up as a profession. But I had reckoned without Penny's determination—and her deviousness. She had a three-part operation lined up for me: first, the setup; then the transfer; then the coup de grâce.

First came the setup. I was still doing all Penny's class registers. She now suggested that I come early enough to assist her in the first class and then do my own class as usual. "Assisting" meant standing at the front of the class and demonstrating the poses so that people could always see what they were supposed to be doing. I did not mind that. It never occurred to me to wonder why a woman who could keep perfect control of a class of up to fifty people, and who could help all of them by herself, should suddenly be needing an assistant. After a while, Penny asked if I could assist her in both the other classes. She also showed me how to make a few hands-on adjustments and asked me to walk around and correct any mistakes that I could see. She said it was because the classes were so full and she couldn't get around to everybody. So I was now spending the entire afternoon with her: assisting in the first class, doing the second, and assisting again in the third. And still I didn't smell a rat!

Something very strange was happening in my life. During my childhood, I had developed into a proficient pianist and would sometimes practice as many as ten hours a day. I had a piano in my room at college, but I couldn't always play it when I wanted. Serenading others with Rachmaninoff or jazz at 7 AM is not exactly the way to win friends in a group of undergraduates. I had also lost interest in my undergraduate degree. So sometimes during the day, I was at a bit of a loose end. In order to occupy my time, I would sometimes practice a few of the things I could remember from Penny's classes. Sometimes I would even pick up the signed copy of *Light on Yoga* that she had given me and practice from that. Gradually, I practiced the piano less and less and my yoga poses more and more. The latter were silent, so I could do them anytime. It wasn't long before I had a real home practice routine going, without really having tried. But even though I was now practicing several hours every day, it was not exactly that I was a dedicated or serious student of yoga. It just looked that way from the outside. I wasn't practicing to get any better at yoga. I was just doing it for the entertainment value—and frankly, because I had nothing better to do with my time.

The next year, B. K. S. Iyengar was back in London and so was I. I didn't really belong in those classes, but nobody had the heart to throw me out. I just kept smiling and maintaining an even demeanor, no matter what was thrown at me. It seemed to be the best policy. All in all, my life was rolling along quite pleasantly. Then Penny struck with the second part of her little plan. One day, she called from London and said that "something" had come up. She couldn't come down that day, so would I please teach her classes for her? I refused and told her that I did not want to, that it would never work. But there really wasn't a lot of choice. It was teach or disappoint a lot of people. In any case, Penny had set it up perfectly. Everybody knew me. I kept the register, handled the money, had been going faithfully every week since the classes had started, and was assisting her anyway. I knew the names of all the poses, and the instructions had slowly sunk in over the years. So I went along, apologized to people that Penny was not there, reassured them that she would be back next week, and taught my first three yoga classes. Some of the people present that day still call themselves my students, and I thank them humbly for that honor.

But a new and disturbing pattern established itself. Whereas previously Penny had never missed a class no matter what the weather or other circumstance, suddenly there were now a lot of days when she had to cancel for one reason or another so that I had to step in and teach all her classes. Still, I suspected nothing.

B. K. S. Iyengar continued to come to London yearly, and I went to every class I could. In 1974, I heard reports that several of his senior teachers had gotten together to form a teachers' association to look after their affairs. It didn't really have anything to do with me because I wasn't really a yoga teacher. But I had finished my undergraduate degree by then, and I was trying to decide what to do for a living—although Penny had already decided for me.

It was time for the third part of her plan—the coup de grâce. Around 1975, she dropped her bombshell. She telephoned and told me that she had decided there was no point in her coming down to teach anymore, because I could run the classes just as well. My pleas were in vain. I was forced to announce the devastating news to all her students. To my surprise, nearly all of them were happy to carry on with me. Since I still couldn't think what to do for a livelihood, I decided that I might as well teach these few yoga classes until what I really wanted to do with my life showed up.

By 1977, the Iyengar teachers had completed all the arrangements. The (now-defunct) B. K. S. Iyengar Yoga Teachers' Association was formed. To my amazement, I was one of the founding members. I even helped write the constitution. The first Iyengar teaching certificates were personally issued by B. K. S. Iyengar himself and did not carry a date. I got one of those. I had also started going to India on a regular basis to study directly with him in his brand-new Institute in Pune. On some days while I was there—apart from his daughter, Geeta, and his son, Prashant—I was the only person in class. I was also taking sitar lessons; had started learning Sanskrit; and encouraged by Guruji, had even translated a couple of ancient texts into English, including *The Yoga Sutras of Patanjali*. So I carried on, teaching a few more lessons here and there, while waiting for what I really wanted to do with my life to appear. From that day to this, nothing has shown up.

Even though it crept up on me unexpectedly, I have had a good life as a yoga teacher. I have met many kind people, and I have traveled to many places. This book started as a way of expressing my gratitude to the man who had made it all possible: my teacher, my Guruji, B. K. S. Iyengar. I figured that there must be a lot of other people at least as grateful to him as I was. Maybe a few of them might also like to thank their teacher for what they had learned from him. I knew most of the likely candidates personally. I had even taught a lot of them over the years. I began to contact them to see what they thought of the idea. As I worked the telephone and the e-mails, word of what I was up to began to spread. I knew then that the whole thing was viable and continued with my labors.

I offer this book to my teacher, my guru, as a small token of my gratitude for all that he has done for me and so that others can come to know him.

KOFI BUSIA

PART ONE

The Embodiment of Practice

B. K. S. Iyengar

T. K. V. DESIKACHAR

If you want to know who someone is, it's often best to start by asking someone who knows him well. Even though the aim of yoga is often said to be to get to know our own selves, the way that others see us is often just as revealing. So we start our journey with Sri Tirumalai Krishnamacharya Venkata Desikachar, Guruji's nephew, and a brother in the devotion to yoga.

B. K. S. Iyengar

Standing tall through your actions
Understanding Body, Breath totally
Never yielding to failures
Destroying all blemishes
Always alert and attentive
Releasing everyone's energy
Applying Asanas with variations
Rejuvenating tired bodies
Action and dedication as the only goal
Joy and Health as the focus
Attending to students' needs
Inspiring everyone by your presence
Yoga expounded by example
Exacting in discipline
Never compromising your teaching
Giving your best to the world
A celebration of your teaching years
Raja Guruave, Namo Namahai

CHENNAI, INDIA
NOVEMBER 2006

&

T. K. V. DESIKACHAR is the son of Sri Tirumalai Krishnamacharya (B. K. S. Iyengar's guru) and the son-in-law of Iyengar himself (Krishnamacharya was married to Iyengar's sister Namagiriamma). In honor of his father, Desikachar founded the Krishnamacharya Yoga Mandiram—a nonprofit yoga center located in Chenna (formerly Madras), India—in 1976 to share and propagate Krishnamacharya's teachings. Desikachar is a household name in yoga, being renowned as a world-class authority on the subject. He has published numerous works, including *Health, Healing and Beyond: Yoga and the Living Tradition of Krishnamacharya, The Heart of Yoga: Developing a Personal Practice, The Viniyoga of Yoga,* and *Applying Yoga for Healthy Living.*

The Beginning of Freedom

RAMA JYOTI VERNON

Rebekah Harkness, the Standard Oil heiress, was one of many of Yehudi
Menuhin's friends who took an interest in B. K. S. Iyengar. In 1956, she
invited him to visit her in the United States to help her with some stomach problems she was having. While there, he gave demonstrations in
New York and Washington, D.C. It was not an altogether happy experience. "I saw Americans were interested in the three Ws," he later said.
"Wealth, women, and wine. I was taken aback to see how the way of life
conflicted with my own country. I thought twice about coming back."

Fifteen years later, Menuhin gave a concert in Ann Arbor, Michigan,
at the home of Mary Palmer. Noting her interest in yoga, Menuhin said
to her, "You must meet my yoga teacher in India. His name is B. K. S.
Iyengar." Inspired by *Light on Yoga*, Mary determined to meet him. In
1973, she asked him to teach a class for about forty students in Ann
Arbor. Meanwhile, Rama Jyoti Vernon was also trying very hard to track
him down, and she was eventually able to find him in his home in Pune.
As Iyengar said, he was not prepared to return to the States until "a student came to my hometown and tempted me to visit." This is her story.

The end of discipline is the beginning of freedom.
—B. K. S. IYENGAR

It was my mother who introduced me to yoga at a time in U.S. history
when the word was known only to a few. There was a handful of texts
and teachers available to help guide those who were thirsty for knowledge of the vast and ancient teachings of yoga. I was asked to teach and
did so reluctantly, always feeling I did not know enough. The classes grew
to such an extent that training other teachers was an organic unfolding

of the growing demand for yoga in California in the 1960s. I sought out sources of knowledge for myself as well as the teachers and students.

Dr. Haridas Chaudhuri of the California Institute for (Asian) Integral Studies became my fulcrum of spiritual exploration. Through the institute, I hosted and studied with a vast array of Indian masters, bringing their teachings of yoga and related subjects from the East to the West.

Some teachers expounded the philosophies, and others, just the physical practices. But none described exactly how the philosophy correlated to the practice of postures and breathing. One teacher shocked me by crossing off *asana* and *pranayama* from the chart of Patanjali's ashtanga yoga, saying they were physical and were not part of the "raja yoga" system. I was horrified, feeling that these two elements were the touchstone of experiential yoga.

One day, Dr. Chaudhuri put a newly published book, *Light on Yoga* by B. K. S. Iyengar, in my hand. I thumbed through it with the rapidity of a card dealer, not knowing that this text and its author would one day change my life. Pictures of a yogi in poses I did not know existed inspired and awakened me to new possibilities of practice. *Could it be,* I wondered, *that the yogi in the picture could be the same one who wrote the book?* The writing was as brilliant and majestic as the poses. I could not believe that the writer could also be the one in the pictures. I thought it was impossible for one being to be so eloquent and yet have such control over the human body. The poses flowed like music; the writing inspired like poetry. The text felt ancient, as if great masters were speaking through the pages to bring the practitioner back to the original tenets of yoga and its vast integration into all spheres of philosophies and life.

I devoured the book, gnarling my aching limbs into replicas of the pictures and fervently inhaling and exhaling pranayamas that cooled like the moon and burned like the noonday sun. I tried to copy the pictures, stretching my arms across the world plane and to the pole star in the night sky. Through the book, I was learning that yoga was known to bring inner peace and harmony through integration of body, mind, and spirit. It was known to bring about a self-realized state of "being," an experience of the world as an illusion in the vast array of universal consciousness. Yoga was also known as a physical culture that could bring good health and superlative energy and vitality. This book filled my heart, showing me that yoga was a doorway to ever-expanded conscious-ness. These were the teachings I longed for. The author alluded to what I had felt but at times doubted—that all limbs of yoga could be experi-enced in asana. Who was this Mr. B. K. S. Iyengar? Where could I find him? We needed him to come to California and train our teachers and students. After many inquiries, someone remotely remembered that Mr. Iyengar taught at times in Mumbai (Bombay) but lived in Pune, a three-hour train trip south of the city.

My husband and I ventured to India with the intention of finding this master who I felt was to be a major evolutionary giant in the world of yoga. We were hosted in Mumbai by a family whom we had hosted in our home in the States. We continually inquired about Mr. Iyengar but finally gave up asking. The very last day, our host's daughter's yoga teacher came to the house and invited me to sit in on the private yoga class. As I watched her teaching and demonstrating the headstand, I marveled at her gracefulness and mastery of the pose, especially in a sari. She offered, "I have a wonderful teacher. His name is Mr. B. K. S. Iyengar. Have you heard of him?" My eyes filled with tears of relief that the journey was not in vain. After rearranging our flights, which was no easy task in India in those days, we were on the plane to Pune. We landed in a grassy field in the middle of nowhere. Thank God, there was one taxi ordered by a young man who, we discovered, was the nephew of a man called Raj-neesh; this man would soon be sending disciples to the United States. He graciously offered us a lift to town, where we were to meet Freny Moti-wala, a long-time devotee of Mr. Iyengar's, who would take us to observe his class.

We searched through the streets of Pune after the taxi left, asking di-rections from passersby who would point in one direction and then in another. We walked back and forth and in circles, exhausting ourselves in the dust of the street, the crowds, and the heat of the day. My husband grew increasingly impatient and finally angry. "We are not going to find him. Our plane is leaving tonight for Mumbai, and tomorrow we leave for Bangalore. We cannot change it again." He began to hail a taxi. I felt tired and defeated. So close and yet . . . There was nothing to do but ask for divine guidance. I breathed a great sigh, looked up to the heavens for an answer, and saw a woman in a yellow dress waving wildly, trying to get our attention. It was Freny Motiwala. Our search had ended, but the journey was about to begin. She quickly bundled us into her car and drove us to the illustrious and elusive teacher who I knew would make this pilgrimage worthwhile.

"Mr. Iyengar lives in a very small dwelling." Freny was preparing us as she sped around oncoming cars, appearing to play chicken. "He sleeps in one room and teaches in the other. You will not be able to join the class, as there is no room and it's already in session." We wound down an even narrower dirt-packed road as Freny gave me hope. "But you may observe and later meet with him in private." My heart was pounding with anticipation. At last, after years of devouring his book, I would meet this great master in person.

My husband and I squeezed into a small, tiled vestibule, where we removed our dusty shoes. With whispered instructions, we were guided a few steps into the main room of the Kutir, where seven students were standing with outstretched arms and legs. The man pictured in *Light on Yoga* appeared smaller than on the pages of his book. With a scowl on his face, his large hands and loose wrists stung one of the students with a blow beneath an outstretched palm and fingers that seemed to snap to attention. "I am not slapping you," he addressed the surprised student, as well as all others in the room. "I am awakening the sleeping intelligence that lies within."

"Head balance," he barked, as students scurried for blankets; aligned hands, feet, and spine; and lifted like parchment flying into the air with only space to support them. Mr. Iyengar worked like a sculptor, moving bodies into exacting alignment, with or against the gravitational pull of the earth. He lifted hips, corrected spinal and neck curvatures, extended ankles, and opened armpits to take the pressure off the neck. "Your armpits have been lying in darkness. Now," he was emphatic, "open them to the light." My heart raced with excitement. He was like a great conductor using his hands and arms like a baton to bring the instrument of the body into a harmonious symphony.

"Paschimottanasana." The word was barely out of his pierced lips when seven bodies folded in two, with foreheads on chest, knees, or shins, depending on the flexibility of their hamstrings. Mr. Iyengar jumped on the back of the student on the far left of the room and walked from back to back, sensitively using his toes like fingers, moving skin to achieve a desired effect in the asana. I glanced at my husband, whose face was colorless with fear as he watched Mr. Iyengar move bodies into a full act of surrender as the upper and lower halves converged into one. "You want to study with him?" he whispered through clenched teeth. "I'll have to take you home on a stretcher." Just then, Mr. Iyengar jumped on the back of the last in line, an American student who moaned under the weight of the yogi. He turned his head slightly to one side to direct his voice upward. "Oh, Mr. Iyengar, how I love to feel the pitty pat of your little feet upon my back." Mr. Iyengar laughed, and his smile lit up the room. He jumped off the student's back and, with what seemed like great affection, slapped him on the shoulder and walked away laughing. "Class over."

My husband sighed, and the color returned to his face. "He's wonderful," he whispered, as we were led into the room where Mr. Iyengar slept and ate. We perused the pictures on the walls until he entered: Mr. Iyengar with the queen of Belgium, with the famous violinist Yehudi Menuhin, with Krishnamurti. My husband was impressed and lit up as Mr. Iyengar stepped through the doorway. We sat on his bed and he in a chair across from us. With tears in his eyes, he showed us a picture of his late wife, who had passed away recently, and shared the desire to build a yoga center that would be a memorial to her memory. We sipped tea and munched on sweets as he shared about his guru, Sri Krishnamacharya, who I knew to be one of the great yogis who walked the earth. It seemed like a dream that would be over way too fast. "Mr. Iyengar, would you . . . could you . . ." I stammered, "come to California and teach our teachers?" I spoke fast as the day was ending and our plane would be leaving soon for Mumbai. I implored him, saying how much we needed the in-depth teachings of not only asana and pranayama, but also of how the philosophy of yoga related directly to the poses and to our lives. He was curious and had never been to California, and he asked us to contact one of his students in Michigan to make the arrangements. Even though I did not know at that moment that this trip would lead one day to my starting his institute in California, my heart was so full that I could not speak, as tears of gratitude swelled in my throat and eyes. I did not know that day how much his teachings would ignite throughout America and the world, transforming and revolutionizing the lives of thousands of yoga aspirants.

I could not foresee how his teachings of alignment would open new pathways of asana, drawing practitioners deeper into the essence and infinite expression of the pose as philosophy and life.

As he walked us to the door, I finally blurted out in anguish, "Mr. Iyengar, I've been practicing and teaching all wrong."

His eyes and voice were full of tenderness. "Did you know it was wrong?"

In silence, I choked back the tears of lifetimes and searched my heart. "No," I whispered.

"Then you did not do wrong." His smile again lit the darkening sky as he accompanied my husband and me toward the waiting car.

"Mr. Iyengar," I could not keep from asking one more question. "There are times I just don't want to teach anymore, but the students keep coming. I never think I know enough."

He smiled as we slid into the car, and a thousand suns lit the night sky. The car door closed and through the open window, he did not say goodbye but, "When you walk into the class, say, 'Thank God, I have someone to teach.' One day, when you walk into the class and no one is there, say, 'Thank God, I am free.'"

RAMA JYOTI VERNON has been instrumental in creating a number of organizations, including the California Yoga Teachers Association (CYTA), the International Yoga College (formerly the American Yoga College), Unity in Yoga, and the B. K. S. Iyengar Yoga Association of Northern California. She was one of the original publishers of the CYTA newsletter, which gave birth to the magazine *Yoga Journal*, and she established a two-year curriculum for the first state-certified yoga teachers' training program through the California Institute of Integral Studies. That program became the Iyengar Yoga Institute. She started Unity in Yoga, an international organization that sponsored seven national, and three international conferences. Vernon is active in peace movements and has met with heads of state around the world. Her International Yoga College continues to offer advanced yoga training for teachers and practitioners.

Your Pupil Is Your God

Agnes Mineur

As so many of Iyengar's students have noted, one of his uncanny abilities
is that of making every student feel extremely special to him, to the degree that each of them is the only student he has and cares about.

Probably the biggest blessing of my life was to be able to study in
Pune, India, with Guruji when I was a young girl. I was very supple
then. Though it was fortunate that I was able to start yoga in my youth,
it worked against me because I could move easily in every direction: forward, backward, not really knowing what I was doing. Thankfully, Guruji
worked very hard with me, and though it took him many months, he finally brought my body and mind to a balanced state.

In Pune, I attended classes every day for many hours. Every day I
worked very hard. Backbends and balancings were worked out in the
minutest of details. There were nights in which I could not sleep because
of pain. But slowly I began to be able to feel my body intensely and
started to understand what was happening. Guruji said that we were
lucky that he was able to teach us the asanas in an advanced way, so that
we did not have to struggle to find out for ourselves how to do them.

Every July for many years, beginning in 1970, I went to London,
where Guruji taught teachers' training courses to the most qualified of
his students. We would stay in London for four weeks of hard work and
learning. Hundreds and hundreds of pupils came to these classes, and
those weeks were very intense work for Guruji. I learned so much by
helping him in these classes.

My studies in Pune began in 1971. While I was there, I began to
get experience that would later help me become a yoga teacher. I was

inspired by Guruji's temperament. When I began teaching, I tried to copy him, but soon I learned to be myself and tried to teach in a calm, strong way. One day when Guruji was teaching a very full London class, he asked me to help a student in sirsasana. I carefully instructed the student, and he began to do the pose very well. Pleased with my achievement, I saw another student having difficulties with the same asana, and trying to be helpful, I walked up to him, intending to give him instruction also. When Guruji saw me, he said, "Stay with your pupil. Your pupil is your God!" These words made a great impression not only on me, but on the entire class. I took them to heart, and I tried to teach every class in that way.

One of the special lessons taught me by Guruji was how to teach yoga to pregnant women. My feelings were that it was important to teach not only them, but also their husbands, how to use asana to ease their condition and how to use pranayama to relax. In this way, I could help both parents prepare for childbirth. I learned from experience that when I taught a woman to do pranayama, it helped her control her emotions so that her baby was peaceful and calm and the delivery went very successfully.

Those years were full of hard work and yoga, but we were blessed in that there was also time for socializing with Guruji and having fun. I remember an evening in Pune when we went with the whole Iyengar family to the circus. We were all very happy and having a very good time together. When an act with a snake girl came on, Guruji said, "Look, she looks just like Agnes!" Everybody laughed because they could see it was true. Some people used to tease me by calling me "Miss Chewing Gum."

Following his teaching visits to London, Guruji would go to Gstaad in Switzerland for four weeks, where he would combine rest with teaching Yehudi Menuhin. We would all travel with him, and several of us would crowd onto the balcony of his hotel to practice with him. We would travel around the country, visit the glaciers, and enjoy the breathtaking mountain views. Once we were sitting in a tearoom having something to eat after a long walk. One of our friends lingered a little and was late. We were already at the table because we were so hungry, and the food had been served. But Guruji said, "We will all eat together, and so we will wait for him." After a few minutes, our friend came and we did eat together. These were wonderful days, with Guruji being like a father to us.

It was wonderful to be treated as a member of Guruji's extended family. His wife, Ramamani, knew how hard her husband was working. As a silent and loving woman, she watched him and his students practicing. She understood Guruji's great gift and the love that he had for his work. She was exceptionally patient both with him and with us students, and I remember with pleasure how she would often make me a cup of tea after the classes in their front room had finished. This gave me the opportunity to chat with her and her children.

Even on vacation, when we were resting somewhere, Guruji would say, "See that person there waiting? He has tremendous pain in his lower back." Or, "Look at those crooked legs." Every minute was a learning experience when we were with our guru. He took every opportunity he could to teach us about yoga. I am very thankful to have been in the right place at the right time. The many lessons I learned from him helped me to grow personally and have enabled me to teach and help so many people in my hometown.

It was even through teaching that I met my husband, Leo. He had had a hernia operation and could not sit or bend forward. I used my yoga to help him, and as a consequence, he did not need any further operations. He was so grateful—and I think impressed—that a year later he asked me to marry him. We now have two lovely daughters; truthfully, I owe the existence of my family to Guruji. Leo attended all my classes and also became a yoga teacher. He cannot do the poses quite as he should because of his back condition, but as a couple, we continued to follow Guruji everywhere. Since Leo is very tall, Guruji often used him as an example in classes and used to joke about Leo's height as a way of breaking the ice in classes.

Guruji gave me yoga and, through that, my husband. We will always be very grateful to him for everything. When Guruji teaches, it is with body and mind, heart and soul. In his seventy years as a yoga teacher, he has helped many to heal and to stay healthy, a difficult feat for most of us. He has developed a way of touching body and spirit that is unique and very precise. He knows exactly where and how to touch on the places that have no life to bring them life. Guruji, thank you for bringing me Life.

§

AGNES MINEUR, a native of the Netherlands, was inspired by her mother to take up yoga at the age of twelve. At fourteen, she met and started studying with Dona Holleman, from whom she received private instruction for a few years. She then moved to New Zealand, where she worked as an occupational therapist, and where she began to teach yoga at nineteen. In 1970, she went to London with Dona and met B. K. S. Iyengar for the first time. A year later, she traveled to Pune to study with him at his home with four or five other people. She was present at the opening of the Ramamani Iyengar Memorial Yoga Institute in 1975 and is one of Iyengar's most senior and proficient students and teachers.

Your Guru Is Your Practice

INEZ BARANAY

One of the attractions of yoga philosophy is its practicality. Sage Patanjali, who systematized it, describes the state of yoga in the famous *Yoga Sutras* saying, "Yoga is the cessation of the fluctuations of the mind." But yoga does more than provide a philosophical goal; it gives a method for bringing this goal about. To achieve yoga, it is necessary to bring the mind to a state of focus and concentration. The philosophy then tells us that yoga recommends five steps to help the mind learn to concentrate:

1. It is necessary to develop an *interest* because the mind cannot focus if it has no interest in some object.
2. *Attention* can then be paid, this being a voluntary focusing on the object directed by intention or willpower.
3. *Practice,* or a regular repetition of focus, must then take place.
4. Once practice is well established, a level of *skill* must be developed. Whatever is being done is done with an alert yet calm body, the breath composed and regular, in a way that displays confidence and competence. In accord with the definition of yoga, it should be possible to attain the set goal without distraction or deviation.
5. Finally, whatever is being done can be done with an air of complete *detachment,* or uninvolvement, as if the task at hand is capable of doing itself without the participation of the actor—almost as if someone else is doing it and it is simply being witnessed. This last phase helps to create the calm, emotionally balanced state that yoga seeks.

Of course, as Inez Baranay now points out, all of this is much easier to talk about than to do.

B*eginning.* You enter the yoga room. You see people doing their practice. They stand on their heads, stand on their arms, and turn their bodies in improbable twists and bends. You think despairingly, *I can't do that!* Then your teacher says, "Once, they couldn't do it either." You start.

You do a little, do what you can. Next time, you do a little more. It's obvious, isn't it? You start. You stand in the first standing pose, tadasana. Just stand. Stand straight. Stand straight and still. And begin to learn all the adjustments you can make—balance, symmetry, alignment, ascension. The adjustments you make, even in this pose, the awareness you bring to it, can be refined infinitely. You only need one asana to understand asana, as you only need one poem to understand poetry.

You start. You remember what Hemingway said: "All you have to do is write one true sentence. Write the truest sentence you know." You write a sentence. You rewrite the sentence. You write the sentence another way. You begin to know the ways just one sentence can be written.

Commitment. So you have taken the first step and another step. Then one day, the next step presents itself. Yoga says, "You can't just 'try it and see' anymore. It won't work until you dedicate a portion, a part, of your life." This is the moment of choice. This is the commitment. You look at the photographs in the yoga school of the guru who taught your teacher. You buy *Light on Yoga.* The inspiration to maintain your commitment is always before you.

Once upon a time, writing said to me, "Get serious! We can't have an on-and-off relationship, waiting for your other jobs to give you time. You might need to earn less money for now. I need all of you. One day I'll look after you, but I can't tell you how long it will take."

Your guru is your practice. "So, are you a guru?" I asked Mr. Iyengar. I had been going to Iyengar Yoga classes for three years, and B. K. S. Iyengar was visiting Australia for the first time. I was making a one-hour radio program on yoga and interviewed the great master. He replied, "Your guru is your practice." The greatest thing a guru could ever say. You learn to do it by doing it. Yoga is learned in the practice of yoga, and writing is learned in the practice of writing. Then what is learned in the classroom?

Teachers. A writer is taught what thought and language are capable of through reading, conversation, reading, life, reading. Yoga is taught through practice, example, practice, reading, practice. A teacher of writing or of yoga shows you what more you can do, what you haven't noticed, where you are cheating yourself by holding back. You teach by learning, you learn by teaching, and each time you find that out it seems like it's *news*.

Masters. Beyond the teachers, there are the masters. There are writers so great that you fall to your knees reading them. If you are not intimidated, you are inspired. Shakespeare—as near indisputable as a writer ever gets—shows you a kind of perfection. Mr. Iyengar, our beloved Guruji, shows us a kind of perfection, a vision of what is possible, a sense that we are participating in something—I want to call it divine, yet I *don't* want to call it divine. In any case, it is transcendent.

Discipline, flexibility, instinct. Once a week to begin. That was more than twenty-five years ago now. After a while, I'd get up and go to the early-morning class even if I'd had a late night, had a hangover, left someone in my bed. Even if I didn't feel like going, I'd find myself showered and dressed and on my way down the early-morning street. After a while, I wasn't having all that many late nights anymore, I drank on fewer occasions, and there were more blue moons than shared beds. Once a week, then twice, then more. During my last few years in Sydney, I went to my yoga school six days a week for a two-hour practice or class. You get the discipline to do so much yoga from doing yoga. Discipline does not mean rigidity. When are there rules, and when are there no rules? It's backbends week, but you have your period so you had better do passive poses. It's forward bends week, but you need the particular energy released by backbends. You had a sequence planned, but the weather has changed dramatically and it will be better to find a new practice suitable for today's conditions.

Guruji himself has written of times when even he finds that "the body refuses." In that case, he says, "I make my body to be friendly with me." He teaches us to watch the state of our selves in order to awaken the body's intelligence. He tells us to find alternatives if we cannot do our regular practice.

Writing begins with irresistible urges. It continues with practice. It's not only when you feel like it, not only when that rare angel—inspiration—comes calling, not only when you're needing to say something or needing to find what you will say. Now it's every day. Now it's the set time and place. No, you're not free to go out for a drink, and no, it's not okay to come by without phoning first—even you, darling. Because I write. I write every day. I don't always feel like it. It is what I do.

In a lecture given in 1997, Guruji talked about the great yogis, who, although they practiced and mastered yoga, kept "the two main pleasures of the world *artha* (material prosperity) and *kama* (sensual joy). These are two of the four main aims in life as defined by ancient *rishis*. While we so often hear that to do yoga we must renounce worldly pleasure, the sages have told us to enjoy them, as long as the other goals—*dharma* (duty, discipline) and *moksha* (liberation)—have equal place. Eventually your discipline is not forced and it is not denial. It is your priority, not your sacrifice."

Plateaus. You are not making any progress. Nothing happens, nothing improves, nothing changes. You can't even do what you did before. Demons called Frustration and Despair crash the party. This is a stage. This is necessary. This you can learn from. This is where you are, so be here. Back to basics. Learn again just to stand still and straight. Remind yourself of all the simplest adjustments. You can't write a new sentence worth writing, so look at the sentence you already wrote. Take it apart and put it together again.

There are times in our lives, I have painfully learned, when we can't expect to make any obvious progress in yoga practice. Simply to maintain is a kind of progress, as it will be into age. And while the progress is not outwardly obvious, there is still a deepening, a refining of the practice, more levels of understanding.

Risk and reward, aim and by-product. It's all risk and no reward at first, and then once again, and undoubtedly some more. All you can do, should do, is get better at what you do. In the *Bhagavad Gita*, we are told over and over that we must perform our actions for the sake of the action and not for the fruit of the action. The reward is not the day you do a headstand at last. It's getting there, it's the importance of each step, each decision. The reward of writing is not publication. (In fact, it has been more truly said that publication is the price you pay for writing.) Anyway, by the time publication comes, the questions of some new work are absorbing you.

You may begin to do yoga for the sake of better health or calmness, to lose weight, or because your girlfriend does it. Guruji has written that while "the aim and culmination of yoga is the sight of the soul,"★ yoga provides beneficial side effects. These side effects—including health and the alleviation of stress, even happiness, self-knowledge, peace, or relief from boredom—might well be the reason we go to class or do our practice.

Writing has what we may call its side effects: publication, major or minor fame, invitations to read at conferences. You may earn enough money to buy a fabulous house, or you may earn enough money to buy a new typewriter. No doubt these rewards are in the sights of many writers, especially (or maybe only) as they begin.

I'm not going to say that the real aim of writing is the sight of the soul. Ask writers why they write, and they will tell you that we write because we must. We write because we can. You go back to Hemingway's first lesson, "Write one true sentence," and you may find that to do so becomes the quest of a lifetime.

The shadow, the unknown. Guruji himself has written in *The Art of Yoga* that the art of creativity is a painful process, with phases of fear, discomfort, tension, frustration, and dejection. These must be accepted, and you have to continue to labor. You are discovering the shadows cast by the light. Whom do you trust when you keep discovering you distrust? Pain and tears! Just when you thought it was getting to be fun, just when you imagined life was sweetness. So it is *because* of the bitterness and darkness, not without them. I'm not sure I'll ever quite understand this, the way "it"—the reason we do it, the reward for doing it—is found in imperfection and not only in perfection.

The body; body and mind; union. The writing body is a body held too long in unnatural positions—cramped, still, hunched, and sacrificed to the life of the mind. The body is a poor, tortured instrument. It has become commonplace to criticize Cartesian dualism or the separation of body and mind, and our health practices and cultural theories continue to develop from the premise of a desirable integration. We understand the body as discursively produced, its actual physical being and the understanding we bring to it as a product of culture.

In its way, yoga also understands the body as a product of past

---

★ B. K. S. Iyengar, *The Tree of Yoga* (Oxford: Fine Line Books, 1988), 85.

thoughts and experiences, and its practice reshapes your experience of your body through a deliberate set of new experiences and thoughts. These are known as *samskaras* (the accumulated residue of past thoughts and actions). Think of the body as a text written by yoga and the self as a text written by you. Patanjali talks of four stages. In this first stage, you work with concentration and determination to try to understand the body. It is only later that the mind begins to feel the action, then becomes more intimately acquainted with it and looks at both the parts and the whole. When that happens, the experience of yoga's famous union between mind and body begins. Do you glimpse the soul? It is extraordinary to experience your self as other than the chattering mind, as other than mind. If the mind is stilled, what or where is the self? If you are observing your self, who is observing, and who is being observed?

Writing depends on the flow of thoughts from the unconscious, and you might wonder which is the truer self—the unconscious or its servant who takes its dictation then edits it. Writing learns from dreams, and dreams tell us we are mysterious to ourselves. Somewhere in this arena, we need an idea we call the soul, that part of us that connects to the mystery.

Reluctance: the alternative-self attempt. The reluctance is mysterious: we just don't know ourselves. I have never regretted a yoga practice; I usually experience agreeable sensations when practicing, and I have always felt "better" in some sense for having done a practice. But if there is a disturbance to my routine, then there is reluctance. I don't do my practice. I put it off, as if it were something to dread and then only endure. There is the self I might have been if I had not taken up yoga, and this self, as if existent in a parallel universe, insists it would have been the better choice. This alternative self might be asserting itself, keeping me from yoga, attempting a coup d'état of the overall self. This other self wants to be more indulgent and escapist, more sociable and socially active, sexually prolific and reckless; to be known for mixing a perfect martini and have a reputation for closing the bar; to have a fiery creativity that manifests in intense spurts of concentrated, rapid, and blazing productivity, balanced by dangerous binges. It is not interested in yoga's control and balance, and it is willing, even keen, to risk sanity. It longs for entropy, or at least trouble; for dissolution, or at least some fracture.

The reluctance is mysterious. It is a necessary relief to lose oneself in writing. It is a necessary drive. I cannot regret all the time I have spent writing. It's good when you're really *on*. I have always felt "better" in some sense for having done some writing. But there is reluctance. I don't do it. I put it off, as if it were something to dread, then only endure. There is the self I might have been if I hadn't taken up—been taken up by—writing, and this self often insists it would have been the better choice. It might be asserting itself, keeping me from writing, attempting a coup d'état of the overall self. This other self wants to have a career that is understandable; be a lawyer, keep regular hours, and get a regular salary; be an academic, work more for other people, do some good, think about real people more, have investments to manage, know a lot about something that matters.

You practice anyway. There is a bodily sensation of need. The body needs the poses: that's what you're aware of first, how you long to stretch and open and turn and balance, and then you feel the need for the effects of the poses. There is a spiritual dimension to yoga, a glimpse of the ineffable and eternal. Many yoga practitioners call this "God" or "the Lord within." To glimpse this is yoga's ultimate aim, yet it is achieved by a complete attention to one's practice.

In writing, the need is also embodied: not specifically in a physical way, but you become aware of a need. You can't concentrate on anything you read; nothing holds your attention fully; you are restless and dull; you take up and drop the TV guide and the movie guide and fashion magazines and the unsatisfactory novels. Then you realize you have been trying to ignore words, phrases, images, insistent words, words that you should listen to, words that you suddenly want to concentrate on, that attract your full attention, that dictate to you. You find yourself making odd little notes on this file and that Post-it, on cards and blank pages and manuscript pages. And suddenly you are *on,* closing in on this idea that's been brewing, this world you need, this phrase that is the way to express it, this chain or web of association you are tracing through these haphazard pages. You stop going out, retreat from the world—sometimes before you've quite decided to. As you begin to write, you do not feel but are a channel for feeling as you become focused and still.

Missing practice. It's not only the episodes of the mysterious reluctance, that reluctance that feels like the denial of the true self. Sometimes there are reasonable reasons not to write, or not write as much, or do less yoga, or not do either today. Though there are those who claim never to miss—up at 5 AM, absolutely daily, in any conditions, in any place. No. You are in the world. There are days when the routines and usual circumstances are altered: travel, illness, guests, fun, and conferences. There is a different energy around you, and you want to pay attention to that or be part of it. This is life and you are in it. Then after a while, you can't bear to be away from your practice. You find that you just do it. In any circumstances. Don't worry if you're missing it; you won't miss it for long. So you learn to trust yourself. At least, accept your own rocky way, the way you keep the practice dangerous by flirting with abandoning it.

Doing it yourself; teaching. You enter the pose, and parts of you automatically begin to make the adjustments, parts remember to make further adjustments, parts will need reminding. Now it is not only parts of the pose that you bring to consciousness, it is the whole, the configuration. Now there's only you; there is no one there to diagnose and click you into shape, pushing or coaxing, giving you the precise instruction. Yoga is DIY (do-it-yourself) maintenance. Taking responsibility for your body. It is a feature of Iyengar Yoga that the teacher gives precise instructions to adjust in the asana and also physically corrects the pose, touches you to do so, pushes, pulls, or just lays a hand here, a finger there, to bring your attention to an aspect you now adjust. In various writings and lectures on his study of yoga, B. K. S. Iyengar talks of the experiments he made to discover the effects of poses and tells us that to really know yoga we, too, must experiment. This is how teachers learn; they learn their own body.

When you begin to teach yoga, you need to pay attention to the asana, to understand what you are doing and devise ways to communicate this. You examine what it is that you do; you research it and reflect on it. The book might tell you to "tuck the sacrum in," but how can you pass this on unless you have learned to tuck the sacrum in and feel how it alters the pose, gives it stability and strength and a center? You can't pass this on until you know your body well enough to be able to see when another body needs this instruction.

When you begin to teach writing, you examine what it is that you do, you research it and reflect on it, and you tell your students. They can find a book to tell them, "Read your work over before you sleep." But how can you tell your students this unless you read your work over before you sleep and can report on how this affects—effects, even—the writing when you wake and begin? "Sometimes you work passively," I tell students. That's what I learn from yoga; sometimes you are active, dynamic, you *do,* you do the pose. Other times you surrender; you "just be" in the pose, just be. When I'm deep into my work, I read it last thing at night, so that my dream time is dedicated to it. Guruji tells us and shows us that yoga is the teacher of yoga, that yoga is to be understood through yoga. Similarly, writing is the teacher of writing; writing is to be understood through writing.

We do it because we cannot not do it. I can apparently perform asana because I've been at it for years, and it looks to a beginner as if I can "do yoga." But I tend to live in my head; my body wants oblivion, distraction; I find it difficult to advance in my practice, to know what my left little toe is doing as I pay attention to my neck. I do yoga because I cannot not do it, because the moment of awareness has barely been glimpsed, because I love this in-between territory—in between doing it for the process and for the product, in between endeavor and accomplishment. I've published a few books, write every day, and teach writing. So a raw beginner might look at me and think I can "do writing." But often I think I am a writer not because words come easily to me, but because they do not. I can rarely write a sentence worth writing at first thought; I must sit over it, pencil in hand, rearranging, adding and subtracting, testing the rhythm. If ever I achieve the effect of lightness, it is hard-won. The work of writing is in rewriting, just as the work of asana is not in striking the pose, but in the adjustments you make to it. The asana is rewritten, the sentence is refined. The work that has gone into the final effect usually remains secret; at best, the clarity and precision achieved make this effect appear natural and inevitable.

Transcendence. The very first yoga sutra of Patanjali says, "Yoga is the cessation of movements in the consciousness."* This seems contrary to

---

* B. K. S. Iyengar, *Light on the Yoga Sutras of Patanjali* (London: Aquarian, 1993), 46.

anything writing could possibly aim for, where movements of the mind are very much what it's all about, and what you really want is for your mind to move right into some wildly wonderful new space of language. But in the absorption of the self into the act of writing, there is a kind of stillness in the frenzy, and who has not read over a piece of writing they have produced and said, awed, "Could I have done that? My god, where did that come from?" Transcendence cannot be an aim. It is like Zen archery, hitting the target when you're not trying too hard to hit the target. It disappears with the thought that you have attained it.

INEZ BARANAY was born in Italy of Hungarian parents who immigrated to Australia when she was a baby. A founding member of the B. K. S. Iyengar Yoga Association of Australia, she has studied at the Ramamani Iyengar Memorial Yoga Institute in Pune, India, and with senior Iyengar teachers in Australia, India, and the United States. She has taught yoga since 1993. Inez began publishing short prose fiction in the early 1980s and has had several critically acclaimed novels published. Her latest book is *sun square moon: writings on yoga and writing*. She is the creator of a yoga and writing workshop for those who practice both disciplines. She has taught writing since 1989 in a range of settings, including universities, community groups, prisons, and mentoring programs. In 2003, she was awarded a PhD in writing by Griffith University, where she occasionally teaches.

A Learner's Journey

Joan White

It is always nice to have a good teacher. It certainly makes learning any subject easy. However, the question of what it takes to be a good student is also important. The fact that people learn at different rates and to different degrees is not always an accident. Not all abilities are innate. Some can be attained through focused and dedicated effort. A keen and genuine desire to learn is obviously something that will increase the chances of success. A willingness to do the work required to gain understanding is another factor. And since almost every subject has its possibly tedious and technical side, the ability to maintain interest when things do not go easily is yet another factor. The latter two are aspects of self-discipline. The intelligent realization of one's own limits plays a role as well. At some point, a good student should also be able to apply what he or she has learned. Additionally, everything learned should become a foundation for yet more learning and the acquisition of further skills.

As Joan White now points out, although there is a definite—though not easy to pin down—set of traits that can characterize a good student, learning is nevertheless a process that occurs between two human beings. It straddles the boundaries of two different visions of that relationship. Sometimes the relationship is subject-object. One person is the subject—the teacher, the donor of learning—while the other is the object—the student or recipient. Other times the relationship is that of subject-subject. The student may well try to define or affirm his or her own sense of being within this relationship and to be an actor in its definition. These dynamics can be particularly telling when the topics linking teacher and student are liberation, enlightenment, and union.

I love to teach. I am passionate and committed to what I am teaching. The subject excites me. I enjoy the challenge of communicating ideas and stimulating the people in front of me to challenge themselves. I teach to those who are in front of me, speaking to my students in a language they will understand. Although I love to teach, first and foremost, I am a student. I teach what I have learned from studying with, practicing with, and observing our beloved Guruji.

The relationship between a student and a teacher has a long, rich history in India. The guru/shishya (master/disciple) relationship is a complicated one and often misunderstood. It involves surrender on the part of the student, and for many, that is an intolerable position to contemplate. Yet in order to receive the knowledge in its fullest sense, to understand nuance and the many levels being taught at once, it requires surrender and giving up intellectualizing and arguing minutiae. This is a very different type of teaching than we are accustomed to in the West, yet the rich, ancient guru/student relationship became the path that I followed. I found Mr. Iyengar to be a yogacharya capable of imparting an immense knowledge of yoga. From the Sanskrit, one can translate the word *shishya* as "one who is willing to learn." I knew immediately that I wanted to study with this person.

In many of the ancient scriptures, and in great detail in the *Viveka Chudamani* by Adi Shankaracharya, the terms *shravana, manana,* and *nididhyasana* are used to describe what is needed to become a good student. The meaning of these words deepens as one's study matures. To start with, they translate as "gaining knowledge by listening to the teacher" (shravana), "wiping away doubts and thinking about the teaching" (manana), and an "absorbed meditation on the subject" (nididhyasana).

At my first meeting with B. K. S. Iyengar, I was suffering from a badly broken back with a poor prognosis for a full recovery. This was in 1973, at an Ann Arbor YMCA gym, in a class of forty students. He set the class up in five rows and put me in the center of the first row. I had met him at dinner the night before, and he knew about my physical problems. He told me to do whatever I could and that he would watch me.

As soon as he started to teach, I felt my intellectual self completely let go. I realized immediately that I must surrender to what he was saying and let my body do the interpreting. It was as if I was in an immersion course in a foreign language, and I decided just to experience whatever I could get. He spoke; I opened my mind and listened (shravana), and my body listened and reacted. Afterward, I realized that I was in the presence of a master teacher. I was then, and remain now, completely humbled. The teaching spoke to me in a way no other teaching had ever done before, and I was determined to learn the art of being a student under his guidance. It was the first of many great gifts I have received from Guruji.

At first, it was difficult to understand the words, not knowing that particular vocabulary. (What exactly *was* this median plane he was referring to?) I knew I needed to do what he was saying and willed myself to let go of the frustration and observe what he was showing. As I am a visual person, through his demonstrations, I understood what to do. His way of demonstrating, vocalizing, verbalizing, and just plain moving his eyebrows resonated with me. He was communicating what he wanted out of me on so many different levels, using so many different expressions, that he caught my attention both as a student and as a teacher.

I was fascinated by his communication skills even when, in those early days, his English was not very fluent. The power of his ability to keep searching for different ways to get his points across showed that he was a master teacher. His fierce devotion to the subject created an authority that I could trust. I had never felt that kind of trust in a teacher before. He was not always exactly kind to the students, but he had a kind of compassion that I had never seen before. He was truthful, which is a quality I had been brought up to believe was of major importance. He told us both what to do and how to do it. For the first time, I felt this teacher was someone who really cared about his students. He taught not for financial gain, not for publicity, not for intellectual prowess, but because he wanted to share his knowledge with us and was willing to find a way to reach us. He would show us repeatedly, over and over, until the bulk of us got what he was trying to impart. I was hooked on the teaching and the teacher.

Since 1973, I have been privileged to have studied many times with Guruji. His command of the English language has become far more sophisticated than in the early days. But his initial idea of "teaching from the known to get to the unknown" has remained the same.

The classes in the 1970s were physically exhausting, and it took a tremendous amount of dedication and willpower for me to keep up. It was almost too much pushing of the physical body without understanding the infrastructure of what and why. It was a period of gathering, when I was lacking in maturity but not realizing it. There was much to learn, to absorb, and to ponder.

Back in 1976, Iyengar wrote an inscription for me on a picture of himself. He said, "May this laugh inspire you in yoga." Although yoga is a serious subject, he wanted me to be inspired by his smile, to see the joyful side of yoga, the playful side of yoga. After so many years, I am still inspired by that inscription.

Mr. Iyengar continued to reveal how important it is to be a listener, a watcher of myself, an observer, a doer. He doesn't give out sequences to practice; rather, he gives guidance about observing, searching, watching the mind, points, points, and more points in poses. Not until I'd been practicing for some time did I realize that it isn't the points, but the principles that matter. I learned from my practice that points may change from moment to moment, day to day, depending on my body, my mood, and my mental state, but the principles do not change.

A guru teaches the student discipline, and the truth does not always make you feel good. I realized that I would have to get out of the approval mentality if I was going to proceed inward. I spent many lonely hours in Pune hotels and apartments working up the courage to go back to class, fearing that I was not meeting expectations, that I couldn't comprehend, that I was physically unable. Then, in 1981, I had a "Eureka!" moment during a class in India and realized that my teacher was playing with my state of mind. Asanas *do* work on the mental plane, and I was responding each time he changed the sequence. Our practices are governed by observation of how we feel at the beginning, what we do during the practice, and how we feel at the end of the practice. I realized that I could actually change my mental state by how I sequenced my practice. I went to Mr. Iyengar and asked him if he had been playing with our minds. He smiled, then laughed and said, "You finally got it."

This yoga fascinated me, and I wanted to learn more about it. So I went to the library that serves as his office at the Institute in Pune and asked Mr. Iyengar if I could begin studying beyond the physical. He looked at me and said, "Yes, you are ready," and gave me a list of texts to start my new studies. I studied them, studied my own practice, and studied my teacher for clues. I observed his practice more closely. I listened when he taught. More and more listening, more thinking.

After 1981, Guruji began to introduce *The Yoga Sutras of Patanjali* to more of us. At first, I resisted learning them. I wasn't ready; I didn't understand the Sanskrit nor the references he was making. I read a couple of different translations but did not really incorporate much of the sutras into my teaching. Later, and now, they have become much more important as I have come to understand them. *Light on the Yoga Sutras* has been a wonderful help along the path. I read the sutras daily now and am constantly finding new depth and meaning in them. I do not just want a disciplined practice; I want a devotional practice.

As I began to explore the meaning of an inner journey (*antaranga sadhana,* according to Patanjali), I began to question myself as to how to go about this journey. I had started as my teacher suggested, working from what I thought I knew, my outer body. I would work with all the points that he had given us, trying to follow his directions to the letter. Each year when I went back to study with him, he would call me up on the platform to demonstrate my trikonasana, and I would dutifully get up and show my pose according to the previous year's directions. And each time he would tell me that I still didn't get it, that what I was presenting was wrong. This became a standing joke.

Finally, I got it. Since I no longer had the same lack of alignment, I was overworking and belaboring "the point." I wasn't feeling what was going on or working from the inside. Instead, I was now imposing directions on myself that were no longer applicable. This was a major lesson. I was, indeed, missing the point. I had gone back to working from my head and not from my heart. Ego is a powerfully stubborn obstacle. I was resistant to experimenting on my own, to finding a state of meditation in the asana. I wanted my answers to come from Pune, not from me.

What I was gaining in flexibility I was losing in actually "being in" yoga, for yoga is not a state of doing—it is a state of being. I was "doing" more poses, multiple times, with less inward movement. Little did I know that inner journeys are not instant things. You don't choose to go on them; they take you when you are ready. I kept being reminded of this by my Guruji and by my injuries.

An injury in 1987 put a definite crimp in my practice. I had no choice but to go inward. Once the injury healed, I had new understandings. I truly wanted a practice that came from my core, my heart, my soul. That means staying in poses longer and penetrating through many layers. Again, I studied my teacher's practice. It's not just about doing a pose; one first has to understand and sublimate the *karmendriyas* (organs of action) and *jnanendriyas* (organs of perception) and then become so involved that it suspends the time continuum. This is the breakthrough into *antaratma sadhana* (the innermost quest). I listened to my teacher with new ears and studied him with new eyes.

I watched Guruji in his backbend practice in 1990, doing a padan-gushtha dhanurasana (inverted bow pose) that left me, once again, in awe. His face was transformed. He seemed to glow from inside, while express-ing a sense of relaxation and total "presentness" in a very advanced pose. His pose had a quality that I knew came from the heart and from the deepest stillness of his being. It was both beautiful and wondrous at the same time. I wanted to feel like that in a pose, to make others feel like that in a pose, to let students know the depth and beauty of this art. I wanted them to understand the relaxation that comes from silence.

I am very grateful to Guruji for sharing with us the process of grow-ing older and internalizing his extraordinary practice. He has taught me the courage to face life. He has taught me that we have to let go of things on one level in order to find new insights on another. Growth is not only about building, it is also about surrendering what you know you no longer need. This continues to be my inspiration for my practice and teaching.

Although I had already begun to teach yoga in 1971–72, after my first week with Guruji, I was full of self-doubts about yoga, about teaching, and about myself. After further studies with Mr. Iyengar, I finally got up my courage to talk to him about teaching. I told him about my doubts, and he told me it was my dharma to teach his yoga. Once I heard him say that, I made it my life's work.

As I grow older, I realize that I have to deepen my inner practice and bring more of this pure system of yoga into my classes to allow people to see yoga as a way of life in a world full of stress and strain. I have gone back repeatedly to the *Yoga Sutras,* as well as other texts such as the *Upanishads* and the *Bhagavad Gita.* I ask my students to examine both their poses and their lives in relation to the eight limbs of yoga, especially the *yamas* and the *niyamas.* I teach from and bring into my classes the important concepts presented in the *Sutras*, not as obscure philosophy understood only by an elite few, but as they relate to daily life as well as what we are doing in the class. Mr. Iyengar began doing this many years ago, and I have studied and learned much since those first lectures on the sutras.

His book *Light on the Yoga Sutras* has been particularly helpful in bringing the philosophical aspect of yoga to my students. His new book, *Light on Life,* is his story of the inner journey. In it, he reinforces the idea that with practice, all of us can stay on the same path, if not the same level, that he is on. I remember a class in the early 1980s in which he was talking about *abhinivesha,* where he explained why death as we know it is not the end. I felt this huge sigh of relief; it was as if someone had taken a massive burden from me. And at that moment, I felt I had a glimpse of enlightenment, if just for a brief moment.

Long ago, I gave up on rigidity: life is fluid, yoga has to be fluid, teaching has to be fluid. One's practice has to depend on one's ability to transform and change—to continue to listen, to remove self-ignorance through knowledge (shravana), to wipe away any doubts with thinking (manana), and to contemplate through a growing abidance in oneself and through removal of habitual error (nididhyasana).

I have learned the art of being a teacher by being a student, and I had the fortune to be a student of a master teacher. Though there are many, many of us in the Iyengar community and classes with Guruji have not been small, I always felt he was talking directly to me. This student offers you her deepest gratitude. Pranams, Guruji.

§

JOAN WHITE is an accomplished and experienced practitioner of the yoga taught by B. K. S. Iyengar, with whom she has studied since 1973. She now trains and helps certify others who seek to become teachers of his pure interpretation of classical yoga. White serves on the board of the National Iyengar Yoga Association and chairs the Certification and Ethics committees.

A Strong Line of Certainty

ROGER LLOYD-PACK

"What shall I do now?" "How should I conduct myself?" Ultimately, these are the kinds of things pondered by those who choose to reflect on the nature of being embodied. No matter what the situation, no matter what the circumstance, learning how to come up with a suitable answer is the purpose of yoga. *Asana* (posture) is a way of asking those questions about embodiment, whereas contemplation and refinement of asana are the way to find the answer. The nature and parameters of the search are clearly illustrated by the story of Bhishma's birth, who some regard as the true hero of the great Indian epic the *Mahabharata,* of which the famous *Bhagavad Gita (Song of God)* is a part.

Bhishma's story began in heaven when Ganga, the river goddess and mother to India's greatest river, reported to Brahma, the Creator, along with all the other gods and beings. While all were assembling, a gust of wind lifted Ganga's thin dress. To spare her blushes, everyone averted their gaze—except King Mahabhisha, who could not tear his eyes away from her body and whose thoughts were impure. For this disrespect toward a goddess, he was condemned to an earthly existence and was incarnated as King Shantanu. Ganga was also destined to be embodied so that she could inflict the necessary discomfitures on him.

Among the denizens of heaven are the eight *Vasu*s (Dwellers), attendants to Indra, king of the gods. They represent eight cosmic natural phenomenona or elemental aspects of nature: *Agni* (Fire), *Prithvi* (Earth), *Vayu* (Wind), *Antariksha* (Atmosphere), *Dyaus* (Sky), *Aditya* (Sun), *Chandramas* (Moon), and *Nakshtrani* (Stars). Their wives befriended Jitavati, a mortal, and Dyaus's wife prevailed on him to take pity on Jitavati and help prolong her life by giving her some milk from Nandini, the divine cow. This would give her another ten thousand years. Under considerable pressure, Dyaus persuaded his seven brothers to help him steal Nandini. Unfortunately, she belonged to the sage Vasishtha who, using his ascetic and cosmic powers, did not take long to work out who the thieves were. He condemned all eight Vasus to suffer a life of embodiment on earth but relented slightly when they expressed suitable repentance and remorse. He then insisted that Dyaus, the ringleader, live out the full term of the curse, assuring the other seven that they would return to heaven within less than a year of being born. Since the Vasus knew that Ganga was soon to be incarnated as King Shantanu's tormentor, they went straight to her and pleaded with her to become their earthly mother. She agreed.

Shantanu and Ganga were eventually embodied. But as is the case with almost all initially divine beings who take on human form, they lost all memory of their heavenly natures and forgot about their divinely appointed destinies. They eventually met and fell instantly and deeply in love. Shantanu pleaded with Ganga to marry him. She agreed but imposed one condition: he was never to question her wishes or actions, no matter how bizarre or contrary they might seem; if he did, she would leave him. He was so enraptured that he agreed.

Shantanu and Ganga had their first child. To his astonishment, Shantanu one day observed Ganga stealing surreptitiously away with their firstborn. He was horrified and devastated when he saw her consign their son to the river. He did not know that, far from drowning, the first of the Vasus was simply being returned to heaven via Ganga's embrace, for rivers originate with her. The same happened to the couple's next six sons as, one by one, they were embodied and immediately restored to their celestial abodes in the same manner as the first. Although Shantanu was beside himself and suffered ever-increasing anguish and torment, he remembered the promise he had made and did not question his apparently murderous wife. However, when Ganga was about to drown their eighth son, he could take no more and importuned with her. She then reminded him of the terms of their agreement and told him that because he had been so bold as to question her, she was obliged to leave him. He was suitably heartbroken and doubly devastated when she took their remaining son with her. That last child was the embodiment of Dyaus who, not having been drowned immediately, was forced to live out a full human existence. His name was Devavrata.

For sixteen years, Ganga raised her son away from his father. He received training in all the arts of kingship and became a highly skilled archer, a great warrior, and the embodiment of all the virtues and attributes of a wise and just king. Ganga then effected an introduction between father and son. That done, she threw herself into her river, and that was the last Shantanu ever saw of her. As for Devavrata, he later took the name Bhishma.

He was respected by all. He understood that his true nature and life were of supreme wisdom in spite of everything. He demonstrated that nonviolence, truth, and forgiveness are powerful enough to overcome all wrongs, for they are the true support of dharma ("righteousness") and thus the way to happiness. He was the embodiment of spiritual insight.

The issues highlighted by Bhishma's existence—being someone whose experiences in life enable him to acquire wisdom and to understand the universal laws of existence—are the same ones now raised by Roger Lloyd-Pack.

Roger Lloyd-Pack was interviewed by Anne O'Brien in June 2006.

ANNE O'BRIEN: Roger, you have been practicing yoga for about thirty years. What has kept you going and instilled the discipline in you to maintain that long-sustained practice?

ROGER LLOYD-PACK: I wish I were as disciplined as that sounds. It's because I don't do so much on my own. When I'm working and acting, I do about fifteen minutes of yoga before a show. It's a very useful warm-up.

But in my daily life, I rely on my weekly classes with my teacher, Ros Bell. Yoga has been a constant with me as a way of being in charge of my body, particularly as I get older and understand how the body works. I love the wisdom of the standing poses. How if I have proper, strong legs, they will support my spine and my spine doesn't get tired. I know which muscles to use, to work, to protect my spine. The real straightening of the legs that you do in the asanas, the real pulling up of the knees—that is what really helps me maintain a healthy back.

I'm able to be in charge of my body and not be a victim of what can happen to my posture if it's not cared for. Yoga gives me an awareness that goes into my life and craft. In my craft, I need a sort of muscle fitness, and yoga helps with that. But it also keeps me oiled; it keeps me flexible. It's very useful to do before any stage work. I enjoy the feeling of aligning myself in these postures when I'm just stretching and feeling. The body feels right to be stretching in that way. It just feels correct. It's a physical meditation because the concentration required makes you stop thinking, makes the inner dialogue cease for a bit.

AOB: You said earlier that you wondered at the process that Mr. Iyengar must have gone through to arrive at the correct positions, a process of trial and error. Can you relate that to your own craft, the honing of it, and Mr. Iyengar's art?

RLP: I suppose I can, of course. One is always more impressed by something that one is not able to master than with something one has done oneself over the years and achieved some mastery. Error in my acting occurs in a rehearsal process. I'll be trying out different ways of saying lines, developing moves, and developing characters. I love the trial and error. I suppose we all incorporate trial and error into what we do. I suppose Mr. Iyengar's understanding of the body must be so minute, detailed, and precise to work these things out, and he's working on them all the time. Refining techniques, always inquiring into the correct way to do, to be. It's rather like early man building temples six thousand years ago, shifting twenty-ton stones. How the hell did they manage to do that? I suppose that's the same sense of wonder I have for Mr. Iyengar. The amount of concentration and inquiry that's gone into refining these postures is very impressive.

AOB: In his latest book, *Light on Life,* he talks about encouraging students and teachers to cultivate that internal inquiry. Yoga is the process. He can give us the tools, but then it becomes an individual inquiry.

RLP: Yes, because it is one's journey. As you say, the teacher can only give you the tools to work, those postures, and help you understand. But you then have to take it on individually, because every person's body is different.

I read once that Jung's definition of intelligence was to be able to monitor the progress of your life, the changing patterns, physically and mentally, as you went through it. I understand what he means by that because nothing is fixed. How many times have I come to conclusions in my life and thought, *Oh, that's it, I've got it now. Now I understand.* And then a few months or a year later, I really have to review that conclusion in the light of other things that shed light on my life. So one's continually changing and reacting to new information. Asana is like that. The asanas you need to do—or are right for you, or better, or easier to come by, or whatever—change at each moment. How you connect with your body is different for everyone. I like the practicality of it. I can feel the physical benefits immediately the next day or that afternoon. The fact that it's doing my organs good as well is a bonus! But I also enjoy the mystic qualities it has. That is always there. The discipline of the postures is an integral part of my life, providing me with a strong line of certainty in an uncertain life.

§

ROGER LLOYD-PACK was introduced to the world of acting as a young child through his father, actor Charles Lloyd-Pack. He received theatrical training at the Royal Academy of Dramatic Arts and went on to perform with the Royal Shakespeare Company in London. He has starred in many televisions roles and movies, including *Oliver Twist, The Vicar of Dibley, Interview with the Vampire,* and *Harry Potter and the Goblet of Fire.* Critically acclaimed and respected throughout the United Kingdom for his work, he was awarded the 1984 London Critics Circle Theatre Award for Best Supporting Actor for his performances in *One for the Road* and *Wild Honey.*

The Practice of Integrity

AADIL PALKHIVALA

In 1937, Krishnamacharya, Iyengar's guru, received a letter from Dr. V. B. Gokhale, a surgeon and a member of the Deccan Gymkhana Club in Pune, Maharashtra State. The letter asked Krishnamacharya to send a yoga teacher on a six-month contract to teach yoga in the Gymkhana, as well as in the schools and colleges around Pune. None of Krishnamacharya's most senior students wanted to go anywhere for six months. Additionally, since they had all studied at the Mysore Sanskrit Patshala, they were all fluent in both Sanskrit and their native Kannada. None could speak either Marathi (the language of Pune) or English. Since Iyengar had attended high school, he was the best English speaker and so was instructed to go and fulfill the contract.

He found himself confronted with students of rare sophistication and education. An immediate difficulty was that Krishnamacharya had never divulged any systematic techniques for achieving the postures Iyengar had learned. He therefore found that he could not transmit the techniques effectively. He tried looking at a variety of books and noted that "The Sirsasana of one person was different from that of another. Each asana was illustrated differently. I thought that the practitioners must be presenting them according to their whims and fancies."* The systematic approach to posture that is the fundamental characteristic of the Iyengar method in yoga was born when he noted that "doubts and confusion led me to experiment with all their presentations to find out by trial and error which were the wrong, which were the right ways."† Iyengar decided that he would only use firsthand, direct experiential information in his new career. Aadil Palkhivala now discusses the implications and consequences of the phenomenal practice routine for which B. K. S. Iyengar is world famous and that lies at the heart of his methods as a teacher.

---

* Light on Yoga Research, *70 Glorious Years of Yogacharya B. K. S. Iyengar* (Bombay: Light on Yoga Research Trust, 1990), 5.

† Ibid.

With respect for my teacher B. K. S. Iyengar's integrity in the practice of asana, I offer this excerpt from my book addressed to yoga teachers, Fire of Love.

INTEGRITY

Be the change you want to see in the world.
—MAHATMA GANDHI (1869–1948)

A wonderful story is told about Mahatma Gandhi. One day, a distraught mother came to him with her rebellious son. She explained that the boy's behavior was erratic and troubling and that this was certainly due to the enormous amount of sugar he consumed. She pleaded with Gandhiji to tell the boy to stop eating sugar, saying, "He won't listen to me, but you are the great Mahatma of the nation; he will listen to you." Much to her disappointment, Gandhiji immediately replied, "Come back and see me in a week."

A week later, the mother and son returned. Without any formalities, Gandhiji announced to the boy, "You must stop eating sugar immediately." The mother, much relieved, couldn't hold in her curiosity and asked him, "Gandhiji, please forgive me for asking, but why didn't you tell him that last week?" Gandhiji slowly lifted his head, looked directly into her eyes, and thoughtfully said, "I had to stop eating sugar myself before I advised your son to do the same."

This story is a portrait of integrity in action. *Integrity* comes from the same word as *integer,* meaning "to be one," "to be whole." When our words and our actions are severed from our thoughts and beliefs, an inner, subconscious stress develops, a pain in our conscience, a disturbance in our soul. We become disconnected. When I say one thing but do another, my buoyant heart sinks, and my inner smile withers. Inevitably, this manifests in the body as illness. On the other hand, integrity, with the strength and calmness that follow in its wake, allows us to sleep peacefully at night. To act with integrity usually causes some initial discomfort, but afterward, the entire body relaxes, the brain enters a state of peace, and we feel whole again. When our beliefs, thoughts, words, and actions all correspond, we are one.

INTEGRITY IN PRACTICE

> The beautiful in music is a by-product of the composer's integrity, a
> function of his search for the truth.
> —ARNOLD SCHOENBERG (1874–1951)

Integrity in our teaching grows out of integrity in our practice. Integrity
in asana is clearly illustrated by Iyengar. Once, we were working on urdhva dhanurasana. Iyengar demonstrated the pose, obviously working very
hard, but I saw that the students clustered around him were not impressed. After demonstrating, he asked for two volunteers to do the same
pose, and they did what to the untrained eye were spectacular poses, their
chests puffed out dramatically, their knees almost straight.

Iyengar wryly remarked, "These are poses lacking integrity." He then
demonstrated the pose again, this time also straightening his legs and
puffing out his chest, making his pose look ten times as magnificent as
the volunteers'. While in the pose, he exclaimed, "Look! I can do that
too!" He then came out of the pose and said, "So what? I'm not educating my body by doing the pose this way. I'm simply falling into the
body's weakness so that I can look impressive. Now I will do the pose
again, but this time with integrity."

Repeating the pose, he unpuffed his chest and proceeded to do the
pose working every joint and every muscle. The trained eye could now
clearly see the difference between the asana done to impress others and
the asana done to develop self-awareness—the difference between van-
ity and integrity.

HUMILITY

> Teach thy tongue to say, I do not know.
> —THE TALMUD

As teachers, our primary responsibility is to be honest with ourselves and
admit our mistakes and weaknesses. To grow as a teacher requires humility and the ongoing willingness to admit that there are infinite things yet
to learn. One of my teachers, Prashant Iyengar, had been teaching in a
certain way for many years, a practice that had been adopted by many of

his students. He used a standard phrase, "including everything physical and physiological," to explain the different aspects of the body. One day, my brother approached him and said, "Sir, I believe that these two words mean the same thing and one can be omitted." Though Prashant was forty and my brother was only nineteen at the time, he paused, thought about my brother's observation, and then said, "I agree." From then on, he never used the second word. To immediately see the truth, especially when revealed by someone less than half your age, then admit your mistake and give up a twenty-year-old habit—that is integrity!

EMBODYING TRUTH

> My life is my message.
> —MAHATMA GANDHI

Integrity in teaching means teaching only the knowledge you have embodied. Thus, when you learn something new, first practice it extensively for a few months, and then teach it only to a few other teachers or senior students. Notice whether you are creating the results you felt inside your own body. Only then do you have the right to teach it to other students. When baking a cake, you can have all the right ingredients in just the right proportions, but until that batter spends time in a hot oven, it will never become a cake. No matter how much we know, no matter how correct we are, it is the fire of practice that transforms us from being knowledgeable yoga teachers into becoming yoga teachers of integrity.

To teach therapeutics with integrity involves cultivating a much deeper understanding of yoga. If I have not felt how my pancreas opens in parsva sarvangasana, then recommending that pose to somebody who has diabetes, just because it was mentioned in a book, lacks integrity. You must study and work with a senior teacher for a period of time until you become familiar with what has to be done for each particular case and each particular problem. In addition, you must practice the postures and pranayamas with integrity to develop your ability to feel their effects in your body. Then, even when you are treating a disease or an imbalance that you have not personally experienced, you will be able to sense the effects that certain postures have on those particular problems and thus be able to customize sequences and practices for individuals.

Be very conscious that you are not teaching from a book or a lecture you've heard, especially when it comes to foundations such as the *yamas* and *niyamas,* or subtler aspects such as pranayama and meditation. The Mother of Sri Aurobindo Ashram used to say that if one teaches something one has not experienced, then the student will not learn it. If your teaching comes from books and not from your own experience, you will not be able to transmit the sensations that vindicate the knowledge, and your students will not be able to feel it enough to absorb it. They may understand it intellectually, but it will not penetrate their very nature. Thus, you must teach from experience and never from knowledge alone.

If we live what we are not teaching, we are liars. If we teach what we are not living, we are hypocrites. Thus, I would never insist that my students practice three hours every day, because I do not practice three hours every day. If I try to persuade my students to do what I am not doing, I create resistance within myself, subconsciously fighting the inner voice of my conscience because I'm preaching what I'm not practicing. Conscious resistance in our students appears only because we are subconsciously resisting our own conscience. This resistance disappears when we teach from integrity.

ALL LIFE IS YOGA

When we live in integrity, a radiance emanates from us, attracting those who desire to live a loftier life. Living yoga with integrity includes practicing the yamas and niyamas on a day-to-day basis and constantly applying the truths of yoga to all aspects of our lives. As Sri Aurobindo said, "All life is yoga." When we embody this noble truth, living all life as yoga, then we are truly living a life of integrity. Our beliefs and thoughts merge with our words and actions, and we become whole.

AADIL PALKHIVALA's experience of yoga and holistic healing was originally prenatal, his mother having practiced yoga with B. K. S. Iyengar throughout her pregnancy. He began observing Iyengar's classes at the age of three, started formal study at the age of seven, and was awarded his Advanced Yoga Teacher's Certificate at twenty-two. Having integrated Iyengar's insights into his teaching, along with the work of Sri Aurobindo and the Mother, Aadil currently works diligently with people who desire a better quality of life through a humanistic approach to wealth and health. He is the founder of the Yoga Centers College of Yoga and president and CEO of The Innerworks Company.

Radical Awareness

My First Class with Sri B. K. S. Iyengar

Judith Hanson Lasater

As everyone must know by now, *yoga* is derived from the Sanskrit *yuj*, referring to the joining of body, mind, and spirit. But yoga is, above all else, practical and experiential. In the opinion of experts, B. K. S. Iyengar has changed how people view and practice this art.

The ultimate test of a visionary or innovator is that of persuading others to adopt his or her techniques. But sometimes those techniques are clothed in such an aura of "obviousness" that it can be very difficult to appreciate their scope. *Light on Yoga* brought Iyengar world attention and laid the foundation for the ceaseless growth in his fame. The photographs often showed him performing complex poses with such casual mastery and elegance that the eyes were deceived into believing that they were simple and straightforward to do. Adding to this impression was the section headed "Technique" that accompanies every asana. There, set out in deceptively simple fashion, was a numbered list. The impression given was that all anyone had to do was follow the steps and they too could reproduce what the photographs depicted. Of course, it was not that simple. This paradox was soon appreciated by anyone who took classes from the master. He made it clear that beneath the apparent simplicity lay considerably more.

The same blend of simplicity and profundity is extolled in the story of the saintly Prahlada, a devotee of the god Vishnu, and his father Hiranyakashipu, the reigning demon king. When Hiranyakashipu became exasperated with his son, who did not want to become the next demon king, he asked Prahlada if he truly believed that Vishnu is everywhere. He scornfully pointed toward a pillar and asked if the god in which Prahlada believed was inside the pillar; his son quietly answered, "Yes." Enraged, Hiranyakashipu struck the pillar to show there was nothing in it—only for Vishnu to emerge as the savior of the world, the message being the paradox that God is in everything while at the same time is nowhere to be seen. As Judith Hanson Lasater now describes, it is one thing for the mind to grasp the meaning of *yoga,* but quite another to experience it. Guruji never lets any of his students forget that yoga is about one subject in particular: understanding our own natures is the method to understand self and the underlying divinity of the universe.

One crisp fall day during my first few months as a yoga teacher, I had just ended a class when a student approached me and asked if I had ever seen the book he was holding. He handed me *Light on Yoga;* I quickly flipped to the back of the book and was mesmerized by the photos. Not only were the asanas shown there some of the most advanced I had ever seen anyone do, they had a palpable quality of beauty and awareness that literally jumped out from the pages as I looked through the book in fascination.

I shook my head at the student as I handed the book back and said with conviction, "No one can do these poses." But I continued to be haunted by the images I had seen. A day or two later, I bought myself a copy, and my interest was again piqued. Unfortunately, the book ended up sitting on my shelf for months.

During those months, I married and moved to the country, at which time I found myself with more time to practice. One day during a session on my mat, I remembered the book and opened it as I knelt on the floor. I began to try some of the poses. Over the next few weeks, I worked with the sequences suggested and now believed my first impression—that the poses were impossible—had been incorrect. As time passed and I practiced every day with the book as a guide, I became a little more convinced that I was actually doing some of them pretty well. Not only was this thought not true, but in hindsight, it became clear that it was quite humorous in its naïveté. I did, however, often have the hope that I could study with the author of the book.

By the spring of 1974, my husband and I were living in California. In the way of all great coincidences, our yoga group had just invited Sri B. K. S. Iyengar to extend his second teaching trip to the United States and fly west from Ann Arbor, Michigan, to teach us for several days. I was confident as the workshop approached that I was ready; after all, I practiced every day and felt I had sufficient awareness and understanding of asana to hold my own in any class. I also felt excited that my wish of several years ago was coming true and that I was at last going to study with the author of *Light on Yoga*.

The workshop was not what I expected. I was surprised first by the fact that Mr. Iyengar had us line up in perfectly straight lines, shorter students in the front, taller ones in the back. He seemed so serious. Wasn't yoga about being relaxed and fluid? What was this urgency and no-nonsense attitude about?

Then the real shock came. He began to teach. The words he used about the poses were electric. Because I am not very tall, I had the blessing of being in the front row. This "blessing" was soon to become a challenge.

Our first pose was tadasana (mountain pose). *I can do this,* I thought. *It's just standing upright before the "real" practice of the "real" asana begins.* Mr. Iyengar began to make comments to me; I don't remember the specific words he used, but I do remember very clearly the way I felt hearing them. He continued to correct my pose verbally and as he did so, I slowly began to notice that irritation arose in my mind: *Why is he picking on me? Am I not doing the best I can? Who is this man anyway?*

We moved on to practicing standing poses with tadasana in between each one. Every time we returned to tadasana, Mr. Iyengar would turn toward me, raise one of those intimidating eyebrows, and instruct me in my pose.

After a few minutes of this, I found my irritation had shifted. Now my inner dialogue became, *Why is he picking on poor little me? I really am trying as hard as I can to do what he wants. Why won't he just leave me alone? Am I the only one not doing it the way he wants? I feel so awful and sad.*

Yet the process continued. Standing pose. Tadasana. Correcting me in tadasana. Standing pose. Not only was he constantly correcting my pose, I did not understand exactly what it was he wanted me to do. Inwardly I was squirming, wishing I could drop through the floor, pass out, anything but keep standing there. Basically, it was hell.

It took longer than I would have predicted, but suddenly I had a blinding flash of the obvious. I realized that he was showing me how I reacted to the challenges of the world by how I was reacting to his challenge of my pose. I suddenly understood that it was characteristic for me, when things weren't the way I wanted them to be, to first go to anger and irritation, then to react with the attitude of "poor little me."

With a smile beginning to spread across my face, I looked up into those piercing dark eyes. He smiled back, and suddenly I felt free. So this was what the teaching and studying of yoga was about! So this was what it meant to use practice in a way that uncovered the hidden patterns of my ego and how they created suffering for me and through me for others in the world. All the irritation and self-pity I had felt just minutes before came crashing down, and all that was left was a taste of wry, self-deprecating humor and a deep curiosity to learn more about myself and my now-suddenly deepened yoga practice.

At last it seemed I was able to hear and learn more. Mr. Iyengar began to describe how all the types of yoga practice were embodied in tadasana, a pose I had basically ignored for years. "The feet," he said, "are bhakti yogis. Do they not caress the earth? Are they not worthy of your awareness? The thighs are karma yogis, holding up the body day after day. This is not just physical practice," he reiterated.

Suddenly I was rejoicing. *A true teacher,* I said to myself. We were still standing in lines, and he was still quite strict, but my perception had changed, so everything had changed. I heard his words as coming from his heart, from his deep dedication to the art and science of yoga, and I grew up a little right there in that class.

I still have my original copy of *Light on Yoga,* purchased decades ago after my student had shown me the book. Of course, it is not at all the same. The cover is faded, roughened with wear, and fraying a little around the edges. There is a stain of unknown origin that breaks the solid orange of the binding. Some of the corners of the pages are turned down, and there are yellow highlights on some favorite passages in the text. Inside the front cover is the bold and inscrutable signature of Sri B. K. S. Iyengar and the date 1974. On the facing page is the equally inscrutable childish scribbling of one my children. Both are equally precious to me.

When I look back to the series of events that have shaped my life, that day when I first encountered *Light on Yoga* is one of the most important, not only because of what I have learned from the man and the book, but also because of what that learning has allowed me to do. Directly because of Mr. Iyengar, I have become privileged to teach others a small portion of what I have been given. I am filled with gratitude and wonder.

Thank you, Sri B. K. S. Iyengar, for your refusal to accept anything but the best and deepest dedication to the practice of the yoga we all love, either from yourself or from your students.

༄

JUDITH HANSON LASATER, PhD, PT, is currently president of the California Yoga Teachers Association and cofounder of *Yoga Journal*. A yoga teacher since 1971, she has studied with B. K. S. Iyengar in India and the United States and helped to found the San Francisco Iyengar Yoga Institute. Judith teaches ongoing yoga classes and trains teachers in kinesiology, yoga therapeutics, and the *Yoga Sutras*. She holds a PhD in East-West psychology and is the author of six books, including *Living Your Yoga, Yoga Abs, Yoga for Pregnancy, 30 Essential Yoga Poses,* and *Relax and Renew.*

"Take an Action"

PATRICIA WALDEN

The word *guru* means "teacher" or "preceptor" in Sanskrit. According to the *Rig Veda, guru* is an adjective meaning "heavy," being contrasted with *laghu,* meaning "light." The guru is the one pregnant or "heavy" with spiritual knowledge, realization, and knowledge. The *Guru Gita (Song of the Teacher)*—a dialogue between Shiva and his wife, Parvati—describes the guru as the one who "removes the darkness of ignorance." The guru's function is therefore to guide the seeker to *moksha* (freedom from the cycle of births and deaths), *samadhi* (the supreme divine bliss), and/or *atma jnana* (a knowledge of the soul based on experience rather than on intellect). As such, atma jnana is often translated as "self-realization" rather than "self-knowledge," for it is redolent of a coming into the light of understanding one's own essential nature through experiencing it within.

> The one who is himself possessed with devotion to his own guru
> And who is a knower of the Self is called a guru.
> The syllable *gu* signifies "that which is dark."
> The syllable *ru* signifies "that which dispels."
> It is on account of this power to dispel that darkness
> That the guru is so named.
> The guru alone is the Supreme Absolute.
> The guru alone is the Way Supreme.
> The guru alone is the Knowledge Supreme.
> The guru alone is the Ultimate Resort.
> The guru alone is the Supreme End.
> The guru alone is the Wealth that is Beyond.
> Because this guru teaches that Reality
> This guru is greater than any other guru.★

★ *Advaya Taraka Upanishad,* verses 14–18.

The guru is an imparter and a facilitator, the conduit through which re-alization of our own true self is transmitted to us as seekers. As now elab-orated by Patricia Walden, the relationship between a student and a teacher can be a very powerful thing.

Patricia Walden was interviewed by Anne O'Brien in June 2006.

ANNE O'BRIEN: Patricia, you have quoted Mr. Iyengar as saying, "Take an action, no matter how small. Just take one action." How has this teach-ing influenced your practice and teaching?

PATRICIA WALDEN: It has influenced me in many ways. When I first met B. K. S. Iyengar in 1976, I had already been doing yoga for some time, but certainly not the way he was teaching it. In the early days, dur-ing at least my first ten years of yoga practice, beginning at age nineteen, I had a very difficult time with discipline, with *tapas;* it was very chal-lenging for me. I remember as a young woman being at the Ramamani Iyengar Memorial Yoga Institute listening to a talk he was giving, and hearing that particular sentence gave me hope. I didn't feel so over-whelmed by establishing a home practice. If I could do just one pose. If I could just take that one action, maybe that would lead to the next one. I took that to heart in my practice and in my teaching.

I have a keen interest in how to use yoga to work with people who are depressed. And that is one of the mantras I use: "Take an action, no matter how small, and take it often." I suffered from depression in my late teens and early twenties, and periodically it comes back into my life, though not very often. I think a lot of people who are depressed suffer from inertia, and then everything feels overwhelming. Sometimes it is just the one small action that makes all the difference.

AOB: Was this step-by-step action characteristic of your study with Mr. Iyengar?

PW: My early relationship with him was literally a baptism by fire. I went to my first intensive with him in 1976. I was in my late twenties, and I thought that I was quite a good practitioner. I went there in a red leotard, dressed to be seen, with a lot of ego, and he said something like, "I'm going to break your ego down." After he made that remark, he didn't say anything else to me for the next three weeks. I came back the next year; he didn't say anything. Came back the next year and the next year; didn't say anything. You know what can happen with gurus and students: we students can be like hungry birds with our mouths open, waiting to be fed, wanting approval, hoping to catch the guru's attention, waiting to be seen. I went through an eight-year period where he said nothing to me.

AOB: Eight years?

PW: Eight years. His not speaking to me just made me more determined and stronger. This is when I really took on my practice. There was a real transformation of practice. What it actually did was teach me how to practice for different reasons. Through this process, I became more confident, more fearless. I learned to practice on my own and eventually to practice not for his approval or anyone else's, but for myself. I finally got Guruji's lessons, this awakening to who you really are. How what you do with your body and your being can really transform all aspects of your existence. That was definitely a crossroads on my path. That was the lesson he was teaching me, and that was a turning point in my life. I have never lost that intensity that developed during that eight-year period of no reaction from B. K. S. Iyengar.

AOB: What happens in Pune that is so transformative for you?

PW: I've been going to study with him yearly since 1976. In the early years, it was to take an intensive with him. In the last twenty years, it's been just to be in his presence, to practice near him or with him. Here's someone who's been practicing since he was eighteen, and that's been his life. His life is very, very simple. He has his everyday ritual. His home is just ten steps away from the Institute. Every morning he walks into the practice room. He goes to the platform in the practice room, to the far corner of the platform. Flurries of his students come, including myself, and do a *pranam* (bow). He takes his dhoti off, his watch off, puts his timer down. His assistants come over, bring him the props that he says he wants that day for his practice, and then he begins. I am always captivated when he begins. He may begin with a ten-minute pose or a thirty-minute headstand. When he goes into a pose, something happens that's really hard to put into words, but many of us who have been around for a long time stop what we're doing, stop our practice, and go and just watch him, because there's such stillness and quiet and light that radiates from his being; it's compelling. He's obviously in a deep meditative state in some of his practices, and when you watch him practice, it's as if you were to enter into that same state with him. There's such power in the stillness and the quiet and in his being that, without any words exchanged, you go right there with him, and you find that you've been sitting there for twenty minutes watching B. K. S. Iyengar do sirsasana. The time goes by very quickly. Watching him practice is one of the many ways that has taught me about yoga and how to practice. There is an energy and a light that emanates from him, and this has changed over time. In the earlier days, in the 1970s and early 1980s, there was always energy and a fire there. But that has changed. The fire's there. The energy is there. But what accompanies that now is this radiance, this light, this silence, and a stillness that's palpable. I've told my students I would go to Pune for one day just to watch him practice. It's that valuable for me.

AOB: So as his practice changes with age, he also candidly talks about the next stage. In fact, in his book *Light on Life,* he refers to his moving on and passing the torch to his students and teachers, saying that it's his profound hope that his end can be your . . .

PW: Beginning. Yes.

AOB: How are you integrating that now?

PW: Well, I'm in process with it. I always knew how attached I was to him as my guru and to his practice. It's been thirty incredible years where I have learned so much. I count on going to India every year, being in his presence, and coming back ignited. And he can say one thing to me or make one adjustment, or I can watch one practice, and that stays in me for a year. I really think I'm a better teacher because of it and certainly a better practitioner because of it. About eight years ago, just before his eightieth birthday, I was practicing with him, and I realized not only was I attached to him, but I was equally attached to his practice to keep my own flame burning, to inspire me, to nourish me. And I wondered what it will be like for me when he's no longer around. So right now, I feel it is part of my work as his student to detach myself.

I am at a crossroads, turning sixty. Fifty was like a little punctuation point. Turning sixty marks the opening of a new phase, with a lot of unknowns. I feel my responsibilities differently. I know that I want to convey the purity of Guruji's teachings to my students—both his vision as a Seer and his methods as a teacher. And I intend to keep up the intensity of my practice.

When I speak of intensity of practice, I am not talking about the physical intensity. I am talking about the intensity it takes to penetrate the refined layers of consciousness.

For example, he may ask in urdhva dhanurasana, "Move your shins back toward your forearms. Move your forearms back toward your shins. What happens when you do that?" And then, "After moving the shins toward the forearms and the forearms toward the shins, lift from the bottom of the navel, and then what happens?" His teaching asks you to question with your whole being, not just your analytical mind. You have to become fully embodied, because the answers don't come from your brain. You have to be absolutely in the present. You bypass the habits of your brain and hear the intelligence of your body and the voice of your Self.

When he is teaching in this way, he is leading you to a subtler level of exploration. At the beginning of a pose, he shows how to create the geometry of the asana. Then he shows how the parts communicate with one another. The ultimate emerges when the rhythm of the asana is established. The parts of the body communicate with one another. Then when your awareness is keen, you feel your consciousness spread evenly throughout your body. The rays of your intelligence permeate your cells. The doer (you, your Self), the instrument of doing (your body), and the asana become one. You are no longer fragmented. You are in a state of integration. You experience the asana as a whole, and your whole being is in a *sattvic* state—a calm state of alertness. This is meditation. Again, it's hard to put these things into words. He wants us to understand that asana is meditation, and he very clearly shows us the path to practice. You start from the *annamayakosha* (the outermost sheath), and you penetrate inward. You penetrate with your awareness. You wake your intelligence. Every aspect of you—mind and body—communicates. The result is integration. You come to know your Self. At the end of the pose, he'll often say something like, "Now you're no longer fragmented. Let the rays of your intelligence spread throughout your asana; let your mind spread throughout the asana; let your consciousness grace the asana so you are in this undivided state. There's no duality." This is a different way of teaching for him. For me, it's another baptism by fire to do this kind of thing with him for an hour. At the end, I just go back to my hotel room and think, "Oh, my god, I just entered into another realm." It's quite extraordinary.

He is currently nearly ninety years old, and he has this life, which I described earlier, going back and forth every day to the Institute, practicing. Whether he's had an injury, whether he's doing a recuperative practice, whether he's doing an intensive practice, whatever it is, he's there day after day. He doesn't hide when he's struggling. I have never met another being who is so absolutely interested in and—incredibly—still so curious about his art. The level of interest, the level of curiosity, and the playfulness is humbling, actually. I'm interested in my art, but his mind—he's of a different ilk. He so embodies yoga and yoga philosophy: it's in every cell. He's taken the practice of asana to a place where I don't think anybody else has. And because his experience has been beyond what most of us can realize, it will be hard to follow him. He goes places inside that we haven't been. So when he passes, how will I keep that motivation up? I certainly don't have what he has, but I'm going to try my best to do as much of it as I can. I believe my devotion to him and the inspiration I draw from him will enable me to do so.

That's what I worry about in my own practice. How can I keep up this level of interested curiosity at the level that he's teaching now? I mean I'm absolutely committed. There's no way I'll ever do anything else with my life. I am more determined than ever to practice the way in which he's teaching me now. I have to go to the level that he is as my role model. His teaching is not for a casual practice: you must be absolutely in the present and be incredibly interested in this art.

AOB: There seems to be a new spontaneity and almost a bhakti quality to his transformation.

PW: A deep, reflective, philosophical side started emerging in him in his late sixties. In fact, many of his major transformations came much later in life. For those of us who have witnessed this transformation and this evolution of this being, it has been extraordinary. One of the by-products of this transformation is the light and the radiance that just emanate from him.

His spontaneity strikes me all the time. Recently, I was at a dinner with him, in my party clothes, and right in the middle of dinner, he asked me to get up and do urdhva dhanurasana! I pointed out that I had a dress on, but his response was, "Who cares?" You have to be ready for anything with Guruji. We could be in the library and he'll be talking about something and we will make eye contact and this outpouring of light just fills my being. I actually start to feel heat from it and teary. This started ten years ago, when I began to have these experiences with him. He has pierced through my thinking mind. He's pierced through my brain and gone right to my heart, and I feel so vulnerable and so at peace. Sometimes it lasts for an hour, sometimes two minutes, and sometimes five minutes.

AOB: Has this fueled your practice in a different way?

PW: Absolutely. Those experiences I have had with him have fueled my practice and teaching, because it makes me see that there's so much more to being a human being than we realize. We read these things about what yoga can do for us. But then when we have the experience and it's different, there are no words to describe it. But it ignites your entire being, and you start to perceive yourself and people in the world differently. That has happened to me, especially over these last ten years with him. It's remarkable, you know, that we've been living these parallel experiences—Guruji's evolution and our evolution as his students. And we feel this tremendous determination to keep his method out there. For me, what keeps his method out there is my commitment to practice, because what makes excellent teaching is the way one practices. So every day I commit myself to a particular kind of practice, knowing that if I don't practice that way, then his teaching, his practice, isn't going to be in me the way I want it to be. I'll move further and further away. Within this, I still find my own voice, allow my own experiences to come forth, and the practice has brought me closer to myself.

AOB: Your authentic self.

PW: Absolutely. In my early days, I would go to Pune and come back and yell at all my students, teaching by imitation. It was an important stage to go through. Often, we imitate the people in our lives whom we respect. They have qualities that we want to embody. Often, those qualities are deep inside of us, but they're obscured by *samskaras*. Then, over time, a wonderful teacher will help those qualities manifest in the student in a unique manner. I feel that Guruji has done that for me. I went through this period of teaching by imitation, and then slowly, slowly, things just evolved in their own time. Over the years, I found my own feminine voice, and I consider myself a strong teacher within the Iyengar method.

There's another phrase of his that I would like to share that is always there for me like "take an action, no matter how small." Once, when he must have been eighty-three, he spoke about still practicing to reduce samskaras that remain in the heart, so that if he's destined to be born again, he may start yoga from where he ended and become more enlightened than at the time of death. Then he said, "I do not want to die as a stopper." I just love that. It's going to stay with me. If I'm having a bad day thinking that I'm almost sixty, can't do 108 dropbacks or can't do jumpings today, that line will come back: "I don't want to die as a stopper." I don't. I want to practice until I die, all my practices: pranayama, meditation, asana. I've taken that on.

I have one last image that I have of him that I'd like to share. He often talks about a river and how it should move freely. Then I start thinking about the banks of a river, and I see this kind of ordinary bank or shore, as a seeker looking for something, and I see B. K. S. Iyengar with this lifeboat filled with his knowledge, inspiration, and light that has taken many of us from this ordinary shore of human existence toward the shore of the self. I don't want to say that I've reached that shore yet, but I feel like that's what he's done for many of us. We have been in his lifeboat, in a lifeboat that's taken us from the ordinary human existence to this magical extraordinary transcendence. That is his practice and life; it's transcendent.

⌇

Patricia Walden's first spiritual teacher was Murshed Samuel Lewis, a Sufi master, who taught dance as spiritual movement—a joyful prayer. This theme of "praying with the body" naturally transformed into her yoga practice in the early 1970s. Patricia met B. K. S. Iyengar in 1976. She was immediately struck by his light, energy, insight, and genius, as well as by the joy and humor that he often projects. She became his devoted student, traveling to Pune, India, to study with him regularly. Under Mr. Iyengar's guidance, she gained a systematic and inspirational approach to practice and teaching. His influence was complemented a few years later when she met Dona Holleman of Florence, Italy. In the mid-1980s, Patricia began to take a more active role in the Iyengar Yoga community, cofounding the B. K. S. Iyengar Yoga Center in Cambridge, Massachusetts, in 1985; organizing the 1987 B. K. S. Iyengar Yoga Convention; and serving as president of the B. K. S. Iyengar Yoga Association of Massachusetts from 1987 to 1990. She has co-authored three books, writes regularly for *Yoga Journal,* and teaches regular classes in Cambridge, Massachusetts, and throughout the United States.

B. K. S. Iyengar: The Man, the Myth, the Magic

Marian Garfinkel

Yoga may mean "union," but it is also practical; it is for doing. If concentration can allow us to be observers of consciousness, then what purpose does this serve if we do not embody that experience? The benefits of yoga surely also depend on why we practice—on how we choose to incorporate it into our lives. For some, yoga remains a physical fitness program, albeit one incorporating some breathing and relaxation techniques. But to others, those techniques are key. They are signs of yoga's method for bringing deeper enjoyment and satisfaction to life. To them, this "listening within" is a way of learning how to grow. The concentration yoga develops brings a heightened inner awareness. That heightened awareness encompasses the mind, for it is the mind that observes awareness and its consequences. This encourages the experiential learning and embodiment characteristic of yoga. As consciousness is observed, we realize that we are something more than just "this"—that is, "this" body, "this" mind, "this" particular existence. The door opens to the fact that there is more to know and appreciate. And because yoga is about practice, a thing can only be accepted if it is experienced as true. On the other hand, if a thing is accepted as true—that is, it is recognized as a principle that should be abided by—then its tenets must be embodied. It must be enacted because it has become a part of the awareness; yogic awareness is practice. Yoga should therefore encourage anyone who practices it to embody its philosophy for living. The sense of oneness that yoga encourages—that unity with the world around us—should become a fulfillment and an experience. Marian Garfinkel now discusses aspects of that embodiment.

THE MAN

I met B. K. S. Iyengar for the first time on a rainy Sunday night in 1974 at the home of William and Mary Palmer in Ann Arbor, Michigan. His poise, grace, ease, and friendliness were obvious. He was charming and interested in each individual. When I was introduced to him, he made me feel comfortable and asked, "How can I help you in the class tomorrow?"

"I need some help with my headstand," I told him.

The next morning I was standing directly in front of him when he called the class to order. He jumped off the table and confronted me directly, "You wanted to stand on your head? You don't even know how to stand on your feet." After thirty years of studying with him, I understand how much easier it is to stand on one's head than to stand correctly on one's own feet. That first brief experience showed me the truth of yoga and how important it is to study and practice correctly under the guidance of a good teacher. I knew he was my real teacher and saw the genius of the man. To learn to stand majestically on our own legs is a life-learning process and a journey that never ends.

I saw Mr. Iyengar in many situations and many locations—London; Paris; New York; Philadelphia; Los Angeles; Washington, D.C.; Delhi; Mumbai; and Pune—and came to appreciate the incredible versatility of the man. He commanded attention and respect and could discourse on various subjects, the true Renaissance man in every setting. After a concert by the Philadelphia Orchestra conducted by Aaron Copland, Mr. Iyengar went backstage and was greeted by the orchestra and Copland himself. Mr. Iyengar generated tremendous excitement and electricity that rivaled that of the conductor. When touring the Metropolitan Museum of Art in New York City, his depth of knowledge and ability to observe, analyze, and appreciate the complexity of Egyptian art was surprising. At Buckingham Palace, his appreciation of the majesty, splendor, and magnificence was impressive. In Washington, D.C., at a reception at the Indian embassy, the ambassador wanted Iyengar to teach him yoga then and there! For more than thirty years, I have known Mr. Iyengar as a man who is comfortable in any situation and, when appropriate, has taken charge, presided, and commanded the occasion.

On his first visit to Philadelphia, Mr. Iyengar gave a demonstration at Haverford College. It was here that he met Robert Engman, an American sculptor. Engman was so inspired by the presentation that he created a sculpture in Iyengar's honor and titled it *After B. K. S. Iyengar.* "Iyengar is a great man—a supreme artist," remarked Engman. "He has influenced how I think about my work. He demonstrated precisely his person, and what he has done with himself and his life from the time when he was eighteen years old to present time. It was absolutely the most incredible physical and mental expression I've ever witnessed in my life, barring none."* On his second visit to Philadelphia, Mr. Iyengar addressed medical doctors at the Philadelphia College of Osteopathy and enlightened them with innovative ways of giving traction to the body. He showed how yoga could be used as treatment for many medical problems. Returning to Philadelphia for the third time, he demonstrated his incredible artistry once again. At the installation of the sculpture *After B. K. S. Iyengar* at the Morris Arboretum, he was more than sensational. He mesmerized the crowd with his own instrument—his body. Through his discipline, Iyengar has achieved balance in his life—the same balance Engman expresses in the Iyengar sculpture.

As the Family Man

I have seen him as a father responsible for providing for and educating his children. After the passing of his wife, he took on the dual role of mother and father to his children. He encouraged the differences in them and now cherishes and supports these differences, having allowed each child to develop according to his or her own interests. He has welcomed his daughters' husbands as his own sons. I had the pleasure of meeting his sisters and brothers and learned of his generosity to them. As a father, grandfather, father-in-law, brother, and friend, he has always been kind, gracious, and nourishing. He lavishes affection on his grandchildren and is guiding his granddaughter with precision and awareness in the pursuit of yoga.

---

* B. I. Taraporewala, *Body Thy Shrine, Yoga Thy Light* (Bombay: Light on Yoga Research Trust, 1978).

As the Student, as the Teacher

At the Institute, Iyengar is always practicing and inquiring. He is focused on his study and learns from his practice. On Friday mornings, he does his standing backbends and intense practice. It is a serious pursuit. In addition, he continues his work by writing, philosophizing, interviewing, and reading. He is motivated and driven to be involved with his environment, his students, and himself.

Iyengar is his own best teacher and his own best student. He has always remained a student—eager to learn, to find out, to question. He is an inspiring teacher who knows how to bring out the best in every one of us and gives freely of his knowledge—if we're lucky enough to understand. To be able to take a class with B. K. S. Iyengar can only make one stronger in life. In my years of study with him, I have learned his lessons of being more critical and searching in my own practice and teaching. This stern discipline and perseverance is necessary to be a true Iyengar student of yoga. The knowledge is subjective, and there is personal clarity and confidence.

Iyengar knows the capabilities of his students and can extend their reach. He demands that the eyes and ears be wide open and alert. This brings awareness and light to the darkness. When asanas are done correctly and the pose is achieved, he will show a student how to still further improve and refine the posture. Whether working with a wide-eyed, innocent, raw beginner or a mature and seasoned student, this outstanding teacher brings out the best.

As the Medical Man

On my first visit to Pune in 1974, I saw him as a medical man. I marveled at his amazing ability and power to treat and even cure medical conditions. B. K. S. Iyengar's genius for diagnosis and treatment is unique and world famous. When he was in Philadelphia, I had introduced him to Robert, a disabled young man, who had been hit in the head with a golf ball and suffered the symptoms of a stroke victim. "Bring him to Pune, Marian, for medical attention," Iyengar told me. Robert's rehabilitation of nearly three months in India convinced me it was not just the benefits of yoga, but the knowledge and expertise of B. K. S. Iyengar that made me want to pursue yoga seriously and validate his work to the medical profession in the United States.

Later, I dedicated and presented my doctoral dissertation to Mr. Iyengar on his seventieth birthday in Pune. With his encouragement and consultation, I had a study published in the *Journal of the American Medical Association* in November 1998, demonstrating the positive effects of a yoga program on people with carpal tunnel syndrome. This was the first time anything on yoga had ever been published in a peer-reviewed medical journal, and I gave him the journal for his birthday. Along with countless people the world over, I have been his medical patient and the grateful beneficiary of his expertise. I am just one of many individuals who have been inspired by the modern-day medical miracles achieved by B. K. S. Iyengar.

As the Artist

B. K. S. Iyengar epitomizes the definition of an artist as defined by Edwin Zoller in his book, *From a Painter's Notes: The Writings and Work of Edwin W. Zoller:* "In the artist's makeup, there is a basic compulsive drive that requires him to continue to probe the phenomena constituting his environment and to find suitable forms with which he can present his reactions to them. In this creative activity he moves from intention to realization through a succession of steps involving the acceptance of some solutions and the rejection of others which help to crystallize the meaning of his environmental influences and offer him some reward for his way of life."★ B. K. S. Iyengar's drive to further innovate and his dedication to find solutions to problems separate him from others. For an artist like Iyengar, the compulsion to satisfy creative urges, as Zoller further states, "... is so strong that it cannot be denied." Through constant practice, he has refined the demonstration, performance, and integration of yoga as a living art, a testimonial to the creative spirit.

★ Edwin Zoller, *From a Painter's Notes: The Writings and Work of Edwin W. Zoller* (self-published, Philadelphia, 1967).

As the Courageous Man

B. K. S. Iyengar is a courageous man, as defined by Rollo May in *The Courage to Create:* "He possesses a willingness to express and develop his own original ideas, to listen to his being, to be true to himself, and to make a contribution to society."★ Courage is the foundation of his values. The manifestation of this courage is seen in his passion for life—his physical, intellectual, and emotional practice of yoga. He epitomizes the example of physical courage, the courage to develop awareness and sensitivity of the body through constant intense practice of yoga. Courage is demonstrated through his personal life. When challenged to endure the death of his wife and later recover from his motorcycle accident, he had the courage and capacity to rise above despair. His own life suffering has enabled him to see the afflictions of others more clearly and be compassionate toward them. Moral courage has its source in such identification through one's own sensitivity with the suffering of one's fellow human beings.

THE MYTH

To look at Iyengar and the many myths that surround him, it is necessary to know what myth is and does. When the ancients told stories to each other about gods, goddesses, heroes, and heroines of legendary fame, they believed in these figures of mythology and made them real. Humans saw life and the universe influenced by heroes of the past; these beliefs had an enduring influence and effect on their lives. The gods could make playthings of human beings. The gods were invincible and strong. They had no limitations and could do anything. All of the stories surrounding B. K. S. Iyengar paint him as a mythical hero—with superhuman knowledge and intuitiveness. In this way, he is part myth. He has the ability to empower people to change their lives—to rise above physical health, to rise above poverty and frailty, to rise above despair. Just as he teaches, he himself exemplifies a man who has risen above poor health, poverty, and personal circumstances. He emerges with a persona larger than life.

★ Rollo May, *The Courage to Create* (New York: Bantam, 1975), 3.

B. K. S. Iyengar is internationally acclaimed for his contribution to yoga, but more than that, he is a man who symbolizes a principle of conscious life, independence. A self-made man, he has never let adversity interfere with the individuality of his thinking. In the Ramamani Iyengar Memorial Yoga Institute and residential compound—all of which came about through his own effort—he can look back over his life, which enters the ninetieth decade, and recall the influence of worldwide travel and famous and not-so-famous people whose lives he has touched, and perhaps those whose lives have influenced his own. Iyengar is a man among men—devoted to his country and his people. He has never forgotten his birthplace. In the town of his birth, Bellur, in the state of Karnataka, he actively works to improve the lives of the people, including contributing to building a temple, a school, and a hospital. He can be recognized as one of the true remaining spirits to grace the nation of his birth—a "national treasure." Anyone who has been fortunate enough to have directly experienced his teachings and personal touch can recognize the spirit of independence in this one-of-a-kind human being.

Our bodies are the most intimate contact with ourselves. We work with them to find our destinies to give these animate objects new life, perhaps a first life. Through the practice of yoga as taught by Mr. Iyengar and the practice of his teachings, we are able to use what we have been given in our lives to release our own richness and beauty and to be independent and live consciously. Iyengar illustrates more than once the inevitable commitment of a brilliant man who is generous in the sharing of his knowledge; of this, there can be no dispute.

THE MAGIC

What Iyengar does and how he does it is magical. He has the magic to create. That magic is something that goes beyond yoga—magic that goes beyond the man himself, magic that can't be questioned with the mind. Whether in the Institute, in medical classes, or in conversation with him, this magic has to be experienced in his presence. His magic creates harmony for those of us around him. When you are with him, you are in the moment. There's no pain, no suffering, no logic, no words. You see it; you feel it; you know it. He puts that magic in the moment.

He makes the magic last.

❦

MARIAN GARFINKEL, PHD, is a Senior Intermediate Iyengar Yoga teacher with more than thirty years of teaching experience and has studied extensively with Mr. Iyengar in India since 1974. She is a member of teacher-assessment committees and teacher-training programs. Dr. Garfinkel is a specialist in the prevention and treatment of repetitive strain injuries and arthritis; a faculty lecturer at Drexel University, School of Nursing and Health Professions; and a clinical investigator at the University of Pennsylvania Medical School. She contributes to various newsletters, periodicals, and journals in the United States and abroad. Her study on carpal tunnel syndrome was published in the *Journal of the American Medical Association*.

Light on Love

JOHN SCHUMACHER

Yoga is a spiritual quest, which makes it likely that we will run into un-familiar thoughts and ideas that ask us to take a different perspective. Moreover, yoga's language can be hard to understand, acquainting us with new concepts, such as dharma, for which there is no easy English equivalent. But we can sometimes be blindsided in our quest to become good yogis for another reason. It is easy enough to call seemingly ordi-nary English words into service and make them stand duty for impor-tant ideas in yoga and Sanskrit. At first sight, they may seem similar enough. But we then come to realize, slowly and painfully, that the res-onances attaching to the English word play little or no part in the San-skrit. *Kama,* generally translated as "love," is such a word. *Kama* looks and sounds remarkably like *karma,* so initially they may be confused. John Schumacher now discusses *bhakti,* a word prone to similar confusion. Al-though most-usually translated as "devotion," the word is difficult to pin down.

Guillame of Aquitaine, born in 1070 C.E., may have been the first rec-ognized troubadour, but the tradition of *fin amors* (courtly love) that he sang about was already well enough established for him to poke fun at it in some of his bawdier verses. Courtly love was a formalized system of flattery, admiration, and courtship based on medieval ideas of feudalism and fealty. At its best, feudalism was seen as an enabler of devotion be-tween a true knight and his lord. As the system declined, a gentleman knight could swear devotion to a suitable—but often unavailable—"fair lady." She could then energize him to express the higher aspects of knightly behavior. The rules decreed that a love of this kind was so pure that it could not be contained within marriage. Some commentators in-sisted that "true love" between a married man and woman could not re-ally exist because, as husband and wife, they were bound by the marriage itself to honor and serve each other. True courtly love existed when sim-ilar agreements were voluntarily proposed between two parties who were not married and therefore not obligated. The *princesse lointaine* was the "princess far away" whom the demure knight could love from a distance, devotion to her being his near-divine inspiration as he sought to do well in her name. To this day, and to most Westerners, the most important form of love and devotion that exists is thought to be that between a man and a woman, which therefore almost always has sexual overtones. Other kinds of love have to be "explained." They also tend to be implicitly measured, usually to their detriment, against this highest of all standards. As John Schumacher now makes clear in his examination of this most profound of all human emotions, it is often only the appreciation of a spiritual quest of a deep and transformative kind that can make us appreciate the many dimensions and kinds of love that can exist within the human heart.

To many of the millions of people who are at least ankle-deep in their yoga experience, B. K. S. Iyengar is a household name. Mr. Iyengar's contributions to the literature of yoga are inestimable. His first book, *Light on Yoga,* has become a classic, a requirement for even the most minimal yoga library, and is arguably the best and most comprehensive book on the practice of yoga available today. His subsequent books—*Light on Pranayama, Light on the Yoga Sutras,* and *Light on Life*—are all essential reading for anyone with any real interest in the subject. His methods of practicing and teaching have influenced the shape of yoga as it is practiced in the modern world, whether the practitioner is an Iyengar Yoga student or from a different tradition. Mr. Iyengar's use of anatomical language to describe the actions of the body in yoga poses, his emphasis on alignment, and his pioneering employment of props are now ubiquitous in the teaching of yoga. Even the idea of group classes as distinguished from individual instruction is an Iyengar innovation. The success of his application of yoga as a therapeutic modality has been instrumental in capturing the interest of Western medicine and science. The imprimatur of the scientific community confers credibility in our society, and that community's growing recognition of the validity of yoga as a means to health and well-being has helped catapult yoga into the public's consciousness. Finally, recognition by the international media of the scope of his influence has increased his visibility and stature worldwide. Thus,

B. K. S. Iyengar's contribution to the rapid growth of yoga in the world today is unparalleled, and he is widely recognized as the world's foremost yoga teacher.

Any attempt to categorize Guruji's approach to yoga always falls short. His method is truly unique. His emphasis on asana and pranayama as vehicles for awakening are characteristic of some of the tenets of hatha yoga, although the absence of the regular practice of *kriyas*, yogic cleansing practices, and some of the other more esoteric aspects of hatha yoga differentiate his approach from that described in *Hatha Yoga Pradipika,* a seminal work in this tradition.

Mr. Iyengar's humanitarian work—especially his huge contributions in time, energy, and money toward uplifting his birthplace, the impoverished Indian village of Bellur—certainly falls within the purview of karma yoga, the yoga of action and selfless service in the world. The path of karma yoga is also exemplified in his choice to live life as a family man while at the same time toiling tirelessly to propagate the message of yoga for the benefit of all humankind.

Jnana yoga, the yoga of wisdom and discrimination, is evident in Guruji's method as well. It appears clearly in his approach to teaching and practicing asana and pranayama. Rather than simply placing the body in certain positions or breathing in particular patterns, the Iyengar Yoga practitioner is trained to apply awareness to the movement of intelligence in the body in such a way as to develop the discriminative faculty of the mind that is characteristic of jnana yoga. Guruji teaches us to mindfully explore our actions and tendencies as we practice, to observe the effects of our actions, and to apply our knowledge and experience toward correcting our errors and refining ourselves. Gradually, through persistent and conscious practice, we cultivate our physical and mental intelligence into spiritual wisdom.

Guruji's method follows the traditions of raja yoga, yoga that seeks to balance all the faculties—physical, mental, moral, and spiritual, as defined by Patanjali's eight-limbed path. In Mr. Iyengar's perceptive commentary in *Light on the Yoga Sutras of Patanjali,* he describes Patanjali as his "Invisible, First and Foremost Guru." Mr. Iyengar's approach is clearly based on the eight-limbed path (ashtanga yoga) Patanjali outlines in the *Sutras.*

Thus far, I have mentioned all of the major traditions of yoga save one, bhakti yoga, the path of love and devotion. Bhakti yoga represents the emotional aspect of the spiritual quest and is classically described as the surrender of oneself through adoration of the divine. In his book *Yoga: The Technology of Ecstasy,* noted yoga scholar Georg Feuerstein describes bhakti yoga as "the self-transcending power of love."* Feuerstein quotes Sage Narada's *Bhakti Sutra* as saying the devotee "sees nothing but love, hears only about love, speaks only of love, and thinks of love alone."

When the scriptures speak of love, they are not referring to egoic attraction, the romantic love usually portrayed in song and story. Rather, they describe a passion for the divine in any of its countless manifestations, a devotion of the heart that pours out toward the One, that seeks to sublimate the individuality of the lover to the will and presence of the Beloved. In *Light on Life,* Mr. Iyengar says, "The Love that transcends the particularity of individual attraction and perceives the soul within the other is the great pathway to God."† Bhakti yoga, then, is not the search for self-gratification through attachment to another person or object. It is instead the complete surrender of the devotee toward that manifestation of the divine that cracks open his heart and consumes him with passionate love for his Beloved.

Perhaps because of its emphasis on the asanas or what appears to be the relatively small role devotional rituals play in its practice, or maybe even because of the powerful and uncompromising manner in which it is taught, I think it is fair to say that Iyengar Yoga is not usually thought of as an exemplar of bhakti yoga. But I must also say that to believe that the qualities of bhakti—love and devotion—are absent from Iyengar Yoga is to misunderstand both the method and the man.

Upon first meeting B. K. S. Iyengar, the words I would have used to describe my impression of him would probably not have included *loving* or *devotional.* I experienced his presence as intense above all else, and because of my own insecurities and inexperience, that intensity intimidated me. He also displayed an occasionally fiery temper that only added to my general apprehensiveness. But I was struck as well by his tremendous energy and remarkable spontaneity. His reactions to situations in

---

* Georg Feuerstein, *Yoga: The Technology of Ecstasy* (Los Angeles: Tarcher, 1989).
† B. K. S. Iyengar, *Light on Life* (New York: Rodale, 2005), 86.

the classroom were immediate and honest, and he was as quick to laugh good-naturedly as he was to shout at or scold someone.

As I spent more time studying with him, I came to see another part of B. K. S. Iyengar, his generous nature. He gave of himself unstintingly in the classroom and outside it. I felt that he held nothing back, that he was giving his all, all the time. This generosity was apparent in the effort he put forth to teach us and in his willingness to help those with particular problems. Gradually, I began to understand that his generosity of spirit is an outgrowth of deep compassion. It is interesting to note that the word *compassion* derives from the Latin words *com,* meaning "with," and *passus,* a past participle of the word *pati,* meaning "to suffer." Mr. Iyengar's work to relieve the suffering of the people with whom he comes in contact springs from his deep empathy toward those in pain. Perhaps this is because of his difficult youth, which was marked by ill health and abject poverty, because of the suffering he experienced in his own body and mind as he struggled to master his art, or maybe as a result of his ability to see the essential humanity of the people he meets. Whatever the reason, compassion is a fundamental aspect of Mr. Iyengar's character.

Although *passion* has its root meaning in suffering, in common parlance, it is usually taken to mean an intense love for, or devotion to, someone or something. In most people's minds, passion, as powerful emotion, is not usually associated with either yoga or the yogi. Rather, one imagines yoga as conferring the epitome of equanimity and conjures up the unassailable calm of the sage sequestered from the vicissitudes of life in lofty meditation. *The Yoga Sutras of Patanjali,* sometimes referred to as the bible of yoga, and B.K. S. Iyengar, through his work and life, put the lie to this misconception. Both are graphic and compelling examples of the place of passion in the pursuit of yoga. Patanjali says that *samadhi* is nearest to those whose desire for samadhi is intensely strong (1:21). The passionate pursuit of the goal overcomes the obstacles that inevitably arise. And anyone who has seen B. K. S. Iyengar practice, demonstrate, teach, or talk about yoga has experienced his unmistakable passion for the subject. His fervor goes far beyond the enthusiasm of even serious students of the art. He is consumed by yoga, and he gives himself to it completely.

Very few have the discipline to practice with the intensity required to penetrate the depths of any art to the extent that Mr. Iyengar has done with yoga. To muster such discipline demands almost unimaginable willpower to be sure, but willpower alone is insufficient to sustain that level of intense practice for the prolonged, uninterrupted time necessary to achieve what Guruji has achieved. Unrelenting discipline of that sort can come only from the deepest levels of devotion. One has to imagine Michelangelo and the Sistine Chapel, or Milarepa struggling to fulfill the demands of his guru, Lama Marpa, or Job persisting through his afflictions to begin to comprehend the fierce devotion Guruji's efforts must have entailed.

Yoga, of course, means "union." Union occurs on many different levels, with the ultimate yogic union being the realization of the conjoining of the individual spirit (*jivatma*) with the great cosmic spirit (*paramatma*). Through yoga, one experiences one's interconnectedness with the One and thus with every manifestation of the One. Evidence of interconnectedness may appear in many ways. One significant example in Guruji's case can be found in his teaching. For the serious and skillful yoga teacher, the relationship with the pupil is a deeply intimate one. It is not a subject-object interaction, but subject-subject instead. As with dance partners or lovers, the distinction between teacher and pupil becomes less and less delineated the more experienced and committed the relationship becomes. During his recent visit to the United States, Guruji said, "Though I have come several times and taught lots of people, this is the first time all my pupils touched my heart, which was unforgettable. When I looked at the faces of the thousands of people I met, I felt that the work I did must have touched their hearts and souls, as if we had known each other for centuries. The work of the past has fructified in such a way that we're all together without difference between a guru and a *shishya,* as if we are friends." The connection that was initiated the first time B. K. S. Iyengar came to America to teach, more than half a century ago, has gradually developed through the power of his teaching into a bond not just of teacher to pupil and vice versa, but of heart to heart, a bond based on mutual love and devotion.

It wasn't always like this. He went on to say, "Before there were always frictions. I had a lot of problems when I came here years ago. There were so many challenges, and having come out of those challenges, the fruit is visible after twelve years." To continue over all those years in the face of such opposition and conflict has required profound dedication on Guruji's part not just to his practice, but to his teaching as well. His pupils can sense his passion for sharing the realizations and joys he has attained, and they respond to it by giving him their love and trust.

Mr. Iyengar's passion for his art is clearly a primary source of the powerful connection he has with his pupils. But this bond is not just an impersonal interaction based on mutual devotion to an ideal or practice. Guruji's intense desire to spare his pupils some of the struggles he experienced and to help them to, as he says, "stand on my shoulders" and take the art to new heights, is an outgrowth of his deep devotion to the students themselves. They feel his passion for their growth and well-being directly and personally. So many times I have heard pupils speaking about their experience of being in class with Mr. Iyengar, saying, "I felt as if he were teaching the class directly to me," though it was in a room of a hundred people. This personal quality of teaching is certainly the mark of a master teacher, but even more, in Guruji's case, the power of that personal experience that they feel comes as a direct result of his devotion to the pupils and his desire to serve their best interests.

I spoke earlier of Guruji's compassionate nature. Many people at first miss the compassionate aspect of his teaching. They see his intensity and feel the force of his passion, but they may fail to understand that one of the points of his teaching is to help them, as Patanjali says, "avoid the miseries which have not yet come." Just as a child may not understand a parent's discipline as an act of love and compassionate care, so the beginning student or the casual observer may not see the intensity of Guruji's teaching as a means to optimize the student's progress toward the joys of health and freedom and avoid the pain of pitfalls along the way. Guruji has set the highest standards in his teaching because yoga itself has set the highest of standards: the realization of perfect freedom. He pays unswerving attention to what his pupils do and relentlessly holds them to that high standard. That attention grows out of love and devotion. Guruji pays attention because he is deeply devoted to his pupils, just as loving parents pay attention to their children because they love them.

Perhaps the most obvious example of Mr. Iyengar's compassion is to be found in the medical classes he conducts and in the individual therapeutic work he does with those who are suffering. When doing therapeutic work, Guruji brings all the vast knowledge of his many decades of practice and teaching into focus with the patient. Even more powerful than that knowledge, though, is the power of his attention. His attention when teaching a class is intense, but it is not the same as the laserlike concentration of attention he directs toward working with someone suffering illness or disease. Suffering seems to call forth an even higher level of compassion from Guruji. Like a bee to a flower, he is drawn to those in pain. I said that attention is love. Attention is also energy, and energy has powerful healing qualities. Guruji directs the energy of his attention to the suffering person, and that energy is itself an important part of the therapeutic process. The patient's own healing energy is bolstered by the energy of Guruji's attention, which inspires the patient to face his predicament squarely and encourages him to take the actions needed to ameliorate it.

The generosity with which Mr. Iyengar gives his time and energy is well-known. Many have seen him, nearly at the point of exhaustion, take still another hour to struggle to help alleviate a student's suffering, using his own body in the process in ways that must be painful even for him. Surely compassion and generosity of the magnitude he so often demonstrates are manifestations of love and devotion of the highest order.

For me, this bond of love and devotion became most evident during Guruji's *Light on Life* tour. I attended an intensive class early in his tour and felt that all of us were thrilled to be there, eager to see again (or for the first time) this man who had touched us all, directly or indirectly. When he arrived at the hall that first morning, the cheer that went up, the sustained applause, the unmistakable love directed toward him, took even him, I think, by surprise. Our love reinforced the love he felt for us, gave to us, and has given to us for years, and so the spiral of love soared upward. After the classes, it was still there in the way people greeted each other on the paths between the classes and spoke to each other in the dining hall.

At every stop on the tour, the experience was essentially the same: adoring crowds expressing their love and affection for a man who had given so much to so many. Seeing this, it occurs to me that Guruji has reached a place in his *sadhana* where he can receive the love that is directed toward him and not get caught in it. He is able to allow the light of love in and shine that light back out with such power and radiance that to be around him is to be in a state of love that comes from the joy of being in the presence of a clear mind and an open heart. More than his innovations and incredible insights, even more than his remarkable compassion and healing skills, the example B. K. S. Iyengar gives of the power of yoga to elevate oneself to a state of loving grace is his greatest gift. He has said it himself: "All the other yogas; karma, hatha, jnana, and raja, all culminate in bhakti yoga, the yoga of love and devotion, the yoga of the heart." He is its shining example. He expresses this eloquently in his wonderful book *Light on Life:* "Love must be incarnated in the smallest pore of the skin, the smallest cell of the body, to make them intelligent so they can collaborate with all the other ones, in the big republic of the body. This love must radiate from you to others."★ The challenge, then, for those of us who would follow the teachings and example of B. K. S. Iyengar—indeed, for all yoga practitioners—is not to get lost in the mechanics of the practice. As important as technique and diligence are, even more important is for us to dedicate our practice and our teaching to opening our own minds and hearts and the minds and hearts of our pupils to the power of Love, to transcending our petty fears and ambitions, and to directing our energy toward awakening the awareness of the divinity that resides within us all. Then, perhaps, we can fulfill one of Guruji's most cherished wishes and create a community based on affection and respect; then, perhaps, we can do as B. K. S. Iyengar says we must and let our love radiate to our students, our colleagues, our friends and families, and to all our brothers and sisters the world over.

JOHN SCHUMACHER is the founder and director of Unity Woods. He has practiced yoga for more than thirty-five years and has taught in the Washington, D. C., area since 1973. He has studied in India with B. K. S. Iyengar many times since 1981 and is a certified senior Iyengar Yoga teacher. He also spent many years studying with internationally acclaimed teacher Dona Holleman, who strongly influenced his practice and teaching. John was cited by *Yoga Journal* as one of "25 American originals who are shaping yoga today." He has written for

---

★ B. K. S. Iyengar, *Light on Life* (New York: Rodale, 2005), 59.

a variety of publications and has appeared in numerous local and national media, including *U.S. News and World Report, W* magazine, *Yoga Journal, Washingtonian* magazine, the *Washington Times,* and the *Washington Post.* Schumacher travels throughout the world, including Europe, Asia, Africa, and the Caribbean, to conduct workshops for students and teachers of all levels.

The Secret Teaching

SHARON GANNON AND DAVID LIFE

Every subject has some question that is very easy to pose but extremely difficult to answer because it strikes at the very heart of what that subject is. It would seem easy enough, for example, for a geographer to define a lake as "a large body of water (or other liquid) surrounded entirely by land." But some lakes are actually regarded as inland seas, while many small seas have to suffer the indignity of being referred to as lakes. Then there is Lake Eyre in Australia, which is actually a dry basin most of the time that masquerades as a "real lake" in times of heavy rainfall. And what about a forest? We know immediately that every tree in any forest is doomed to die at some time. So what is the exact relationship between each tree and the forest? A forest can hardly depend on any one tree for its definition, nor on all the trees within it at any one time, because every one of them will eventually be replaced. Since no two trees are identical, in what sense (if any) does the forest remain the same when one tree dies and another takes its place? Just how is a forest to be defined when all the trees that make it up are impermanent and they all change?

Yoga can certainly be written about in books, but can the knowledge that yoga strives to impart really be explained in any of them? By tradition, the knowledge sought in yoga can be attained only within the lineage or heredity of yoga. This is a tradition dating back to ancient Vedic times and is called *guru parampara* (the succession of discipleship). It is the handing down of the knowledge of liberation through the ages and from one generation to the next. Somehow, in guru parampara, the knowledge transmitted is supposed to remain unchanged and inviolate, even though every teacher and every student who participates in it are as different as two lakes, two trees, and two forests. This contradictory and paradoxical situation is now reflected on by Sharon Gannon and David Life.

Mary Dunn was standing in her short, elasticized-leg shorts, with a big smile on her face that never altered when Mr. Iyengar repeatedly interjected into her presentation. Elise Browning Miller, John Schumacher, Patricia Walden, Manouso Manos, and others were no different. In each case, when senior Iyengar teachers—people who are celebrated and honored teachers in their own right—were put into a situation that could have threatened their egos, they were not threatened. With hundreds of aspiring yoga students looking on, documentary digital footage catching each nuance of facial expressions, their positions on a stage in plain view, each of these prominent yoga teachers took the opportunity to show that their dedication to their teacher was more important than any feelings of losing face in public may have been. As a result, the entire space was enveloped in an atmosphere of awe and beauty.

Like Mary's elasticized shorts, the innovations that have grown out of the work of B. K. S. Iyengar are ubiquitous. He was a pioneer who went into the wild territories and established pathways through the dense undergrowth of ignorance, making connections and creating safe passage routes. The overwhelming sweep of those innovations is awesome. The props that he pioneered are found in yoga rooms of all stripes around the world. His conceptual framework for physical alignment that would lead to complete liberation is drawn on yoga mats from Pune to Pittsburgh.

Still, what stands out as his most profound contribution has been in the area of the student/teacher relationship. It is so easy these days to relegate the position of a yoga teacher to that of a mere instructor rather than that of a guru. That shirking of responsibility, on either part, can block any progress toward yoga. Of course, each generation of lineage receivers must be able to engender the same relationship toward their guru as they would have with their students in turn. That was the magical occurrence that lay before us. In the same room, we were witness to the transmission of the secret teachings through many generations of yogis simultaneously. There was a force of nature being conducted through the ceiling, walls, and floor of the room; through each heart; and into the hands and feet, the nervous system, and the bodies of knowledge and vitality. Any force that is being transmitted need only arrive at a receptive channel to be realized. Recognizing and nurturing that receptivity is the job of a good student. The main job of the guru is to acknowledge the student as a realized being and to seek ways to remove any obstacles to that truth. Through the unique relationship of guru and student, the student is given an opportunity to relinquish attachment to his or her own ego and glimpse real yoga. No one lost face because everyone saw one face, and they saw themselves reflected in that face. The faceless face.

When we look back at the lineage of teachers, we can easily see Mr. Iyengar's pivotal and relevant place for us. We know some of the difficulties that were confronted when he was spending the short time he did with his guru, Sri Krishnamacharya. We know that Mr. Iyengar has held his guru in the highest regard and never failed to acknowledge and appreciate him. We know very few details from our history of the social, psychological, intellectual, and physical hurdles that constituted the relationship between Sri Krishnamacharya and his guru, Rama Mohan Brahmachari, in the Himalayas. We know absolutely nothing about the relationship between Rama Mohan Brahmachari and his guru, or his guru and his guru's guru. We know absolutely nothing, that is, if we are not having that same experience now with our own guru. The experience may seem to be different outwardly. There may be infinite landscapes and costumes, but the methods for getting to the root of the problem have not changed. We are experts on the relationship between ourselves, as students, and our guru. We are empowered to conduct the perfect consciousness through our teacher to resonate with our bliss and propel our minds and bodies into virtuous action. As good students, we are empowered to work for the liberation of our own teacher as a method to reach that enlightened state ourselves. As gurus, we know that the way we were taught must be upheld as the way to teach others. Our own relationship to a lineage of teachers informs us that we are not the source of consciousness, but consciousness itself. Mr. Iyengar is more than an "instructor of yoga" and his students are more than casual acquaintances. As we witness the baton being passed in the lineage of teachers, whom do we cheer for more? The one holding the baton or the one receiving the baton? We ask ourselves questions: What if the baton is dropped? What if it is never given over? What if it is never grasped? What if it is thrown away? There can be obstacles to the direct perception of the truth.

The problem, the main obstacle today, seems to be a lack of humility. A humble one realizes that once you stand before the eyes of the guru, his or her gaze is always upon you. When we obstruct that gaze coming through our own eyes by means of lenses tinted with reluctance and fear, we stop the transmission. When we look upon our yoga gurus only through the cool shades of pride and the smirk of self-importance, we stop the transmission.

What we saw during those days filled with joy was an unbroken line of transmission humbly passed from teacher to student, resulting in a diverse forest of bounty spreading out from one very ancient and wise wish-fulfilling tree that grew out of the bedrock of yoga philosophy.

Having received the great boon in life of receiving the holy teachings, the prize is to have our greatest wish fulfilled. Like a wish-fulfilling tree, the guru allows us to flower and come to fruition in a way that would benefit the lives of others. In a forest of trees—of pine, of oak, of maple, of ash, and of many others—all grow out of the same fertile soil, through the same methods, having similar karmas—advantages as well as setbacks and difficulties—and manifesting in a forest of lush diversity. Each of these trees becomes a wish-fulfiller in turn. They are rooted in the bedrock and as they make more soil with their roots, they shade the young from the harsh weather and whisper the secret teachings.

ॐ

SHARON GANNON AND DAVID LIFE are students of Brahmananda Saraswati, Swami Nirmalananda, and Pattabhi Jois. They cofounded and codirect the Jivamukti Yoga Center, founded in 1986. Together and separately, they have published articles in several publications, including *Yoga Journal,* and they cowrote the book *Jivamukti Yoga.* David has received advanced certification in the Ashtanga Yoga method of Pattabhi Jois. Together, he and Sharon are recognized internationally as adept, creative, and knowledgeable yogis.

Iyengar Yoga?

MANOUSO MANOS

Iyengar (noun) a type of hatha yoga focusing on the correct alignment of the body, making use of straps, wooden blocks, and other objects as aids to achieving the correct postures. ORIGIN named after B. K. S. Iyengar (born 1918), the Indian yoga teacher who devised this method.
—OXFORD ENGLISH DICTIONARY

The story of how the word *Iyengar* made it into the *Oxford English Dictionary* is an interesting one. Those who compile Oxford dictionaries try to record how the English language is being used by a large number of people over a reasonable period of time. A word is likely to be included if it appears five times, in five different printed sources, over a period of five years (although in some cases it is clear long before the five years is up that the word is a fully accepted part of the language). But as Manouso Manos tells us, there is much more to the story behind the noun *Iyengar* than that.

What is Iyengar Yoga, and why has this phenomenon spread so widely? I personally do not know how to answer that but have seen its growth run like wildfire across the globe.

Many years ago, I was lucky enough to be traveling with B. K. S. Iyengar. One of our stops on the trip was London. When the time came to leave for the airport, there was not enough room in the car that was to take us there, so I volunteered to take the underground to Heathrow. Upon arriving and not seeing any of Guruji Iyengar's entourage, I decided to check in. I had no idea if I had arrived before or after the group. When the woman at the counter asked me for my seating preference, I said that I had an acquaintance on the flight and would like to sit beside a Mr. B. K. S. Iyengar. Her reply was, "Like the yoga," and I said yes, that it was in fact that same man. Her instant reaction was "Oh, I would very much like to meet him."

B. K. S. Iyengar has dedicated his entire adult life to educating the public on the glories and nuances of yoga. He has invested untold energy and hours in its practice and propagation. He has modernized this very ancient subject and made it available to the general populace of the entire world. He has integrated not just individuals, sects, creeds, and classes together under his tutelage, but he has also brought this most ancient subject into line with modern-day scientific understanding.

The definitions of *yoga* are many. The historic texts of the Vedas call it "skillful action." Anyone who has seen Iyengar's demonstrations or studied photos of him in the asanas would say that his physical actions are skillful, but is that what these ancient texts are implying? No, the Vedas are talking about right living and doing the right thing in one's decisions. They are pressing the students of life to find the moral path in all situations. B. K. S. Iyengar has always been a man of strong moral character and leads by both word and deed. He has long pressed his students to follow a righteous life. His exemplary life and strong writings on the subject are a beacon for all to find the skillful action that will be the best for humankind, even though it may come at a personal cost and require bravery and tenacity. He is the embodiment of "skillful action."

Another definition of *yoga* that has been passed down is "subject and object merge to become one." Imagine what Iyengar means when he says that he "becomes the pose." When the rest of us take asanas, we push our bodies into these positions. B. K. S. Iyengar finds his way into the depths of the pose until he and the asana are one, neither independent of the other. His thoughts, feelings, and actions become part of the same entity. The doer, the doing, and the done are inseparable. B. K. S. Iyengar absorbs into the subject, or the subject and object become one.

Sage Patanjali defines *yoga* as the suppression of the fluctuations of the mind. Anyone who has seen Guruji Iyengar's asana practice will attest to his determination. You can watch as his mind becomes absorbed.

Imagine having your life's work, your life's subject, eventually bearing your name. Imagine that your name becomes synonymous with that concept. Imagine that your name could not be spoken out of the context of that subject. The woman at the airport counter related a name to a common subject for a reference point, but Iyengar is yoga and yoga is Iyengar. Subject and object are united.

MANOUSO MANOS, one of the most senior Iyengar Yoga teachers in the United States, has traveled to Pune, India, for more than twenty-five years to study with B. K. S. Iyengar. His understanding of the body, skill in therapeutics, and energetic and motivational teaching style provide both a challenging and energizing experience for his students.

A Tribute

ERICH SCHIFFMANN

The purpose of yoga is to make visible that which was previously invisible. Things must, in other words, be seen from a different perspective. But chance and serendipity are not the only reasons we can sometimes see things freshly and uniquely. The ability to see things in a bright new way is surely also a property of thinking, of outlook. If we develop flexibility, a willingness to enjoy unknown things, and a tolerance of ambiguity and unpredictability, are we not then doing a great deal to help this process along? As Erich Schiffmann demonstrates by both his account and his person, creative individuals of this kind have a lot of energy, but they are also capable of long periods of profound rest and quiet. They are highly intelligent, but they also display that childlike simplicity of insight that allows new discoveries to be made. They are serious and disciplined, but they are still playful and near feckless. They have excellent imaginations, but they are simultaneously grounded in the reality of the attainable. They are passionate and committed, but they can look at everything they do with the necessary dispassion and disinterest that allows all prior achievements to be cast aside at a moment's notice as if they were nothing. They are rebellious and independent, yet they are able to use all available resources as a foundation stone for their new offerings. They seem irresponsible and beholden to no one, yet they conduct themselves according to the letter of a law laid down by some higher authority known only to them at the present time—but it is available to anyone who will follow their example.

What an honor to be writing about one of the most important men in my life. And what a challenge. The simplicity of it, though, is that Mr. Sri Sri B. K. S. Iyengarji had a tremendous impact on me in my formative years. He made a difference in my life, one for which I am eternally, publicly grateful. I have not spent as much time with him as many others have, but I have studied with several of his senior students, most notably Dona Holleman and Vanda Scaravelli, and I did spend six months with him in Pune in the summer of 1977. I took two classes a day with him; I watched him do his morning and afternoon practice for months; I took many, many notes; and I have watched him teach in Mumbai and took classes with him in London. And, of course, I have all his books and know many people who have studied long and hard with him. He may remember me. I rather doubt it. He might remember my association with Krishnamurti. But that does not matter. I remember him, and I remember what I learned from him.

As a teenager, I had been a student at Brockwood Park, the Krishnamurti school in England. Krishnamurti had been a lifelong practitioner of yoga and had been taught personally by Mr. Iyengar for more than twenty years. Yoga was taught at the school, and these were my first formal yoga lessons, but at that time, they were taught in the Krishnamacharya-Desikachar tradition. I knew of Iyengar, of course, and I had a worn copy of *Light on Yoga,* but I had not yet met anyone who had studied with him or could tell me much about his style.

When I was twenty, I made a pilgrimage to Madras (now Chennai), India, and spent a year studying yoga with T. K. V. Desikachar, the son of the legendary Krishnamacharya, Iyengar's guru. At this point, I had no plans of becoming a yoga teacher. I just wanted to learn yoga and was fortunate enough to be in the right places at the right time. On my way back to the States, I stopped in England to visit my friends at Brockwood. They told me that the previous yoga teacher was no longer there and asked me, since I was recently trained, whether or not I would like to be the resident yoga teacher at Brockwood. I said, "Of course!" It was perfect. I couldn't have orchestrated a better plan. I began teaching immediately. I was twenty-one.

Toward the end of my first year of teaching yoga at Brockwood, the father of one of the students came to visit. He was a Frenchman named J. B. Rishi, and as luck would have it, he was teaching Iyengar-style yoga in Paris. He came to my class, offered feedback and sage advice, and showed me a number of incredible ways to work the poses. I was thrilled and in awe, and I became acutely aware of just how much I didn't know.

I knew I needed to study Iyengar-style yoga, but I couldn't afford another trip to India and was not quite sure how to proceed.

That next summer I was in Saanen, Switzerland, near Gstaad, at the annual Krishnamurti gatherings. A chance introduction brought Dona Holleman into my life. Dona lived in Italy, and though she was still young, she had been with Iyengar for a long time and was his senior teacher in Europe. I did yoga with her several times that week in her room at the hotel and at a chateau in the hills above Gstaad. Dona was amazing. She opened up a completely new world and awareness for me of what it meant to do yoga. She was precise, articulate, fun. She could do the poses better than anyone, and she was an excellent teacher. She had a way of being able to explain the poses that made them seem magical. I subsequently visited her during Christmas, Easter, and summer breaks when Brockwood was on holiday. I learned a tremendous amount from her, but witnessing her love, admiration, and devotion to her teacher left an even bigger impression on me. I remember her saying his touch was "divine."

During the summer of 1976, Iyengar was teaching in London, and because of my associations with Dona and others, I was allowed to attend. The class was full, however, and since I could not actually participate in the Friday night class, I sat in the bleachers and watched. It was extraordinary; I loved it. There was such a buzz surrounding the whole event. And there to the side, before class started, was Mr. Iyengar himself warming up with backbends such as dropovers from headstand, mandalasana, ekapada viparita dandasana, vrschikasana, and so on. He was beautiful. It was magical. And luckily, I was able to attend class the next day.

All I remember is that the class was packed, that Mr. Iyengar had an enormous amount of energy, and that during virabhadrasana 1, he came over and slugged me in the chin. Apparently, I was pulling my chin down too much. I never did that again when he was around! In spite of this, I was very impressed by this man. He was an extremely creative, brilliant teacher, and I wanted to study with him.

I went to Pune, India, during the summer of 1977 to study with the great Iyengar. I was apprehensive about going to India again because I had gotten very sick the first time I was there. I vowed to be more careful this time, not to drink the water or buy any food off the streets. Someone was generous enough to pay my way. I was there with friends from England, Scotland, and Australia, and I had a blast. I would arrive at the Institute every morning at seven to watch Iyengar practice. I observed him closely and wrote down everything he did. Class would begin as soon as he was finished and would last three hours. We would then walk to town, eat, go to our room and take notes, then nap. I would then walk to the Institute again to watch Iyengar do his afternoon practice, an hour of headstand and shoulderstand variations. This was followed by a pranayama (breathing) class, which was followed by the evening class that was open to the public. We would then walk back to town, eat, return to the hotel and write down everything we could remember, and then sleep. It was a lovely summer.

One incident I remember most clearly occurred at the end of class one morning. It had been a very intense, difficult class, and during savasana, I went particularly deep. I remember being very quiet, very centered, and yet very wide awake. Iyengar must have noticed this, because he came over to me afterward and said, "You see! It takes Krishnamurti twenty years to get your mind quiet. I can do it in one class." He had a point. His methodology worked. It was not just physical, as his teaching was commonly criticized of being. At that time, many people attempted to discredit him by saying his yoga was not spiritual. But here it was! Spiritual in the most practical, grounded, obvious way. It was equally obvious from what he said to me that his intent all along was to impart the *experience* of yoga—not just put everyone through the paces, physically speaking. The whole point of all this physical hard work—and it was very physical and very demanding—was to get into a deep meditative state. And for me, it worked. I am extremely grateful to have learned this from him. Interestingly, what I remember most is watching him practice.

I arrived early every morning at the Institute before class, and I would just sit there and watch him practice. I watched him every afternoon as well. What a treat. I had been in his classes, and I had watched him teach, but to watch the real thing, live, was special. It was an even more powerful teaching than the actual teaching. I sat to the side of the room and watched him closely. I watched his every move from the moment he appeared in the doorway until the moment he left. I studied the way he practiced and the way he was. And I wrote it all down. I wrote down everything he did. I also wrote down what Geeta was practicing and what Prashant was doing. It was different every day. This was interesting in itself, but even more interesting, more valuable, was the way Iyengar practiced. He was so internal, so introverted, so immersed in his experience, and so obviously allowing himself to be guided from within, such an excellent student of a subject with which he was in love. This obvious love and passion of his became the most profound teaching for me. He was just the master doing his yoga. He was the student honing his craft and learning masterfully. It was inspiring to watch. It is still inspiring. It has stayed with me to this day.

I never did become an "Iyengar teacher," but I try my best to teach with the same self-mined wisdom I observed Iyengar mining every early morning and every afternoon in the yoga room. I love him for being so genuinely who he is—a luminary in the yoga firmament and a shining example of a principled life.

❦

ERICH SCHIFFMANN is an internationally renowned and accomplished teacher, known for his best-selling book, *Yoga: The Spirit and Practice of Moving into Stillness,* and his award-winning video, *Yoga, Mind and Body.* He began practicing yoga as a teenager and started teaching after studying with T. K. V. Desikachar and B. K. S. Iyengar in India. Besides his classes in Los Angeles, he regularly teaches workshops and retreats throughout the United States and abroad.

Light on Knowledge

ALAN GOODE

Yoga, we are told, should be learned at the hands of a good teacher. Assuming we can find a good teacher, a guru, what is their job? What can we expect them to do? To answer this question, Shankara wrote a famous mantra that is often chanted before the start of a yoga lesson or practice session:

Vande gurunam caranaravinde
Samdarshita svatma sukhavabodhe
Nihshreyase jangalikayamane
Samsara halahala moha shantyai.

I honor the teachers with their two lotus feet;
who have revealed to me the joy that is mine;
most excellent sages, my refuge in the dark impenetrable thicket;
who bring peace from the poison and illusion seeking ever to exist.★

As Alan Goode now reminds us, the teacher we seek is the one who can help us to forget the things we should never have remembered and to remember the things we should never have forgotten.

IYENGAR'S IMPRINT

Much can be said about Guruji's method of practice and his teaching style. Through his books, he has demonstrated the depth and understanding of the subject of yoga—the beauty of his practice and his ability to articulate the subject and its relevance to a modern society. His words and his works leave a legacy that cannot be measured by the man alone.

Another aspect of Guruji's genius is the imprint he has left on his stu-

---

★ From "Yoga Taravali" by Adi Shankara.

dents. The depth of this imprint can be seen in their lives—their willing-ness to dedicate their lives to this practice and vision of yoga. I would like to explore this method of absorbing knowledge: imprinting.

Most learning is an act of cognition, that is, an act of understanding something initially through explanation followed by comprehension—an act of mind. Access to and proficiency in the activity are then devel-oped through applying the principles described to achieve fluency and competence in the activity. The important thing to note in this sequence of learning is the starting point of explanation: a process of mind. Learn-ing is undertaken through the process of understanding what the teacher has said. It therefore involves rationalizations and the vocabulary of lan-guage, and it can be limited by these same factors. Communication be-comes possible by rendering the activity into something that can be recognized by the student. By the same process, it implies that if some-thing is not explainable, it is not understandable. If something is not ra-tional, it is not cognizable. This is far from true, however.

Imprinting is the act of placing a set of images in the storehouse of our impressions—to develop a background on which we draw each time we practice. It does not necessarily require comprehension in order to pro-ceed, and oftentimes, it defies comprehension initially until it is fully in-tegrated. For his students, studying with Guruji has left an intense set of experiences that are initially indefinable but are gradually unraveled as they are reexamined through the student's own practice. Working directly under Guruji has required that the student develop their own practice in order to locate themselves within the experience they have had.

To understand imprinting in more depth, we must first examine memory. Memory is the way we handle an impression, not the impres-sion itself. We assume that when we remember something, we cast our mind back and look at the image of what happened. We assume that the memory is fixed and that the act of remembering is somewhat akin to re-viewing a video library of our past experiences. Yet in reality, it is clear that remembering is not a fixed process. We remember different aspects of an experience at different times, and by mulling something over re-peatedly, we can even shape the way we remember the event. The event becomes what we remember. This observation recognizes the role that our mind plays in memory. We bring the event into our frontal brain to recollect it. In effect, we get the impression out of its store and turn it over in our mind.

Memory recreates the event and reshapes it each time we handle it. If we follow this thread, then what do we draw on when we remember something? Any experience is held in the body, in the emotions, and in the mind. These impressions sit beyond our memory and are what we reach into to touch the experience of the event now passed. This would explain why our memories are not devoid of emotion. In practical terms, when a student does trikonasana, for example, that student draws on their mental image of the way the asana looks, their past experience of the asana, the points they have been taught, the energetics of the asana, and much more. It is not a simple act of reproduction. Different students experience the same asana differently, depending on how they hold the image of the asana. When teaching, the teacher does more than instruct the asana. The teacher sets an image of what to aim for within the student. Teaching should broaden the experience of the asana to encompass the totality of the student. Working with Guruji, the student is made to work beyond thought and often to defy thought as they are forced to act intensively in the moment.

Guruji comments on the way memory should be used in the practice of asana:

When memory is completely cleansed and purified, mind too is purified. Both cease to function as distinct entities; a no-mind state is experienced, and consciousness alone manifests itself, shining unblemished without reflection of external objects. This is called nirvitarka samapatti.

Memory is the recollection of past thoughts and experiences. It is the storehouse of past impressions. Its knowledge is reflected knowledge. The *sadhaka* should be aware that memory has tremendous impact on intelligence. By perseverance in yoga practices and persistent self-discipline, new experiences surface. These new experiences, free from the memories of the past, are fresh, direct, and subjective; they expunge what is remembered. Then memory ceases to function as a separate entity. It either merges with consciousness or takes a backseat, giving predominance to new experiences and bringing clarity in intelligence. For the average person, memory is a past mind. For the enlightened person,

memory is a present mind. As memory is purified, intelligence becomes illuminative and moves closer to the seer, losing its identity.
This is *nirvitarka samapatti*. Even for the unripe mind, there is a
right and a wrong use of memory. It is not for recollecting pleasure, but for establishing a fund of experience as a basis for further
correct action and perception.

In asana, for example, we start with trial and error. The fruits
of these experiments are graded by the discriminating intelligence and stored in the memory. As we progress, trial and error
decreases, and correct perception increases. So memory provides
foresight against error. In headstand, for example, something that
usually goes wrong is that the upper arm shortens. Memory warns
us to be aware before it happens. Discriminating experimentation
awakens consciousness. Awareness, with discrimination and memory, breaks down bad habits—which are repeated actions based on
wrong perception—and replaces them with their opposites. In
this process, the brain must be creative, not mechanical. The mechanical brain questions only the external phenomena, bringing
objective knowledge. The creative brain calls into question inner
and outer phenomena, bringing subjective and spiritual knowledge. In asana, understanding begins with the inner skin; in pranayama, with the inner membrane of the nose. These are the starting
points of the spiritual quest in asana and pranayama.*

It is clearly stated in this passage that memory should not be used for
the re-creation of past experiences. If memory is cleansed and purified
by new experience, it does not mean that we no longer remember, but
that we do not merely re-create old experiences and that memory is used
to discriminate between what is known and what we have not experienced before. Memory effectively helps us identify what is known so that
subtle shifts of new experience can be identified.

Again, when Iyengar is commenting on Sutra 1:44, he says,

". . . In Nirvitarka samapatti, the sadhaka experiences a state without verbal deliberation. All the subtle objects reflected in savichara

---

* B. K. S. Iyengar, *Light on the Yoga Sutras of Patanjali* (London: Aquarian, 1993),
136.

are extinguished. He is free from memory, free from experiences, devoid of all past impressions. This new state of contemplation is without cause and effect, place or time. The inexpressible states of pure bliss (ananda) and pure self (asmita) rise to the surface and are experienced by the sadhaka."*

A state of nonverbal deliberation is where there is no internal dialogue. The degree to which we normally follow our inner conversation is astonishing. When engaged in talking to ourselves, we are not present to the experience directly because we are more involved with the interpretation of what is happening. We get caught up in what we think is happening, will happen, or did happen. This is an essential step in the development of a practice. It involves moving beyond explanations and talking ourselves through asanas to a point where the asana is observed and contemplated even as it is performed.

Guruji tells us that memory can also be used to clarify and discern. Memory can show us what is the same, what is different, and what is new. Memory can be the basis of fresh experience, not merely the repetition of our past. As a methodology, it is an avenue to orient ourselves within the subtle internal world so that we are able to identify the more repetitious patterns of thought and experience and to clarify our perception.

RESIDUAL IMPRESSIONS—SAMSKARAS

Throughout our lives, we experience reactions that are disproportionate to a situation. An image may trigger a flush of anger, fear, or grief linked to some past experience. Not linked to what is currently happening, the experience brings back a flood of emotion. Imprinting is the act of placing a set of images in the storehouse of our impressions. Each act in daily life leaves an imprint that influences the next act. Each practice forms the imprint for the following practice. If our experience is continually negative, then the cumulative experience is negative. I am not speaking of positive and negative feedback in this instance—of encouragement or discouragement. More important than these affirmations of good or bad

---

* B. K. S. Iyengar, *Light on the Yoga Sutras of Patanjali* (London: Aquarian, 1993), 91.

is whether the experience can be read and built on. Does the experience clarify perception or merely produce more thought? What is the residual impression? These imprints are not to be mistaken for perfecting the form of the asana. I am not speaking of refinement, but of proficiency.

The term *samskara* (past impressions) refers to the way we carry the past; the way it shapes our present and can be seen in the way we hold our bodies, the way we think, the way we feel; how our habits and history are formed and reformed in our day-to-day lives. Whether conscious or sublimated, these impressions color our outlook on the world. Likes and dislikes, fears and desires are interwoven in the fabric of all our actions. When we listen to a familiar piece of music, nuances and subtlety gradually come to light as we start to hear the underlying weave in the background; we uncover greater understanding through intimacy with the piece. Similarly, all our actions have attributes connected to the intention behind the action. This is the "background" in asana. Through the repetition of asana work, we observe and uncover these influences. Our desire to further a forward bend, for example, may cause us to exert greater effort. Greater effort or force causes the muscle to trigger and contract. Thus, not only is the asana less effective, but we are also in the contradictory position of trying to go further while simultaneously having to suppress or ignore the intensity of sensation aroused to achieve the perceived aim. We are desiring and rejecting at the same moment. An action, then, is not one-dimensional and may mean different things in different situations or at different times. *Samskara* is the term used to describe the residue of our actions that carries over long after the event is finished. These imprints propel us to further action through craving, desire, fear, and aversion. Yogis attempt to cleanse their actions of mixed messages and intentions so that their actions become free of generating future imprints—pure action.

B. K. S. Iyengar writes,

ACTIONS
Depending on their provenance, the fruits of actions may either tie us to lust, anger and greed, or turn us towards the spiritual quest. These residual impressions are called Samskaras: they build the cycles of our existence and decide the station, time and place

of our birth. The yogi's actions, being pure leave no impressions and excite no reactions, and are therefore free from residual impressions.

DESIRES AND IMPRESSIONS

Desires and knowledge derived from memory and residual impressions, exist eternally. They are as much a part of our being as is the will to cling to life. In a perfect yogi's life, desires and impressions have an end; when the mechanism of cause and effect is disconnected by pure, motiveless action, the yogi transcends the world of duality and desires and attachment wither and fall away.★

With this in mind, it is important to recognize that the quality of our actions is as important as the outcome of each act, as all actions leave residual impressions. It is not merely an act of getting the asana right. It is equally important to resolve the asana—to resolve one's motive in the asana. This resolution is the component that allows us to stay in the asana. The teacher directs the student in the quality, the tone, of the action as much as the technique. It is difficult to convey, as it is the inexplicable component of teaching where an asana is transmitted from teacher to student. By way of example: A teacher through their explanations and demonstrations, through adjustments and variations of each asana, will develop an understanding of the asana within the student. Explanation may not always be the best method, as more words often generate more thought. It may be better to show an asana, have the student perform and then adjust the asana. This nonverbal form of learning is valuable because it is not constrained by words. The student is trained to know the asana physically, intellectually, energetically, and emotionally, so that the imprint of the experience is clear and not clouded or cluttered by too many variables.

So what, then, of imprinting? Imprinting is the laying down of a body of experience that allows us to access something greater than the stretches and breathing exercises. These practices are the vehicles by which we experience and clarify our perception, not merely perform

---

★ B. K. S. Iyengar, *Light on the Yoga Sutras of Patanjali* (London: Aquarian, 1993), 37.

and recreate asana shapes. Memory is what we draw on to commence our practice, but if we go on memory alone, we merely recreate what is already known, what has been done. Each asana is the experience—we shape the experience physically, mentally, and emotionally. Physically, it is the precision with which we act. Accuracy and observation do more than shape the pose, they also bring us into the moment to experience directly. Guruji's method is to bring the student into the moment through precise instructions, acted on immediately. The impact of this is to cleanse the student of all memory traces and to encounter and identify new experience. In this moment, we become free of time, of memory, of personality. We stand outside the normal experience of our internal dialogue and ourselves. This method sits totally aligned with Patanjali's *Yoga Sutras*, where transformation is described as a gradual developmental process. The term *kriya yoga* is used by Patanjali to define a process in the practice where sustained action (*tapas*) leads to self-study (*svadhyaya*) and eventually surrender (*Ishvara pranidhana*) of "I-ness," the giving up of ego.

Just as each asana requires different qualities of concentration and application, Guruji articulates these asana imprints in the mind beyond the rational (articulated) experience. In doing so, he helps us establish a template to draw on which is a form of knowing held outside of words. Once a quality is recognized, it does not need to be analyzed by the student—it is known.

§

ALAN GOODE has been practicing yoga for thirty years and teaching for more than twenty years. He holds a senior teaching certificate in Iyengar Yoga and travels to India regularly to study. He was the cofounder of both the Newtown Yoga Studio and the Blue Mountains Yoga Studio in Australia, and he now runs a school (Yoga Mandir) in Canberra, Australia. Alan has extensive experience in teaching remedial classes for those with injuries and medical conditions, beginners' courses, and general and experienced-level classes. He trains teachers, conducts workshops, and runs professional support and development services for teachers. He is passionately involved with the practice of yoga and its application to daily life. Through his writing and newsletter, he unravels the themes of the *Yoga Sutras* and demonstrates their link to daily practice.

The Evolution of Practice

Or How Our Truth Changes

PIXIE LILLAS

Is there such a thing as ultimate truth? Does that final answer to all possible questions exist? Is there a magical formula that, when we have found it, allows us to solve all our problems and live "happily ever after"? Suppose that all human knowledge could indeed be encapsulated into one extremely powerful incantation of everything, ready to be intoned at any time. Whoever knew that incantation could then resolve all issues and would never have to learn anything else ever again.

But if such a formula existed, to whom should it be given? Surely to someone who is worthy to receive ultimate truth. Who would that be?

The ancient texts suggest that, formula or not, all seekers of ultimate truth should be intelligent, perceptive, sincere, and familiar with the metaphysical and ontological issues involved in knowing and possessing ultimate truth. They should not only be moral and ethical, but steadfastly inclined—from the very depths of their nature—to the good, the true, and all that accords with ultimate truth. They should have complete purity of heart and mind. This means being free from any desire for material gain. They should be able to overcome all temptations stemming from lust, greed, anger, pride, envy, and the rest. They should have no desire to dominate others for, as Lord Acton (1834–1902) said, "Power corrupts; absolute power corrupts absolutely." Ultimate truth is the source and property of all.

Although these requirements set high standards, they are traditional for seekers of ultimate truth. They prepare those seekers, or students, to be due recipients of that truth.

Yet the doctrine of ultimate truth also suggests that all seekers are already vessels for it. So what happens, as Pixie Lillas wonders, to the seeker as he or she is gradually transformed from a person who is *already* fit to receive ultimate truth to one who is *at last* fit to receive it? Also, what happens to ultimate truth itself? If the seeker is a vessel and the seeker changes, does ultimate truth also change, or does it remain the same?

As Pixie Lillas observes, there seems to be another dimension involved. Since the demands made of the seeker are so high, what are the chances of maintaining them unless the seeker receives some help and guidance? So an old theme recurs. By tradition and in practice, it has always been maintained that the most important qualification for a seeker of ultimate truth is constant association with—and receipt of personal instruction from—someone who has already seen that truth and can instruct the seeker by example, practice, and by embodiment of the lifestyle it demands. What of that?

At my first meeting with Guruji at the Ramamani Iyengar Memorial Yoga Institute in Pune in 1977, I was young in yoga and in years, and I was going to the Institute without any real idea of what time spent learning from Mr. Iyengar would involve. I thought perhaps that it would be more "yogic" to go with as few preconceptions as possible, believing myself to be open-minded and without set concepts. As soon as I arrived, I began to see that this was just one of the many fixed beliefs I held.

The only real expectation I openly allowed myself was that I would have a demanding physical experience. In this, I was not wrong. What I naïvely did not anticipate was the intellectual, emotional, and even psychological challenges that this thing called Iyengar Yoga was to present and the way in which the classes would upend my perception of how things were and what I believed myself to be.

I fancied myself passionate, strong, and open to learn; Guruji found me proud and a bit stubborn. I wanted certainty, the facts, what exactly was required in each posture. Guruji said that "the truth changes" and presented us with a multifaceted approach to the postures that required engagement and what he called "yoga intelligence." This was not something you could learn by rote or in books, I discovered, but was an understanding that came only through experience and observation in practice.

These were new ideas, and they had me completely baffled. They form a large part of the foundation of an approach that I continue to love, admire, and wrestle with to this day. Over the last thirty years, throughout all the transformative milestones of my life, the challenges of a body changed by those many events, and by time itself, I have looked to Guruji and his continued practice for inspiration and guidance.

His daughter, Geeta, once said in a talk she gave during Guru Purnima that Guruji and his practice were two inseparable things. When he had money and fame, he practiced; when he had no money, no food, no acclaim, he practiced. When he was young, he practiced; when he grew old, he practiced. It seems practice was not just the key, but both a tool for life and life itself. In my own experience of perplexing or difficult times or of a physical problem, I have learned, from Guruji's example, to just practice, and something will change, even if simply, to give rise to some small shift of perception. Even if what I do makes something worse, that in itself is further understanding. How can we learn what to do with a problem if we avoid it or just think about it? Considered action, gaining some tangible feedback, brings about a different understanding of what we are dealing with; that is the key. From the level of raw beginners, Guruji has said that, as teachers, we must "get them moving," give even new students an experience in their own bodies of what yoga can be. Talking about it, giving a lecture about it, brings a very different result. The mind, Guruji has said, can be a treacherous friend. It may give us illusions of what we think we need, want, and understand.

The body, on the other hand, is tangible and concrete and can show us without any room for doubt whether we are doing what we thought. It clarifies our perception of ourselves. In simple terms, is the arm straight or crooked? There can be no confusion there if we just look. The body is full of messages, of hints, if we just listen more attentively or even a little. Recently, Guruji pointed out that the body tells us so many things, all the time, and we do not pay attention. I used to be a little amused to hear him tell us about something his body said to him, things like "Kind sir, can you not see that the knee is bent?" or "Why are you seeing only on the right side? Should not the left also be straightened?" I have now seen that his body seems to be forever telling him things. There appears to be a constant dialogue and stream of information coming into his awareness. The beauty of it is, according to Guruji's teachings, that this is true for all of us, the main difference being that we generally do not take heed. We tend to ignore the basic precepts of action and reaction, cause and effect, pose and repose, that can lead us closer to "meditation in action." Yet that is exactly where the key to intelligent practice seems to lie.

What to do then if we listen but hear only a garbled message, one that seems to leave us with more confusion and doubt? Here again Guruji has given us guidance. He said once that if we feel doubt, let it be there and just continue to practice, letting it sit side by side with us and see which one wins out.

I have certainly had many periods of doubt, with uncertainty not just about the techniques of the postures, but even more about whether my approach was useful, helpful. Was I going in the right direction or making things worse for myself? How was I to know, to find out which direction to move in? According to Guruji, nothing can change if we don't act, pull out our mat and learn something through trial and error. Of course, we sometimes risk seizing our newfound wisdom vigorously and then make it the next dogma to follow. I often feel I have discovered the absolute solution to some pain or have found something essential in a backbend, only to learn that it is just one aspect, one small part of the deeper understanding required. Nothing is absolute, written in stone just to be copied day after day. This would be to deny the very premise of yoga itself, to hinder any self-awareness and obstruct any self-knowledge of even the most basic kind.

It would seem, then, after all these years, that "the truth" does change, that it is not a constant we can grab hold of and parrot from then on. Maybe there are certain realities that are solid and immutable, but we as humans are not, so it is perhaps more that our perception of things changes along with our continuing experiences in yoga. This can be disconcerting, but in many ways, it can also be a comfort. There is always something we are missing, another approach, blank or dull areas to be discovered and illuminate us a little more.

There is one particularly vital thing I have learned from Guruji, among the many hundreds of lessons received, and it is something that seems to have seeped into my existence almost subliminally over the years: he never stops learning, he never stops practicing and experiencing in one form or another. This passion and search for excellence make him more than just a master in yoga, but a teacher on many levels. Yehudi Menuhin called him "my best violin teacher." In a class, he almost forces us to be alert and alive in his presence, and this allows new perceptions to arise even as we outwardly practice the same old poses. I have often had a sense of soaring, of reaching something beyond my own capacity as he gives the perfect instruction at exactly the perfect time. He takes us step-by-step through postures and a sequence in a way that brings us to a point where we can receive new understandings, observe them objectively, and then reflect on our next action. He gives us the method by which we can learn to practice, just as at times he has been known to "give" us a pose. In 1977, he "gave" about forty of us kapotasana, physically taking us all into the full pose, as one by one, with many astonished grunts and gasps, we found our heads on our heels for the first time. He then explained that we now had the experience of the posture and therefore had the tools to learn it as we knew what we were looking for.

Classes with Guruji entail a sort of surrender. He has often encouraged us to give over during the class and to leave any questioning for later so that we can fully experience what he is teaching. During his eightieth birthday celebrations held in the Ambrosia Center outside Pune, after many repetitions of virabhadrasana II for at least five or six minutes per side, we thought that surely by the next day we would be unable even to raise our arms in urdhva hastasana. But on the contrary, we were fresh and ready to start again. When some months later I tried to do the same poses following the video from those classes, I was unable to return to the joyfulness or even find the will to hold my arms up for that length of time. Guruji has explained that we don't get sore in his classes because we surrender ourselves for that time, another useful reminder of the connection between mind and body. It is something in our attitude that either hardens us or leaves us free. I have heard talk of a mythical thirteen-minute parsvakonasana in Panchgani that was sustained in the same incredible way by most of the students present.

Geeta recently pointed out that it is so simple for us as students of Iyengar Yoga: we only have to "do it." Guruji has done the discovering, the sequencing, the piecing together of techniques to help us avoid some of what he has called his earlier mistakes, helping us on our path of learning. He has presented us with a structure, an art, and our job is just to commit to it. If we practice with openness and intelligence, changes occur. When some modification takes place in our body, we gain a new experience of ourselves, and this in turn alters our perception of who we are, of what we can do, and of the world we live in. We re-create the kapotasana; we have something to work with, a new starting place.

Some would say that this is tantamount to an act of faith. Perhaps, at times, it comes down to something like that, if that is what we would call a practice we come to believe in, something we trust will make us the best people we can be. I feel that yoga, both its practice and its teaching, brings out the qualities that are most positive in me; at times, it helps me be closer to what I aspire to be. In years gone by, we used to call it finding a "path with a heart." Guruji said once that if something helpful crosses your path, seize it and learn from it with joy.

There is no greater gift we could receive than that of being alive to ourselves and our surroundings, of finding a willingness to see and to learn and to be transformed. It is something for which we, Guruji's students, owe him our deepest gratitude and love.

Whether we are in his presence in class or far away in our own homes and yoga centers, he is always there with us in his teachings, in his example, in the brilliance and sincerity of his yoga. He is, and will always continue to be, side by side with us on our mat.

᠔

PIXIE LILLAS started practicing yoga in 1976 with Dona Holleman in Italy and first went to the Ramamani Iyengar Memorial Yoga Institute in Pune, India, in 1977. She cofounded the Balmain Yoga Studio (BYS) in Sydney, Australia, in 1980 and has been director and principal teacher there ever since. As well as teaching at the BYS, Pixie runs teacher-training courses and workshops in Australia and Europe. She has been closely involved with the B. K. S. Iyengar Yoga Association of Australia since it was established in 1985 and with the running of assessments for teacher certification since that time. She continues to go back to study with Iyengar on an almost-yearly basis.

The Totality of Experience

ALAN FINGER

An *adhi* is an anxious reflection or mental agony, such as a painful thought we may be having. There are two kinds. *Samaya adhi* is a product of the mind or the emotions. *Sara adhi* is a more deep-seated spiritual or psychological malaise that involves such long-term issues as our karma, lifestyle, belief system, and general outlook on life.

A *vyadhi* is a disease, sickness, or ailment. It is a physical expression of a disequilibrium in our energy and is caused by disturbances, corruptions, and/or obstructions to our energy. A vyadhi represents patterns of energy that have become disrupted and distorted by the degeneration and dissipation of the body, thereby bringing pain, stasis, disease, suffering, and even death.

Alan Finger now wonders whether adhi and vyadhi are connected. Can the one be transformed into the other? If so, how? What would be an effective therapy for any and all vyadhis? Would it be one that removed the source of any potential disturbances, blocked pathways, and inimical energy patterns? If all vyadhis are caused by adhis, how can we destroy all adhis so that vyadhis no longer arise?

Although Sri B. K. S. Iyengar probably does not remember me, his influence on me and the Integrated Science of Hatha, Tantra, and Ayurveda (ISHTA) yoga system was profound. When I first studied with Iyengar on one of his visits to South Africa, it was the early 1960s and I had been practicing with my father, Kavi Yogiraj Mani Finger, and his primary teachers for several years. Focused on the subtle body, my father's physical practice was approached almost entirely metaphysically, with little consideration of physical alignment. As our daily practice consisted of a half-hour of headstand—with a full hour once a week—and holding most other asanas for five to fifteen minutes, the lack of form led to many aches and pains for me! As this situation continued, I became more and more curious about how to pursue the physical practice without injury or pain.

My fortune in this life has always been to have the right teachers appear to me at the right time, and sure enough, it was at this point that Sri B. K. S. Iyengar arrived to give a series of lectures in Johannesburg. I attended the lectures and was totally inspired by Iyengar's wisdom of anatomy and alignment. It opened a whole new view into the yoga practice.

I began to see how I might be able to combine the subtle body practices of my father and his tantric teachers and the soundness of Iyengar's inspiration into the practice of asana. For the first time, it became apparent to me that the physical body and the energetic body were just different densities of our essential selves, and therefore, what occurred on one level had everything to do with what happened on another. Physical obstacles could result from emotional or energetic blockages and vice versa, and working wisely and consciously with the physical body profoundly influenced the movement of energy in the subtle body.

I clearly remember Iyengar's passion and clarity. It was as striking and powerful then as ever! As we would say in ayurvedic terms, he had a very high *pitta* (fire) constitution, and I recall explaining this to fellow students who found his strict approach a true challenge. Mr. Iyengar was so fervent about getting the point across rather than *how* he got the point across. His rigor was, in fact, part of his genius—how clearly he saw the work that must be done and how passionately he felt about it. This perspective helped me and my fellow students open ourselves to Iyengar's skill and wisdom.

It was these meetings with Iyengar in South Africa, more or less forty years ago, that were the foundation of my inspiration to merge the subtle body and the physical body in yoga practice. This integration became the fundamental understanding of asana practice in the ISHTA system: that physical alignment and energetic opening must coexist simultaneously and nourish and inspire each other.

Iyengar's mastery and wisdom not only revolutionized my understanding of the physical practice of yoga for the ease of my own asana, but also inspired me to explore anatomy and how the body works. His genius for the body became the keystone to the understanding of the body in ISHTA Yoga, and an essential element of the union of the physical and metaphysical practice; the union that in the ISHTA philosophy is the total experience of yoga.

I honor Sri B. K. S. Iyengar for his role in my life, my system of ISHTA Yoga, and most of all, for his tremendous role in bringing yoga into this *kula*.

S

ALAN FINGER is a second-generation yoga master who has been practicing yoga for more than thirty-five years. His path began as a teenager in his native South Africa under the tutelage of his father, Kavi Yogiraj Mani Finger. His father studied both at home and on regular travels to India, a study that transformed his own life and that of his son. From the age of fifteen, Alan has dedicated his life to an in-depth study of all traditions and a scientific exploration of the exact blend of postures, breathing, and meditation that accesses human potential to the fullest and benefits all levels of being.

The Secret Gift of the Bandhas

GODFREY DEVEREUX

> Some divide asanas into those which cultivate the body and those which are used in meditation. But in any asana the body has to be toned and the mind tuned so we can stay longer with a firm body and a serene mind.... Space must be created between muscle and skin so that the skin receives the actions of the muscles, joints and ligaments....The skin then sends messages to the brain, mind and intelligence which judge the appropriateness of those actions. In this way, the principles of yama and niyama are involved and action and reflection harmonize. In addition the practice of a variety of asanas clears the nervous system, causes the energy to flow in the system without obstruction and ensures an even distribution of that energy.
> —B. K. S. IYENGAR, *Light on the Yoga Sutras of Patanjali*

> If *yoga* means "union," referring to the union of body, mind, and spirit, then who and what is it that practices? Who and what is it that learns? Who and what is it that comes to fill the spaces created between the parts described? Godfrey Devereux inquires how that energy is to be grasped, and who and what does the grasping and the benefiting.

I discovered yoga at sixteen years old, in 1973, and spent the next five years practicing from a very informative and well-written book. It was not until I finally attended a class that I realized the neck and back problems I had developed were not the result of bicycle riding but faulty yoga practice. I had stumbled into an Iyengar Yoga class, and for the next twelve years was to seek them out whenever I could. As I familiarized myself with the subtleties of alignment in standing postures, inversions, and simple floor postures, I lost the ability to put my feet on my head, my leg behind my neck. At the same time, I lost the pains in both my neck and my back. I was neither complaining nor concerned.

Eventually, I stumbled into an Ashtanga Yoga class in Hawaii. All of the fifty-five postures were familiar to me, but their context was not. The breathing method, the *bandhas,* the jumping style, the physical and psychological continuity, the sweat, and the surrender provided a context in which my body began, at last, to express more fully and deeply the alignment my Iyengar teachers had been trying to instill in me. The effect of the *vinyasa* practice on me was to shift that knowledge from my brain to my body. At last, I felt I was practicing yoga. Despite my enthusiasm for the practice, I did not become an Ashtanga practitioner, just as previously, I had never seen myself as a practitioner of Iyengar Yoga. The vinyasa techniques were there; the alignment of Iyengar was there; and for me, they served only to clarify, enhance, and expedite each other. As a student of both the Iyengar method and the vinyasa method, I am simply a practitioner of yoga.

However, once I discovered vinyasa, my passion was to get the better of me. I was soon doing varied sequences of up to three hundred asanas in six-hour practices. It was not long before my leg was behind my neck, my feet on my head again, as I floated in and out of handstands in between. However, I completely abandoned the nourishment of inversions and the settling of stillness. Eventually, all the jumping, heat, and sweat were draining me of moisture and energy. I became dehydrated, depleted, and physically exhausted. But worst of all, I became psychologically exhausted and lost the ability to recognize the imbalances I was creating, until finally, at the point of breakdown, I stopped. My body refused to allow me to practice anymore and insisted that I sit in meditation or lay myself over a chair in supported postures.

During the respite my body imposed, I took to exploring, especially what I had been taught were the bandhas. It soon became clear that impetuosity had not been my only problem. By tightening my anus and pressing my abdomen back for up to six hours a day, I had generated a deep and tenacious hardness in the core of my body. No wonder I could not sleep. I took my explorations to my students and the teachers I was working with. It soon became clear that whatever my Ashtanga teachers may have understood, my understanding of the bandhas was wrong. It so obviously feels wrong to create the hardness in the core of the body, especially the cranium, which tightening the anus and pressing the abdomen back generates.

Thus began a long, obsessive exploration of the bandhas. It began with clarifying what *mulabandha* and *uddiyanabandha* are not. It took a few years, with plenty of guiding feedback from my students, to clarify what mulabandha is. Even more time was needed to clarify exactly what uddiyanabandha is. On the way, *jalandharabandha* was also clarified. The first thing that became clear was that there is nothing mysterious or esoteric about the bandhas. They are nothing other than specific sets of muscular contractions. What eventually became clear was that they are simply the muscular response of vertebral verticality to gravity. Without them, the vertical integrity of the human spine and of the breath would be deeply compromised.

The key to this exploratory process was basing it on a classical hatha yoga *shat kriya* practice that I had been doing daily since my yoga journey began: uddiyanabandha. I learned this as a practice to do before asanas or pranayama. I had also come across it in advanced pranayama descriptions. Even though there seemed to be little clarity about what uddiyanabandha meant relative to asana practice, there was no doubt about what it was in pranayama practice. It is the opening of the rib cage when the lungs are, and remain, as empty as possible. This creates a pressure differential that sucks the abdomen back and up. It is a suction that is done *to* the abdomen, not *by* it; just as orange juice does nothing to get up a straw.

It seemed obvious to me that I would need to breathe during my yoga practice and would not be able to keep my lungs empty. Yet having been told that Desikachar teaches that mulabandha is triggered by exhalation, I could not help but notice the symmetry. I found that by breathing out deeply, the pelvic floor responded with a rotation of the anal mouth deep into the pelvis. As it rose into the pelvis, it met resistance and narrowed. The pelvic floor muscles remained relaxed and passive; no hardness was generated by this process. Could this be what "contract your anus" really means? Not contract it actively, but do something that narrows it passively? B. K. S. Iyengar states, in *Light on Yoga,* that mulabandha is done in the lower abdomen but not what exactly is done.

Mulabandha is done in the lower abdomen and affects the pelvic floor. Uddiyanabandha is done in the rib cage and affects the abdomen. When the lungs are opened by lengthening the spine and expanding the ribs, even without holding the lungs empty, the abdomen is sucked in and up passively. The muscles that we use to do this are accessory muscles to inhalation: spinal and intercostal muscles. Likewise, the muscles that we use to engage the pelvic floor into the pelvis are muscles accessory to exhalation. If we keep the accessory muscles of inhalation continuously active, the spine remains long and the chest remains open, even during the exhalation. Likewise, the lower abdomen remains withdrawn, flat, and engaged, even during the inhalation. In other words, uddiyanabandha is the continuous activation of accessory muscles of inhalation. Mulabandha is the continuous activation of accessory muscles of exhalation. At the same time, uddiyanabandha contains mulabandha. If the spinal and intercostal muscles are strong enough, the opening of the rib cage will reach the throat muscles also. Then jalandharabandha, which involves the accessory muscles of respiration in the throat, shows up too, in a single muscular process that activates all three bandhas together.

If the rib cage is opened by first lengthening the spine and then opening the chest, muscles in the lower abdomen spontaneously engage. This is an organic response, mediated through the nervous system, to the vulnerability that lifting the rib cage creates by raising the center of gravity. To keep the body as stable as possible by keeping the center of gravity as low as possible, muscular contraction is required lower down. This is always in the lower abdomen (pelvis). When standing, it is also in the thighs, calves, and feet. Exactly where and how much in each place depends on individual muscular availability. If there is weakness or tension in the feet and legs, it can come in the buttocks instead, in which case the bandhas and structural integrity—what I define as the greatest possible freedom in the spine and breath—will be compromised.

Within the unity, or yoga, of the three popular bandhas, a number of interesting phenomena take place. At their heart is the lifting of *uddiyana* (flying up) producing *mula* (root) below. While the rib cage, neck, and shoulder girdle lift, there is a balancing downward momentum. This stabilizing response can be felt in the skin of the upper back sliding downward and gripping inward as the shoulder blades rise with the rib cage.

It can also be felt in the skin of the upper abdomen pulling down toward the pelvis as the deep abdominal muscles engage. This tucks the rib crests downward and inward relative to the lift of the rib cage. These external events are mirrored internally by a potent sense of momentum going simultaneously upward deeper inside and downward at the surface, both front and back. This can be interpreted as a double spiraling dynamic in the trunk—a subtle, though obvious, energetic response to simple muscular activity.

Eventually, it became clear that the bandhas had been participating differently in both strands of my yoga learning. From my Ashtanga teachers, I had learned the names and the supposed purpose of the bandhas but not how to do them. From my Iyengar teachers, I had learned the sets of muscular contractions that constitute the bandhas but no words or concepts to define or integrate them. Yet while my Ashtanga teachers made no mention of *padabandha* (in the feet and legs) nor *hastabandha* (in the arms and hands), their constituent actions had been provided by B. K. S. Iyengar himself.

While doing an Iyengar teachers' intensive in Pune, I finally had the good fortune to encounter his teaching directly. In his teaching, the role of opposition became clear, though not yet its significance, especially in the arms and legs. It took me many years to realize that opposition is the key to structural integrity. Without it, there is no factor limiting the opening of joints and protecting them from harm. When the activity in related parts of the body are opposed to each other, they limit each other. In that limitation, they fertilize each other by preventing excess movement.

An obvious example of this is the differing momentum in the upper and lower arm so fundamental to my experience as an Iyengar Yoga student. More subtly, it can be found equally in the legs. Yet it was not until I understood the principle of opposition functioning as a spiral dynamic that I was able to use the legs as effectively as the arms, finding, of course, that the key was in the feet and that the power of the thighs must be used with great care if the knees are not to be damaged. So not only do the muscular actions in the trunk that generate integrity create a spiral dynamic, but so also do those in the limbs. Within this dynamic, the whole body is unified as each part is integrated into the whole.

If the unification of body and action that activating bandhas in each part produced was not enough, there was more to discover. Central to what I received as an Iyengar Yoga student was the phenomenon of feeling each part of the body simultaneously. This was the key to yoga postures being a spiritual, as well as physical, practice. This also was only possible for me once I had discovered the integrating spiral dynamic of the bandhas. Now, rather than addressing myself to multiple parts of the body, I need only concern myself with the constituent elements of the spiral dynamic—the lengthening of muscles, openings of joints, and broadenings across the skeleton that are organized and integrated through opposition.

The three active elements: broadening, lengthening, and opposing absorb my total intention, replacing the need for individuated awareness of the particularities of the body parts that are experiencing them. My attention remains sensitive to the openings in my joints without needing to locate or name them. As the body parts melt into broadening, lengthening, and opposing, these three elements dissolve into the singular dynamic of the bandhas. In this way, I discovered, on the basis of organized muscular contraction, the deep and full significance of the word *yoga,* and this significance goes far deeper than the physicality of the body. Yet the depths to which the word *yoga* points can be accessed so easily and effortlessly through the judicious use of muscular contraction. This use brings about what the yoga world now knows as "alignment" but also brings about much more without any need to lean on borrowed esoteric concepts.

Often I am asked where I discovered the spirals. Though my interest in spirals was inspired by Michio Kushi, my recognition of their presence in my body was the gift of B. K. S. Iyengar. Like all great gifts, it was not obvious at first. It took many years to unwrap. But in the end, I find that once again, as I did to my surprise in Pune, I must bow to the feet of B. K. S. Iyengar, the man who leads us to the full significance of yoga.

§

GODFREY DEVEREUX's Dynamic Yoga has its roots in both Iyengar and Ashtanga Vinyasa Yoga. He inspires as a precise, sensitive, and open teacher with a good understanding of yoga's profundities. His approach contextualizes practice in the five elements by using five fundamental techniques as lenses to clarify the inherent integrity of body, mind, and spirit: asana, vinyasa, bandha, pranayama, and drishti. Movement is used extensively to sensitize, awaken, and prepare the body for the stillness of yoga postures, within which the bandhas are used as the inherent key to structural, functional, and energetic integrity.

The Universal Yogi

Andrey Lappa

> True knowledge has no other source other than the One....Those who
> have realized the path of yoga . . . are oriented towards the preservation
> of the ideals of unification.
>
> The true pathway implies complete freedom of choice. It is for those
> who are capable of loving only one Master and receiving lessons in any
> form.
>
> —Andrey Lappa, *Yoga: Tradition of Unification*

My path toward yoga began at the age of twelve, when I spent a year in Mongolia. It was 1977 and my father, a programmer working for the Soviet Union's space program, was sent on a business trip to Mongolia to build the first computer system in the central government building of the capital Ulaanbaatar.

Mongolia was quite undeveloped. Fortunately, there was a Russian school in Ulaanbaatar where I was able to continue my secondary education. As there were no after-school activities for children, my father arranged for me to visit a Mongolian Buddhist monastery (*dazan*) where one of the monks, who spoke flawless Russian, could tutor me twice a week. Over the course of a year, I learned the fundamentals of Buddhism, the meanings of the images and symbols on the walls, and the Mongolian language, and I was invited to the traditional Lamaist rituals (*pujas*).

In 1978, we returned home to Kiev, the capital of the Ukraine, at that time still a part of the Soviet Union. I returned to my regular activities in various social clubs: sports, music, model building, and folk dancing. At this time in Communist countries, such activities were of high quality, well taught, and free for children. However, despite having plenty of friends and hobbies, I realized at the young age of thirteen that something vital was absent in my life. I began to miss the beautiful spiritual culture that I had been introduced to in the Mongolian monastery. I felt strongly that I had to follow a spiritual path and needed a principal goal and a sense of purpose in my life. At that time, there was no chance of finding a Mongolian Buddhist school in Communist Kiev, but I began to search for something similar.

My Buddhist teacher had told me that Mongolian Buddhism was similar to Tibetan Lamaist Buddhism. So I began to research cultures connected to Tibet and discovered both Indian yoga and Chinese martial arts. These systems were not similar to Mongolian Buddhism, but I found satisfaction in starting a personal spiritual practice in these alternative directions. At the same time, I was determined to discover my destiny in life, and I tried my hand at a variety of different subjects, in addition to yoga and martial arts. I attended secondary school, graduated from schools for the piano and accordion, built aviation and ship models, and trained myself to become an expert swimmer. At the age of sixteen, I became a Master of Sport for the Union of Soviet Socialist Republics and spent the next eight years on the Ukrainian National Olympic swim team. After three years of martial arts training, I realized that the spirit of yoga corresponded much more closely to my peace-loving nature. I made the final decision to conclude my martial arts training and to concentrate my energy and abilities on yoga alone.

At that time, information in the Soviet Union regarding yoga was both limited and restricted. Only a few books were made available, and the Communists carefully controlled their content. I knew one man in Moscow who had spent five years in prison just for teaching hatha yoga. The Communists were aware that yoga had a philosophical basis, and no philosophy other than Communism was allowed to be taught.

Fortunately for me, one of my friends managed to transport B. K. S. Iyengar's book *Light on Yoga* over the border illegally, and he translated this book into Russian. It was the best book about yoga I had seen up until then. It is hard to believe, but some people in the Soviet Union had such a hunger for yoga that they translated books from English to Russian without any commercial intent, just for the opportunity to improve their personal practice and to share this unique knowledge with their friends. During that period, many yoga books were illicitly translated into Russian by enthusiastic yoga practitioners for their personal use and had to be kept hidden in their homes.

I remember one unpleasant incident that took place when I was eighteen. By then, I had an extensive yoga library and was attending university. One day, I was called to the office of the university's Young Communists Organization. Their leader asked me whether or not I practiced yoga. I understood very well what the result of an honest answer could be and therefore chose not to answer at all. He said that if they were to search my home unannounced and find even one illegal book about yoga, they would make sure that my university education would cease. Fearing these consequences, I hid my entire library under the floor of our second house in the village for a long time, but such political pressure made me even more dedicated to the practice of yoga.

Light on Yoga was one of my best teachers at that time. I followed each word of B. K. S. Iyengar's instructions in that book, not only for my practice of asanas, pranayamas, and meditation, but also to lead my daily life, following all principles of the *yamas* and *niyamas*. *Light on Yoga* was an inspiration for my practice for many years, and I practiced almost all the asanas in the book by myself before I had reached the age of twenty-five. At this time, I did not have a conceptual understanding with regard to principles of alignment and was not aware that I was not performing the asanas entirely correctly, but in general, they looked very similar to those in the book.

I accumulated a great deal of information and practical experience in yoga, and many of my friends asked me to teach them. In 1984, still a student, I agreed. Because it was dangerous at that time to refer to my classes as yoga, for several years, I labeled the training "psycho-energetic gymnastics." In 1988, I graduated from the university and worked as a military engineer in a scientific institute in Kiev, all the while teaching two yoga classes each night. I already had nearly three hundred students at that time.

The political reforms of Mikhail Gorbachev in the Soviet Union began in 1986, and over the course of the next few years, there was significant political liberalization. I was very happy to learn that international yoga conferences were being organized by the Russian Yoga Association and Rama Jyoti Vernon in Moscow in 1990 and 1991. Many yoga teachers from India, Russia, the United States, and Europe took part in these conferences, which were called Unity in Yoga. I participated, and it was there that I met B. K. S. Iyengar for the first time. It was a joy to take classes with him and to get a deeper understanding of yoga during his lectures at the conference.

In 1993, I finished my doctoral dissertation in the field of underwater technology for navy submarines and promptly decided to end my engineering career. I had no interest left in working just for material benefits, and my personal interest in human nature became the central focus in my life. I became a full-time yoga teacher and yogi and left the engineering world behind.

In 1992, Ukraine became an independent country, and nations around the world opened their embassies in Kiev. The first Indian ambassador to our country was Mr. Deware. He was very active in trying to popularize Indian culture in the Ukraine. He organized regular traditional Indian celebrations, including Divali and Holi, in Kiev, and invited local groups and organizations that had an interest in Indian heritage to take part. There were Indian dancers, musicians, and theater artists at these celebrations, and my students and I were invited to do demonstrations of asanas.

I took part in these programs regularly during the next two years, and in 1994, Mr. and Mrs. Deware decided to finance a trip to India for me with the intention of improving my level of education in yoga. They asked me what school I would like to visit, and I replied that it had been my dream for many years to study with B. K. S. Iyengar. They were delighted to hear my answer because they had known Guruji personally for a long time. If I remember correctly, they told me that they had been neighbors of B. K. S. Iyengar's until 1976 and resided in the same building as his family.

Mr. Deware wrote a letter to Guruji, asking him for permission for me to come and study free of charge in his institute in Pune. Guruji kindly agreed to provide this opportunity for me, and Mr. Deware paid for all of my expenses: Indian visa, round-trip tickets, and lodging in India as well. I was truly blessed to receive this generous support from both Mr. Deware and B. K. S. Iyengar.

I studied at the Ramamani Iyengar Memorial Institute in Pune for two months. I wanted to study longer, but the length of time had been fixed between Mr. Deware and Guruji. I was hungry for yoga knowledge, and two months of studies only increased my hunger. Therefore, I chose to extend my stay in India and travel for four more months, studying in other schools of yoga as well. I studied with Yogacharya Rudra at the Shivananda Ashram in Rishikesh, and Pattabhi Jois and B. K. S. Iyengar in Mysore, among others.

After this visit, I made a practice of going to India each year, and I visited the Ramamani Iyengar Memorial Institute in Pune three more times. I studied with B. K. S. Iyengar, with his daughter, Geeta Iyengar, and with his son, Prashant Iyengar, during that time. During the course of these visits, I received a great deal of important information regarding principles of alignment in asanas, individual corrections, ways to develop asanas with the use of props, and pranayama and meditation techniques. I have never come across a higher quality and conscious practice of asanas in any another school of yoga, which is why I still make use of these methods and techniques in my personal practice and my teaching of yoga.

All this was completely new for Russian yoga practitioners, and I dedicated myself to spreading this important information within the territories of the post-Soviet countries, especially in the Ukraine. In 1996, I opened my own yoga studio in downtown Kiev, one of the first yoga studios in the country. The next year, I opened a second yoga studio in the city, occupying a three-story building. It was the largest yoga studio in all of the post-Soviet countries, with a total space of more than ten thousand square feet, including five large training rooms and a swimming pool for practicing pranayama in the water.

During my studies with B. K. S. Iyengar, I was deeply immersed in and inspired by his ideas and concepts through his creativity and yoga consciousness. I was fortunate to be able to combine these qualities of his with skills gained from my modern Western education to see and develop some essential aspects of yoga. For example, Guruji taught principles of the main directions of joint mobility at the Unity in Yoga conference in Moscow. I learned from his teachings how a joint could be moved in multiple directions: forward, backward, bent to each side, twisted to each side, extended, and compressed. I applied this concept to my own yoga practice and attempted to use this idea with all joints of the human body; I extrapolated a complete system of new asanas based on this principle.

Later, I analyzed all the well-known asanas that existed in different schools of yoga throughout the world, and I realized that there was an inordinately small number of arm asanas in yoga compared to the ones that existed to develop mobility in the legs and spine. There are thousands of the latter, but very few (no more than six) for developing mobility in the arms, and these were only for stretching rather than strengthening. Believing in the necessity for a more balanced yoga practice, I began to develop a number of asanas for developing directions of mobility for all arm joints that would allow them to parallel the well-known asanas that developed mobility in the legs.

This research and the addition of new and vital components to the total compendium of known asanas made it possible for me to reach a standard of unified development for all parts of the human body and to achieve a well-balanced effect from the yoga practice. This is a very important step in the development of conscious yoga. I owe that first spark to Guruji, a spark that was ignited during the conference in Moscow and that kept burning throughout my studies with him at the Ramamani Iyengar Memorial Yoga Institute in Pune.

B. K. S. Iyengar has been a very important influence on my personal yoga practice and teaching. I have received knowledge from him that I have used, and continue to use, in my life. Guruji has had a powerful influence on the evolution of all yoga throughout the world. Most asanas used by practitioners in different schools of yoga are taken either from his book *Light on Yoga,* from him personally, or from his disciples. The majority of yoga teachers in the world now use his principles of alignment in asanas, and you can find props developed by Guruji in almost every studio in every country. But even more important, from my point of view, is the beautiful, correct, deep, and conscious yoga practice and teaching that Guruji Sri B. K. S. Iyengar has passed down to future generations of yogis all over the world.

§

ANDREY LAPPA is one of the most influential yoga masters of the post-Soviet countries. He has studied with teachers both famous and unknown, including

B. K. S. Iyengar and Sri K. Pattabhi Jois, and has practiced meditation in many monasteries and temples throughout the East. After many years of exploration into the most esoteric and challenging practices of yoga, Andrey developed the incomparably powerful and effective Universal Yoga, a comprehensive approach to spiritual evolution. He has taught yoga since 1988 and is president of the Kiev Yoga Federation in the Ukraine. Currently, he conducts teacher-training programs around the world and has reintroduced hatha yoga to the monks of his Tibetan Buddhist lineage in Nepal. He is the author of *Yoga: Tradition of Unification*.

The Great Gift

JULIAN SANDS

> If a well-toned body works better each day, surely the same is true for a well-toned intelligence. For our bodies, the fruit of our sustained, intelligent effort will be, in its widest sense, health. But at another level, what we are really gaining (and this is the cause of our satisfaction) is self-control.
>
> —B. K. S. IYENGAR, *Light on Life*

As was the case with so many others, Julian Sands first started yoga reluctantly and at the behest of another, only to have things develop from there.

Julian Sands was interviewed by Anne O'Brien in July 2006.

ANNE O'BRIEN: When we talked earlier, you stated that you see yoga as the great gift. Why?

JULIAN SANDS: Actually, it is a term that was used by my first yoga teacher in Los Angeles, Diane Gysbers, who is one of the great Manouso Manos's students. She described yoga as a gift when I very, very reluctantly had my first lesson. For me, yoga was something I had a consciousness of during most of my adult life but never really encountered, preferring instead to climb mountains and run marathons. But when my wife was pregnant with our first daughter and had also sustained a back injury, her doctor recommended yoga lessons. Just as providence is the only thing in life you can really trust, Diane came along to work with her at the house. I very quickly saw the benefit, not just in my wife's health, but also in her overall well-being. And the benefit in our familial well-being was undeniable. I wanted to be a part of it, even if reluctantly. I agreed to have a ten-minute session with Diane, which then worked into a half hour, then an hour, and then to an ongoing practice. That was more than ten years ago now. Great breakthroughs came in workshops with Diane and Manouso, Karin O'Bannon, and others. But as we know, it is doing yoga in your own life in a daily practice that is the significant thing. Although I still run marathons and climb mountains, every aspect of my life personally and professionally has been improved by my encounter with yoga and yoga becoming a part of my life. If things start wobbling a bit, by doing more yoga, equilibrium is restored. The benefit is wonderful. To be introduced to yoga is a great thing, and yes, ultimately yoga is a gift.

AOB: I wonder if there are any specific lessons or discoveries in your own practice of yoga that help you with your craft of acting?

JS: There are practical things. I've always believed that a certain holistic fitness in mind and body was essential to be an actor. For me to be an actor in the English (Olivier) tradition, it was essential to have a sort of military fitness. Yoga—specifically headstand, virabhadrasana II, and trikonasana—somehow harnesses a martial fitness and combines it with an emotional and intellectual balance that puts me in a good position to go to work. It is something Diane said: "Whatever time you have for practice is what you have. If you can just do three poses, it is important." Not that she or I advocate doing only three poses in a practice, but if there is only that much time before going to work, those three poses somehow, for me, get everything stimulated and give me a much keener perception of the character I want to present and a much keener understanding of how to present that character. Headstand has been the great revelation; it has opened the doors for me probably more than any other single pose.

AOB: Is there something specific to the headstand? Is it that you literally are looking at your world upside down, or do you think it is more related to the physiological dynamic that occurs in the body?

JS: I think it is both. The actual physical pose allows the consciousness to break out of the restraints of normality. When I climb mountains—especially if I have been on remote, upper mountains for a few days—when I come back down to the world I left behind, I feel not quite there and that some sort of adjustment must be made. In other words, my perspective has been shifted. Before I am reconsumed by the normality or regularity of life, there is a period of detachment, perhaps enlightenment, of seeing things afresh. To some degree, being in sirsasana has the same effect. When I come out of sirsasana, there is this sense of seeing everything afresh, as if one were coming back to one's normal condition with a heightened perception. The really wonderful thing I like to do when I get to the top of a mountain is do a headstand. It is really an amazing experience, partly because of the geophysical energy present at the top of a mountain. To experience that energy directly in your head is rare. I have enjoyed headstand on mountains all over the world and thoroughly recommend it!

AOB: Does that seeing things afresh also help you deal with fame? It is thought that the Buddha once said something like "Fame is the deadliest poison." Are there aspects of the yoga practice that help you negotiate what may be the negative and transitory side of fame?

JS: Yoga helps one deal with the transitory nature of everything! I have a very minor level of celebrity. Yoga is the great leveler. It requires humility; the practice insists on it. To go to a class, stand with others in tadasana, listen to the teacher, and follow the practice—everything else just slips away. If fame develops or perpetuates ego, or if it creates desire, the simple act of just going to a class can be the antidote. I have described yoga to people as being hugely self-negating as well as self-affirming. It is the practice of finding that balance. Practice is anti-ego. And since I have been practicing for more than ten years, I can see that my practice is always in flux. The personal consciousness of practice has become much more developed, even if there have been declines in some aspects of the physical practice. However illustrious any pose may have become, I am always a beginner and will always be a beginner.

AOB: What is inspiring you in your practice these days? Is there any particular path of inquiry that is calling you?

JS: I suppose what inspires me today is what has always inspired me— the opening up of myself and the letting go of myself. That is something that, as an actor, I find both beneficial and extremely interesting. My work has become far more confident and more interesting to me as a process, because through yoga I have had a deeper feeling for the energy that goes into being an actor—whatever the psychology and emotional life of the characters. There has been much more substance to my ability to wrangle all of the components of a character.

I find Mr. Iyengar a source of inspiration. I have only seen Guruji once, when he gave a talk in London. That was an amazing and revelatory encounter. I was so struck by his elegance; there was such obvious reconciliation between being and body. He was such a man; he wasn't spirit. He was human, not a bodhisattva, although that argument may be made. It was his corporeal presence that was so impressive. I thought, "My God, he is eighty years old!" That luminosity isn't an abstraction— you feel it very powerfully. It was so inspiring. I am very, very grateful to my teachers and to B. K. S. Iyengar for harnessing, structuring, and making accessible everything Patanjali was trying to put out there as everybody's gift.

JULIAN SANDS is a British leading actor who has enjoyed a twenty-plus-year career in Europe and the United States. He has appeared in numerous plays, films, and television projects. His many film credits include *The Killing Fields, A Room with a View, Gothic, Naked Lunch, Boxing Helena,* and *Tale of a Vampire.* He makes his home in London and Los Angeles.

Yoga and Sound: A Passion, A Prayer

RAMANAND PATEL

When we first begin yoga, there are so many new things to contend with. We soon run into Sanskrit, the language of India. All its ancient texts are written in Sanskrit. The names of the postures and the fundamental concepts all come from Sanskrit. Immediately, we run into the problem of translation. Does *posture* really get across the meaning of the Sanskrit word *asana*? Slowly we begin to suspect that, in some essential way, it doesn't. Then we think that since words don't always match up exactly, maybe concepts don't either. Some words, such as *karma, mantra,* and *dharma,* have been imported wholesale into English. Is that because there is no English equivalent? If not, how can we be sure that we've understood those words accurately, rather than allowed our understanding to grasp some conceptually mongrelized version? The Sanskrit word *akasha,* for example, is generally translated as "ether." When the planets were thought to rotate gracefully on celestial spheres around a stationary sun, "ether" filled up the space beyond the moon. It was a rarefied substance permeating all of space; that is, space existed, and space contained ether.

Akasha is very different. Before all of this existed—indeed, before Time itself existed—there was only the possibility to be, which we can call God. All objects, all energy, all space, all time issued forth from that. However, since that primordial possibility for being was the only thing that existed, was not our ability to perceive objects made from the identical substance? What else was there?

This is the immediate problem with translating *akasha* as "ether." *Ether* does not include the "space" inside our awareness in which the perception of the object occurs. It also does not encompass the fact that we can perceive that we are perceiving that object. The Western understanding of space does not conjoin object-perception to awareness-perception. In the West, these are regarded as completely distinct; in Sanskrit, they are not.

Another issue is the method used by the Creator to produce this universe. The word *Creator* is not appropriate because Sanskrit has no concept of a creator. *Manifestation* is not the same as *creation,* for the world was made manifest from itself by itself and was not created by anyone or anything.

At some point, everything was made to vibrate—resulting in sound. The power inherent in mantras lies in their recognition of the ability of the primordial manifestation—that potential harbinger of consciousness—to impart and impose its essence into everything. This immediately leads to the majestic properties of music, a subject here taken up by Ramanand Patel. As human beings, we can hear and create vibrations as music. An instrument is played and it "does" something to us—our consciousness is "stirred." Every musician wonders, is it really possible to play the same song twice? When we play a piece and are creatively inspired, what passes through us and becomes music? What is the role of consciousness? What is the relationship between individual consciousness and the primordial manifestation of consciousness? How does the latter transform itself, through us, into sound? Who are we in this process—beings affected by sound, beings who create sound, beings who have become sound objects?

While visiting my sister in Pennsylvania in 1991, I was invited to teach yoga at Swami Dayananda Saraswati's ashram. There, I had the great fortune of meeting Pandit Mukesh Desai. Mukesh was the resident music teacher at the ashram, a foremost gifted disciple of the world-renowned North Indian classical vocalist, Pandit Jasraj, and my sister's music teacher. I found him to be an ordinary, unassuming character endowed with the not-too-enviable gift of telling poor jokes with good delivery. His physical posture and general demeanor were rather poor from the yogic perspective, although he was a very friendly guy. As he was a family friend, my sister invited him home to spend the weekend with us.

I woke up early that Saturday morning to do my daily yoga practice. No sooner had I started, than I heard the voice of Mukesh from the next room: "GA GA MA MA DHA DHA." Not having had much exposure to North Indian classical vocalists, I felt he was going to disturb my quiet, penetrating practice. Although Guruji had crowned me with title of his "most senior student in the United States," I had accepted that as a statement of Guruji's love rather than as a comment on my prowess. Remembering that blessing, I decided that it was up to me, as a yogi, to change my attitude to *kshanti* (accommodation). Rather than tolerating the sound, I began to accommodate it. As my resistance dropped, I found my breath getting more relaxed and my mind more perceptive to how that breath was affecting my body. The practice became subtler, more penetrating. I began to be aware of some of the resistances I was unknowingly holding in my body. To my delight, I seemed to gain energy to go further and hold my poses for longer duration. I found my conclusions of his demeanor incorrect as far as his music was concerned. He was obviously a very serious and gifted master vocalist.

Over breakfast, I discussed my experience with him. The jokes stopped. We had a very interesting and insightful exchange. I wondered if the effect of the sound on my yoga was perhaps partly a result of my Indian upbringing, a culture bias, a pride, a prejudice. We decided there and then that I would gather a few of my American yoga friends and try this out on them. The effects were nothing short of electrifying.

As this was an accidental discovery, I wrote immediately to Guruji, asking for his blessing. His response was, "I am glad you are starting where I left off." I read nothing more than his love in that statement. Mukesh also talked to his guru. Over the years, we have read of this kind of work being mentioned in the sacred books of India. In the early days of my study with Guruji, I constantly heard the words "find out," "discover," and "learn to penetrate." It was heartening to hear Prashantji's comment, "There is no yoga without sound nor sound without yoga."

To me, our beloved Guruji is enshrined with divinity: GOD. Where there was listless life, he became a *G*enerator of confidence; an *O*perator in the selfless, untiring service of humanity; and a *D*estroyer of illness and disease. Everything good that comes out of the work in *Yoga and Sound* would never have happened without confidence, the discipline, and the foundation that he imparted. I am sure Mukesh would say the same about his teacher.

Guruji told me he did not mind my being innovative, but he was insistent that there must first be a good foundation. His intention is certainly not to suffocate free exploration and the passion of the true discovery of ultimate freedom offered by yoga. It is my fervent hope and prayer that we who are responsible for administering this grand vision are worthy. I remember Guruji saying many years ago, "I am not interested in numbers; I just want a few good students." He certainly has the few good students. However, he admits that the numbers have grown far beyond his imagination. And these numbers continue to grow. Let us embrace with a large heart those large numbers who wish to practice, who wish to honor Guruji for his contribution.

When RAMANAND PATEL was twelve, his father introduced him to yoga philosophy and asana, and he learned early on to embrace yoga with a childlike joy and delight. In 1968, Yogacharya Sri B. K. S. Iyengar profoundly influenced the strength, discipline, deepening, understanding, confidence, and enthusiasm of his practice. In 1984, Ramanand intensified his pursuit of truth and knowledge by studying Vedanta philosophy under H. H. Swami Dayananda Saraswati. He also considers J. Krishnamurti to be a major influence on his thinking. Ramanand is recognized and respected internationally, and many in the yoga community regard him as one of the world's foremost yoga instructors. He actively encourages both learning and the sharing of ideas among his students and peers. He is especially skilled as an innovator in the use of props and working with students who have special needs, and he has a special interest in the effects of sound on yoga practice.

Ears: The Corridors to Heaven

SHANDOR REMETE

In order for things to exist, they must first be set in motion. Vibrations must be initiated by something. Music is not the only entity carried as and by sound, nor is it the only thing created by and affecting consciousness and our intentions and sensations. As human beings, we are also endowed with an ability to speak, hear, and understand.

But exactly what do speaking and hearing represent? What happens when we "understand" something? How has our consciousness been propelled from ignorance to knowledge through and with sound? Creativity and consciousness are again involved. As an individual, you are certainly creative, for no one has put together a string of sentences quite like you. Furthermore, among all the sentences you have spoken, many have been unique, and no one—not even you—will ever speak them again. But every one of those sentences has been uttered within the confines of some language possessing rules of grammar, syntax, prosody, and the like. Shandor Remete now explores the significance of the Indian understanding of consciousness, sound, language, and understanding, as well as the tension that language sets up between the need to express ourselves creatively and individually while respecting the conventions imposed by the need to be understood. Throughout this process, the light of understanding stands supreme—a light that is the very heartbeat of the universe.

Pranayama is done with the ears!" As Guruji hissed these words across the classroom, it was as if they issued forth from the mouth of Adishesha himself. This pronouncement came at the conclusion of a pranayama class at the Institute in Pune in 1981. We had just spent two hours learning the proper arrangement of the fingers and wrists and the correct elbow and shoulder activity for the proper manipulation of the nostrils. It had been a step-by-step instructional class on the skillful manipulation of the nasal passages for the proper movement of wind during the practice of pranayama.

You can imagine my reaction after two hours of seemingly endless instructions on fingers and nose when we were told that pranayama is done with the ears! It came with the shock of a volcanic eruption, creating an utter tumult and bewilderment within my mind. In the midst of my confusion and mistrust, I thought perhaps I had misheard him. At the end of the class, I asked my trusted and beloved Guruji if the last instruction given had been some kind of misconceived joke. I received a look, without verbal confirmation, that assured me no joke was involved. What I had heard was the hard truth of the matter.

Little did I know at the time that this last instruction would be the beginning of a long journey of inquiry. Over the next twenty years, my struggle to decipher the information behind that hint would set the course for the rest of my life.

Before I continue with my story, I should explain that my father taught me that if I decided to learn any art or craft, I should only do so from a teacher in whom I had complete trust. He said that I should feel deep respect for that person but be without fear in his or her presence. He also told me that there are two sides to any master craftsman: the practical side that is openly expounded, and the hidden side that carries the secrets of mastery. This hidden knowledge is either hinted at through apparently absurd statements or is revealed through the skillful gestures of the teacher's actions. These messages will only be picked up by apprentices who have a deep love both for the teacher and their chosen craft and who remain forever alert with eyes and ears fully open and mind attentive.

The heavy hint I received at the end of the nasal torture was to interact deep in my mind with an insight I had received a few days before. In the *Yoga Yajnavalkya*, Sutra IX:22 states, "One should only proceed with the practices of meditation if one is well versed in the sciences of marma, nadi and vayu, if one is devoid of the knowledge of these sciences, one should not proceed."

Charged with these two hints concerning marma and pranayama with the ears, I began a study of ayurvedic and *siddha* medicines without which the understanding of marma, nadi, and vayu is not possible. At first, these studies were purely theoretical, but later I had the good fortune to study under a practical guide in South India. He not only demonstrated how this knowledge could be applied in therapy, but also how to use the principles of marma when using one's own body in action. This is achieved partly through the skillful manipulation of the limbs through specific patterns of muscular action in asana and also by using the mind to guide the vayu through the appropriate nadis during the practices of pranayama and the combined process of *dharana, dhyana,* and *samadhi* that Gorakshanatha terms *pranasamyama.* It is through these studies that I have come to fully understand and appreciate the guidance of Guruji, which was given freely through his practical explanations and hidden hints.

From my study of *marmasthana* (or *varma kalai,* as it is called in Tamil), I have come to learn that there is a location inside the cavity of the mouth, directly behind the point at which the teeth close, where mental speech manifests as spoken word. After many years of study and practice, it is from observing this point that I have come to understand my guru's hint that pranayama is done with the ears. Any audible sound that is heard within the body rises at this point. By tuning one's ears to this point within the mouth cavity, one automatically draws the energies of the other four organs of perception to the same point. One can easily test this while lying in savasana, when the mind is quiet and the body is at ease, by gently curling and raising the tip of the tongue into the space behind where the teeth meet and experiencing the energies of all the organs of perception drawing to this point. One not only hears the sound, but also feels it, sees it, tastes it, and smells it.

The *Maheshvara Sutra* explains in detail the process of the manifestation of language. Language is a symbolic yet crude form of communication and can therefore become a barrier to the expression of our innermost experiences. This is why mystics never bother to explain their inner transitions. The crudeness of the symbolic exteriorization of language does not allow it. According to the theories of yoga, the mind must be reduced to silence before it can go beyond the barriers of language and perceive the supersensory world.

The formation of any language begins as an appearance of an idea, which is formed in the substratum of consciousness and is referred to as the *para* (beyond); the seat of the para within the human body is in the region of the coccyx. The formation of a *pashyanti* (vision) from that idea occurs in the area of the navel, while its mental formulation into language is known as *madhyama* (intermediary) and takes place in the heart. The exteriorization of the mental form into a sound is called *vaikhari* (exteriorized). This occurs in the throat, but the final exit point into the audible world is in the oral cavity, as described earlier. This is the seat of the struck sound. Since in yoga one is engaged in the energetic reversal of the manifestation of life, one must learn to direct the attention of the ears to that point within the mouth and the energy of the other senses will automatically be drawn there.

The return journey begins in the practice of pranayama, where attention is drawn from the seat of the struck sound to the seat of the unstruck sound within the heart. In the heart, the mental formation as language is dissolved, then the sound regains its visual appearance at the region of the navel and subsequently is reabsorbed into its causal point (the *karanasharira*). The causal point is the coccyx, which is the dwelling place of the lady of phonemes—or as she is more commonly known, Kundalini Shakti.

By observing the appearance and formation of language and the four locations and stages of its systematic manifestation, one gains a good view of the practices of pranayama, since the science of *sahita kumbhaka* also consists of four corresponding stages: *puraka, antara kumbhaka, rechaka,* and *bahya kumbhaka.* Together with the application of the three *bandhas,* these give us the key to the beyond.

Guruji's two hints have disclosed for me the secrets for the development of skillful and sensitive means without recourse to any of this terminology. All was contained in the simplicity of "pranayama is done with the ears."

Guruji, I have never swerved from what you have taught me. I have taken the practical with the hints and worked it quietly over the years. I thank you for showing me the corridors to heaven, and may the gods give you a safe passage to the world where all the great yogis still roam.

With my deepest reverence and love for what you have given me, a debt that can never be repaid,

SHANDOR REMETE (NATANAGA ZHANDER)

§

SHANDOR REMETE (NATANAGA ZHANDER) has been practicing yoga since the age of six and is the founder of Shadow Yoga. For more than four decades, through his practice and study, he has researched the common principles shared by yoga, the martial arts, and the ayurvedic and siddha systems of medicine. He runs courses and workshops in Europe, Russia, Israel, Asia, the United States, New Zealand, and Australia.

Yoga Is Beyond Religion

H. S. ARUN

> Yoga is not a religion but a religious subject which enhances the religiousness of mankind. Yoga is a subject which cultures the mind and the intelligence of the individual to develop religiousness through practice. It has nothing to do with the man-created religious order; yet it is a religion of human beings, a religion of humanity, as it is filled with the message of goodwill to one and all.
> —B. K. S. IYENGAR, *Astadala Yogamala*

We speak with an easy confidence born from the conviction that we know exactly what words mean. It can therefore be interesting to learn how a word was used by others who felt the same way. It can also be interesting to know how the word was derived, for that can tell us what people used to think of that topic. But a word's etymon—its ancient or derived meaning—rarely bears any relation to how it is used now. A historical derivation can only rarely indicate the current meaning; that must be gleaned from the context. If one's goal is to communicate, then every word should convey its current meaning, because that is invariably what is expected. Since the meanings of most words change, sometimes quite considerably, to suddenly advocate the use of an etymon or pretend that that is how we currently understand the word is to undermine the attempt to communicate. This is "the etymological fallacy"—the attempt to justify ourselves by referring to a word's irrelevant etymon.

Nevertheless, light can be shed on "the true reality" behind a given word, particularly when its meaning is difficult to pin down, even though most speakers use it confidently. The word's history, as well as how it is used in other languages, can reveal a great deal about how others have understood the topic and therefore about the topic itself. Such a word is *religion,* now examined by H. S. Arun.

Nowadays, on my travels, I am sometimes disturbed by what's happening in the world of yoga outside India. While I am very impressed with the level of commitment, the eagerness to learn, and the intelligence of the students in countries such as the United States, Chile, Peru, Argentina, Bolivia, and Israel, I have also seen that they are trying to create an atmosphere for yoga that is often alien to their culture. They may put up pictures of Hindu gods and goddesses, burn oriental incense sticks or chant mantras, perform so-called *homas* or *havanas* (fire sacrifices), or even change their names to Indian-sounding ones. Some even seem to think Buddhism and Hinduism are one and the same and may put statues of Buddha in the classroom.

By itself, that is not bad. But often the pictures are hung in places we would consider inappropriate or highly inauspicious, such as on bathroom walls or where people may put their feet on the yoga room walls. On a more practical level, the incense sticks they use may sometimes cause an allergic reaction among practitioners during class.

Often, I have heard mantras being distorted, and the pronunciation can make them quite hard to understand. People may take just a part of some mantra and rename it "the antistress mantra," "the relaxation mantra," and so on. Recently, I found a CD that has a single phrase, *pratipaksha bhavanam,* said over and over as a *japa.* This seems to come from *The Yoga Sutras of Patanjali* (II:34) which reads, *Vitarka himsadayah krita karita anumodita lobha krodha moha purvaka mrudu madhya adhimatra duhka ajnana ananta phala iti pratipaksha bhavanam.* This translates roughly as "uncertain knowledge [vitarka] which comes through perverse actions and thoughts, will result in violence, whether it is done directly or indirectly, whether it is caused by greed, anger, or delusion, in mild, moderate, or intense degrees. It results in endless pain and ignorance. Such behavior may be corrected by its opposite, that is, introspection, proper thinking, and proper action." If someone only chants the last bit, that the behavior can be corrected by its opposite, it may not be as meaningful.

These things are done with very good intentions, as students want to reach the heart of the yogic tradition. They try to get there by adopting the rituals and practices associated with yoga in its birthplace. Yet perhaps students need not get caught in these ideas. These are all trappings external to the core idea of yoga. The rituals developed from local traditions that were relevant in ancient times. Some are kept up in India because they are still richly imbued with meaning. For instance, we still pray daily to our favorite gods and goddesses and burn incense sticks in offering to them. But these gods are more than just pictures and idols for us, and each aspect has deep spiritual meaning for the worshipper. Such prayer and rituals are part of our religion and our way of life.

But yoga itself is not a religion. Yoga is beyond religion. It can be practiced universally by anyone, without recourse to the religious symbols of Hinduism. After all, Patanjali, in the *Sutras*, which we believe to be the first text of yoga practice, did not prescribe any specific rituals and practices. The Patanjali *Sutras* lay down norms, the *yama*s and *niyama*s, in order to improve the effectiveness of practice. These norms are also universal values. They describe the human aspirations for good comportment and self-improvement such as cleanliness, contentment, self-study, nonviolence, truthfulness, and so on. By understanding the importance of these virtues, practitioners prepare themselves for the right practice.

Also, in the Patanjali *Sutras,* the God (Ishvara) referred to by the author is not an external manifestation of divinity such as in the Hindu pantheon—not Ganesha, or Shiva, or any particular *avatara* or *dashavatara*. Patanjali's Ishvara is explained in 1:24: *Klesha karma vipaka ashayaih aparamrishtah purusha visheshah Ishvarah:* "God is a special unique Entity [Purusha], who is eternally free from all afflictions and unaffected by actions and their reactions, or by their residues. He abides undisturbed in His own Being. He is eternally free and always Sovereign." Patanjali goes on to say, in 1:25, *Tatra niratishayam sarvajnabijam:* "God is the seed of Omniscience, Omnipresence, and Omnipotent. All creations are created by God." And in 1:26, we have *Sa eshah purvesham api guruh kalena anavacchedat:* "God is the foremost Teacher who is not bound nor conditioned by place, space, or Time. He is all and All is He."

This God is not the one of this religion or that. This God is instead the universal truth as understood by all religions. By practicing yoga, we are not subscribing to any particular religion. In fact, yoga can help us deepen our belief in our own religion, whichever that may be.

One tool available to us in this deepening of our spirituality, which all practitioners seek, is the use of the *pranava,* or AUM. In 1:27, Patanjali explains that *tasya vacakah pranavah* ("God [as explained above] is identified with the sacred syllable AUM"), and AUM has thousands of representations and meanings. When repeated constantly, it becomes a japa. All the chantings of mantras start with AUM and end with AUM.

If you study Guruji B. K. S. Iyengar's *Light on Yoga,* you can come to understand that all asanas similarly start with tadasana and end with tadasana. So for all Guruji's students, tadasana in fact *is* AUM. Yet at heart, AUM is only the resonance of the universal sound. It is the sound from which all creation began—three syllables at the root of sound irrespective of any given language. It is therefore a secular articulation of the supreme indivisible energy that resides in all human beings. It is also considered the tool by which we can experience the divine. Modern science says vibration is the source of all creation. It is the subtlest form of God's creation. The AUM sound resonates with the very vibration that is the source of this creation. It is the root of all existence.

Patanjali says, in 1:29, *Tatah kshetana adhigamah api antaraya abhavah ca*: "Repetition of AUM with feeling and understanding helps to remove physical, mental, intellectual, and spiritual impediments, leading the student on to self-realization." So if students want to retain some connectivity with the traditions of yoga, maybe they can stop worrying about representations of gods and goddesses and the complications of chants in a foreign tongue. If they are keen to chant something in order to tune their minds before yoga practice, let them just chant the universally easy and universally pleasing sound of AUM. Or if they can understand Guruji's idea that tadasana is the source of all asana, just as AUM is the source of all creation, let them just allow tadasana to resonate throughout their practice. This is perhaps the "*mula* mantra" of the Iyengar Yoga tradition.

HONNEDEVASTAHANA SHAMRAO ARUN has totally dedicated his life to the propagation of Iyengar Yoga. He takes a personal interest in each student to understand his or her strengths and weaknesses. His continuous research into all aspects of yoga and its relation to the mental and physical well-being of people has helped him to introduce innovative methods of teaching asanas, while staying true to Guruji's basic principles.

True, Auspicious, and Beautiful

EDWARD CLARK

Truth, goodness, and beauty are often called "the three fundamental values." Our ability to appreciate them is sometimes regarded as a defining characteristic of what it is to be human. The agenda for the Western understanding of them was initially set by Plato who felt that "the Good," "the True," and "the Beautiful" had an ultimate unity. Aristotle, who had a far greater influence on subsequent Western traditions, accepted that they were related but felt that there was a clear distinction between them. Looked at one way, Aristotle felt that *sophia* (wisdom) could be seen as the highest virtue regarding these values. Was wisdom then, in Aristotle's view, better than any of them? Or did he mean that none of them could be properly appreciated without wisdom? Some say one, some say the other. Looked at another way, the governing virtue was surely *phronesis,* a word that is hard to translate but can be thought of as a variant of "practical reason" or "prudence"—a due sense of proportion that is both intellectual and ethical regarding the merits and circumstances of a situation. So was this slightly more prosaic phronesis similarly better or necessary to appreciate the three virtues?

Following this tradition, the ancient Western philosophers felt that all human activities fell into three broad groups: the pursuit of truth, the pursuit of beauty, and the pursuit of good and right. Paralleling these, human beings exercise three kinds of judgment that require three kinds of intelligence: the intellectual or cognitive, the aesthetic, and the moral. These in turn permit the existence of the three great branches of Western philosophy: metaphysics, aesthetics, and ethics. Metaphysics deals with issues of truth regarding the universe and the reality and manner of its existence; aesthetics focuses on beauty and related concepts such as the tragic, the sublime, the poetic, and so forth; and ethics deals with "good" and "bad," right action and wrong action. What can these topics mean to a yoga practitioner? How should they be regarded, and what should yogis do to express them in their lives—if, indeed, they should be expressed? Edward Clark now turns his attention to these critically important subjects.

In his book *The Tree of Yoga*, B. K. S. Iyengar writes that "if as an artist (dancer) you also practice yoga—if you are in touch with the internal levels of your being—you will develop a vast range of expression and your art will become what is known as *'satyam, sivam, sundaram,'* true, auspicious and beautiful. Art then becomes divine."[*]

While I am unsure if I have created art that is divine, I have been artistic director of Tripsichore Yoga Theatre since 1979 and have had the opportunity to consider and test Mr. Iyengar's succinctly expressed ideas. His simple words contain complex notions that I hope to address from an informed perspective. In particular, I will focus on beauty, for though everyone has their own intuition about it, I have found that many are deceived about this seemingly simple idea.

This current generation of Western yogis has presided over an unprecedented growth of yoga, including the aesthetic appreciation of it. As recently as the 1890s, a yogi was displayed at the Westminster Aquarium as a freak and was ridiculed by the public and press. Yet today, some hundred years later, gorgeously photographed asanas grace the pages of yoga books, and calendars are adorned with yogis balanced atop rocks or on fantasy island beaches. For groups like Tripsichore Yoga Theatre, yoga has provided a choreographic vocabulary as well as the subject matter for live performances. In the East, there may have always been a taste for the beauty of yoga postures and the poetry of its philosophy, but as the yoga phenomenon has hit its global stride, its postures are now embraced in the West as signifiers of health, peace, and beauty.

Yet some yoga purists find themselves uneasy about these developments. They feel that there may be something distasteful about combining yoga with commercial interests, regardless of its artistic merit. Whether or not a calendar, book, or performance consists of beautiful imagery is immaterial. However, others might argue that throughout history there has usually been some commercial dimension to the creation of art. If artists' work (and this would include everyone from the graphic designers of calendars to performers) is informed by yoga, can they make art that is "satyam, sivam, sundaram"—even if it is commercial?

---

[*] B. K. S. Iyengar, *The Tree of Yoga*, ed. Daniel Rivers-Moore (London: Aquarian, 1994).

Let us try to shed some light on the terms *truth, auspiciousness,* and in particular, *beauty.* In his brilliant essays in *The Dance of Siva,* the philosopher Ananda K. Coomaraswamy makes the exciting claim that the experience of beauty is the same as that of religious experience, that "we are justified in identifying beauty with Brahman—and that in this experience, the distinction between individual and Brahman is transcended."★ If this is so, artists who study yoga as Mr. Iyengar suggests will be making art that uses beauty as a way for their public to engage actively with *brahman.*

First, though, what is meant by *true* and *auspicious?* While notions of absolute truth (and beauty) have been debunked by much postmodern literature, the thought-provoking writer Felipe Fernandez-Armesto trenchantly observes that "any repudiation of truth is self-contradictory."† Still, truth is pretty hard to nail on the head. However, as far as asana goes, it has something to do with how well one embodies a posture. How truthful a posture is might depend on a variety of measures: (1) the degree to which the posture is stable over the time it is held (not to mention how stable the mind is); (2) the degree to which the concentration is single-pointed for the duration of the asana; and (3) the overall degree to which the practitioner has "been" the posture. Similar measurements could be attempted on the flow in vinyasa techniques—ascertaining the degree to which the breath and movement have demonstrated evenness in the transition between postures. All these standards are subject to relativity ("the degree to which"), and perhaps some absolute truth could only be evaluated were the practitioner to become a beam of light.

Auspicious is not a word that enters the vocabulary of most daily discourse. It is a special word and certainly denotes a special state—one that somehow encompasses notions of timeliness and prosperity and that has favorable connotations. It is the "specialness" that counts. While enlightenment (as yogis construe it) may be something that is going on all the

---

★ Ananda K. Coomaraswamy, *The Dance of Siva: Essays on Indian Art and Culture* (New York: Dover, 1985).

† Felipe Fernandez-Armesto, *Truth* (London: Black Swan, 1998).

time, there are few who recognize it on a consistent basis. Doing a yoga practice is special and marks a time when we attempt to recognize the specialness of existence. To do so, we concentrate with a variety of yoga techniques. We notice; we really pay attention; we are deliberately mindful to try to perceive how special reality is. This concentration, when written about, may seem simple and clichéd, but when experienced, it is special beyond words. Yoga is a canon of techniques that can reveal the auspiciousness of any and all times.

It may surprise the reader when I claim that unlike truth, there is no relativism in beauty. Here is my idiosyncratic take on it: beauty is an intuition or experience of reality (or brahman, the universal soul) and our identification (as *atman,* the "individual soul") with it.

The Artistic Process

Beauty is a phase of brahman. Brahman is the totality; the sum of utter unity, the imperishable; the all-pervasive; or in the poetry of yogaspeak, the essential reality that the veil of *maya* (cosmic illusion) prevents us from perceiving. Beauty is a phase that circumstances bring into being and that gives perspective on brahman. It is a possible touchstone from which we can gain insight into the true (and auspicious) nature of reality. Beauty is inherent in all things. But what about things like destruction, crime, or poverty? Where is the beauty in that? The eruption of a volcano might wreak great destruction, but you could take a photograph of the plumes of fire and smoke that showed it to be beautiful as well. Beauty is present in everything, but we need a "technology"—like yoga or art—to be able to perceive it. The role of the artist is to create a vehicle through which the appreciation of beauty (or brahman) can be understood. Note that an important distinction is made here: Art and beauty are not the same thing. Beauty is inherent in all things; art is the technology that reveals beauty. Coomaraswamy presents a useful template for the "history" of any work of art:

> An intuition of matter/subject
> Internal vision
> Externalizing the vision into a technical vehicle
> The stimulation of the perceiver

The first three of these are the province of the artist and the fourth is the realm of the audience wherein the connection is made between the artist's vision and the perceiver who is given an insight into the nature of beauty/reality/brahman. This is the moment when the aesthetic emotion is awakened in the viewer and has nothing to do with analytical capacity. This emotion may be likened to the experience of looking at a fabulous sunset. The observer is struck with a sudden awe at the magnitude of what they notice, and this has nothing to do with their possible analysis of whether they are looking at cirrus or cumulonimbus clouds. What they experience is beauty; they cease to examine internally the concepts that explain a sunset to themselves as they become immersed in the experience of the sunset. There is a self-forgetting.

If beauty can be discovered in anything because it latently exists in all things, an artist may find inspiration in any subject. Beethoven wrote about Elysian Fields; the Sex Pistols were interested in anarchy. Cézanne chose apples; Mondrian, skyscrapers. They then chose to render the subject in their own unique way as music or a painting. But beauty is in neither this technical rendering nor its analytical associations for the observer. For what is attractive to one observer is unattractive to another. Some like Beethoven and despise the Sex Pistols and vice versa. Rather, beauty is in the moment of recognition, the awakening of aesthetic emotion in the viewer. Beauty is the latent phase of brahman that comes into being when this happens.

Most yoga practitioners have an "expert's" response the moment they see a yoga photograph or see yoga done in a studio, because they recognize that the posture signifies, in that moment, the large range of yogic lifestyle and philosophy through association. They are efficient reminders of some underlying truth, and that moment of recognition—before analysis of meaning begins—is where the knowledge of beauty exists. The closer the rendering of the posture is to the "truth" of the posture, the more the observer is inclined to view it with satisfaction and not fret about its alignment or other aspects of technical execution. If the posture was so badly performed that observers were in no way reminded of the underlying truths of yoga—even so poorly done that they could not recognize it as yoga—the moment of beauty would probably not exist. Just as there are degrees of truth, when something does not strike us as beautiful but seems ugly, it is probably because the technical rendering of it was not sufficiently congruent with the content or intention. In the same way, art that stimulates the aesthetic emotion has a unity between the technique and the intention. But beauty may be perceived without the intention (as in the earlier case of the sunset where there is no intention on the part of nature). Art is a technology. Beauty is an experience.

Why is the recognition of beauty important? Recognition of beauty is spontaneous, a pure reaction to the subject without analysis. But our taste in art is somewhat informed by our culture, which means that different people will find different things beautiful and also that through acculturation one becomes able to find things beautiful that were previously incomprehensible or possibly ugly. Just as you might have thought that eating some particular food was exotic or just plain weird in your youth, you come to find it rather tasty as your appreciation of food matures. You might find Mozart finicky and senseless until, for whatever reason, one day you begin to perceive his music as pure, simple, and beautiful. The piece of art has not changed, but your taste has perhaps become more refined. Does this mean that the "beauty" was always latent in the work of art? The obvious contention is that beauty is latent in all things, but we sometimes require a particular exposure to recognize it. I confess I still have a problem wrapping my mind (let alone my leg) around "leg-behind-the-head postures." But the point is that beauty does not happen until it is experienced. When that phase of brahman happens to the perceiver, they recognize it, and it is important because it gives them insight into the underlying nature of reality.

The nature of art in depicting beauty is to somehow show the impossible—an "impossible" that stares us in the face in the mundane aspect of workaday reality. Here, the artist and the yogi have much in common. The nature of practicing yoga postures is to reveal something ineffable. When the practitioner is really there, really doing the posture, and not just working on a technique, this shows through. There is a wholeness, a unity, that moves the yogi to recognize wholeness and unity—the experience of the aesthetic emotion that is the insight into the nature of the totality, of brahman.

What the Artist Does Regarding Beauty

In the first phase of Coomaraswamy's template for the history of a work of art, the artist is drawn to their subject matter by an intuition that this is something they can render. What appeals to one artist will not necessarily be of interest to another, just as their chosen forms of ultimately rendering the subject will be unique. One may be drawn to depict nobility, and another may be impelled toward the gutter. In the second phase, they begin to develop an inner vision (or sound)—some ideal rendering of the subject. In the third phase, the inner vision is then made manifest through their technical means: the choreographer sets the moves, the painter puts oils on canvas, and the composer has the music played.

There is certainly something fascinating about watching someone who is deeply engrossed in an activity, whether it is a construction worker digging up the street or a performing artist at the peak of his or her form. They are utterly consumed in their activity. In addition, while digging up the street may seem prosaic, there is a consonance between the activity and the intention, and this consonance may make the movement seem poetic or even lyrical. This is the assumed notion behind Swami Andy Warholananda's *Campbell's Soup Can*—something becomes art when you notice it as such. Beauty is to be beheld in everything if we have not conditioned ourselves to see it as otherwise.

In the *Bhagavad Gita,* Krishna tells Arjuna, "Those who know, see the same thing in a wise and disciplined brahman as in a cow or elephant, or even a dog or outcast."* But if Krishna chooses to incarnate as a leprous dog, how many of us are capable of beholding the true nature of this being? The spiritual role of the artist is to shed the light of understanding on this hidden beauty. For the performing artist to achieve this, they must deliberately sublimate their own personality so that they can embody some other phase of the universal truth. For instance, actors playing villains need not be cunning, thieving, or murderous cads themselves, but if they do not wholly embrace this state of being, we find their performance unconvincing. The artist does not try to be liked for being

---

* W. J. Johnson, trans., *The Bhagavad Gita* (New York: Oxford University Press, 1994), v:18.

himself; he tries to be appreciated as the vessel through which some idea or vision is portrayed. Yet almost paradoxically, one cannot embody this unless one is capable of moving one's mind and body to a place where one identifies completely with what is being portrayed.

Along with the idea that there may be something distasteful about mixing yoga with anything commercial, there is a not-unfounded misconception that when an artist enters the realm of public exhibition, it reveals an ambition for self-aggrandizement. Certainly, nearly every artist would prefer to be liked, but the real thrills lie elsewhere and cannot happen unless one does the yogic thing of renouncing attachment to the results of one's actions and instead tries to sacrifice oneself wholly to brahman—or what we might call the "present moment." When creating a piece of choreography, I often wait for the happy accident, a point where something goes wrong and produces something much better than anything I could have planned. This is a moment when the choreography takes on its own life. For instance, one second the artist is doing a balance on top of someone else, and the next, he or she is falling over and landing in an unforeseen way. This is great in rehearsal—suddenly new choreography has occurred. But when it happens onstage, there is a real thrill. Artists relish those moments when things go wrong because—in front of maybe eight hundred people—they must suddenly deal with the present moment. To react with fear is a betrayal of the art; it shows only that this whole event was about "you" and not making a fool of "yourself" or about receiving the plaudits of the audience. But real artists do not care much for what the audience thinks while they are performing. For having turned themselves over to the "action" of being in the present moment, they are abandoning (at least for that time) attachment to the result. The *Bhagavad Gita* puts it like this: "Know that action exists in Brahman—Brahman whose source is imperishable. All pervading Brahman is established in the sacrifice."★ All that exists for them is what is going on in the "right now" of the performance. The same would be true of painters as they paint or musicians as they play. This is a state of mind that accords with the yogic notion of detachment, experiencing the purity of brahman comes from renouncing the result.

★ W. J. Johnson, trans., *The Bhagavad Gita* (New York: Oxford University Press, 1994), III:15.

What the Audience Does Regarding Beauty

A work of art succeeds in the revelation of beauty when viewers enter into it, when they empathize. When they engage in the aesthetic emotion, they experience a degree of self-forgetfulness. Again, recourse to the *Bhagavad Gita* proves illuminating: "The person whose self is disciplined in yoga, whose perception is the same everywhere, sees himself in all creatures and all creatures in him. For the man who sees me in everything and everything in me, I am not lost for him and he is not lost for me. That yogin grounded in oneness, who honors me as being in all creatures, whatever his mode of life otherwise, exists in me."[*] This may be likened to a knowledge of God or a melding with the absolute. One's identity is lost because it is the same in all creatures and all things; it is identical to the absolute.

So why not just see brahman by the practice of yogic renunciation of the external world? Why the need for stimuli like art or perhaps by the easier method of experiencing nature? The answer is that for most people working alone, this kind of self-denial (seeing one's self in all things and all things in one's self) is hard to do. But learning to see it, having circumstances like seeing art (or yoga performed) or being in nature, gives one an opportunity to ease into this state of self-forgetfulness—to find God or brahman or the true nature of the universe not by retreating from it, but by engaging with it, by experiencing it through artistic creation or nature.

The experience for the audience works like this: If you see a dancer execute a fabulous leap, part of you participates in that exhilaration. Watching someone in a sad scene onstage or in a film, you also may feel sad. You empathize with what you see—not necessarily because you imagine yourself as the character or because of the semblance between their situation and something in your own life, but certainly because there is participation between you and the work of art. This is quite remarkable. How does it happen that someone playing a role out on a stage or screen some distance away from us makes us identify with what is

---

[*] W. J. Johnson, trans., *The Bhagavad Gita* (New York: Oxford University Press, 1994), VI:29–31.

happening to him? Earlier, we observed that performers endeavor to have a malleable inner life; they can be villains even if they are not like this in real life. There is an outward movement of this inner life that reaches the audience. I liken this to the Tripsichore definition of the seventh limb of Ashtanga Yoga—*dhyana*. In the fifth limb (*pratyahara*), there occurs a directing of the senses, by withdrawing or controlling or focusing so that in the sixth limb (*dharana*) consciousness becomes single-pointed on something, perhaps a vision of a flower or the sound of a mantra. The movement from there to the seventh limb, sometimes defined as "absorption," is typically described as becoming one with that single point. For the actor, the size or location of this single point is the present moment and occurs in the theater space. Therefore, for dhyana, an alternate definition might be "the expanding of the mind to the volume the consciousness contains." In the case of the actor, the volume that his consciousness contains is the theater. He plays the scene in a way that is *meant* to reach the back row because that is the size of his awareness. The volume of the viewer's consciousness is ideally what is going on on-stage. If an audience member is instead noticing the person with a cough three seats away, they are not completely absorbed and hence are less likely to experience empathy with the actor's inner life. To participate with the actor, that audience member's focus and concentration must, like the actor's, be engaged in an outward movement. Likewise, in watching Yoga Theatre, members of the audience may feel some sort of spiritual thrill if the performers are endeavoring to bring the choreography into a dhyanic state. The audience and the performers become aware of the beauty of the postures and their inherent meanings of balance, proportion, harmony, equilibrium, or mysticism. Yoga and art can be used to make it easier to see the underlying and universally shared absolute.

In the discussion of individual works of art, much is often said about moral stance, whether a work appeals to your personal moral sensibilities. I don't think the same can be said of beauty, for it is something that immediately strikes you. Discussion of the object of beauty may or may not enhance that sensation, but it can only be an attempt to fit it into a moral and cultural framework with which you are familiar. If you look at art from another culture, it can be difficult to fit it into that framework, and your response to it may not be the experience of beauty, for beauty occurs when you see yourself in all things and all things in yourself. Curiously, you might experience beauty in something morally dubious to your sensibilities if you respond to it before the analysis of its meaning sets in. A viewer does not get the meaning of a work of art. A work of art has many meanings and those are particular to the acculturation of each individual, but the *experience* of beauty is singular.

PERFORMING YOGA AS ART

As someone who regularly performs yoga as art, I would like to share some observations that I believe have ramifications for the yogi who seeks, through an asana practice, to do that which is satyam, sivam, and sundaram. While there are some differences between what one does in rehearsal and in performance, it is still necessary to give one's all in practicing for a part. You try to do in the rehearsal room what you intend to do onstage. As a dancer, it is possible to do something in rehearsal known as "marking," wherein you merely give an indication of what you will do onstage. This happens less frequently the closer you come to performance, but it simply is not always necessary to go full out. I have found that it is virtually impossible to "mark" in yoga theater because the breath has to be done in the real time it takes to do it when you do it full out. It cannot be marked. Without the breath, the indications of the movements are too inaccurate. Each posture requires a specific breath. Marking a full breath for a performance does not seem to work as an option any more than it would in a yoga class.

The deliberate focus of the performer and the yogi is an important and shared element. The yogi who mistakenly shows off is suffering from the distraction of wanting to be liked or appreciated for their prowess. The intention really should be to embody the form of the asana, to become it, renouncing all care for the result of the action. This means being perfectly in the present, so focus is not just what you do with your eyes, but is the thing to which the entirety of your being is dedicated. This, too, is what the performer does moment to moment or thought to thought. If someone else happens to be observing the yogi in their practice, the conditions for revealing the underlying beauty of the posture are met by the practitioner because he is participating in the absolute. There is possibly another level to this as well. If no one is watching, if the yogi is alone in a studio, he (as witness) may also experience the revelation of beauty, truth, and auspiciousness through his participation in it. Moreover, if what he practices is wholly an embodiment of truth, beauty, and auspiciousness, this hopefully influences his actions in the rest of his life.

When an asana practice is done in a studio, the intensity of one yogi's practice has an effect on those around, just as the intensity of an actor's performance influences the degree of audience attention. One person quietly practicing off in the corner of the studio may not stop the rest of a class from goofing off, but if that one person perseveres, the room quiets down and people get on with practicing. So even though there seems to be a tacit acceptance that asana practice is not for public consumption, it does have an effect on those nearby. If this works in a yoga studio, why would it be profane to do it in a theater or as the subject of a photo for a book or calendar? Why should something that has the potential to reveal the true nature of the universe remain a secret? There are certainly enough injunctions in the medieval yoga texts stating that this is a most secret knowledge and should not be revealed to those who are not ready. Is the world ready for yoga? Why might it not be? If the truth of yoga is "the nature of the universe," it has been staring us in the face all along, but we were not ready to see it. Beauty is a form of experience that makes the nature of the universe manifest to us. It happens when we are ready to see it.

Yoga is a canon of techniques used to aid the practitioner in coming to an understanding of the absolute. Beauty is a phase of the absolute that occurs when the aesthetic emotion awakens. An artist who practices yoga is equipped with techniques than can influence the awakening. B. K. S. Iyengar has succinctly expressed a great truth and prophecy about yoga and art, and it may be that it is not yet auspicious for our generation to perceive it. Yet even a hundred years from now, attitudes toward a yoga calendar or a book of yoga photos or the film of yoga theater performance from our era will be informed by different cultural perceptions. It may be that our artifacts will influence new generations to appreciate beauty and the underlying nature of the absolute.

More than this, in any time and place, yoga is a technology for any of us—artists and the public—to apprehend the true, auspicious, and beautiful nature of ultimate reality.

❦

EDWARD CLARK is the creator of Tripsichore, the London-based yoga performance group that has delighted audiences around the world. He began studying yoga in 1979. Notable among his teachers are Narayani and Giris Rabinovitch, but he also admires Ashtanga Vinyasa, Shivananda, Iyengar, and Viniyoga practices. The Tripsichore group has practiced daily for the past twelve years, devising and refining its techniques for asana, pranayama, pratyahara, dharana, and dhyana. Edward fuses his keen artistic vision with a deep understanding of the essential pursuit of yoga practice. He was the director of movement at Weber Academy in London, a world-renowned school for the arts.

Gravity and You: Perfect Together

Mel Robin

Yoga, once again, makes an important distinction between intelligence and mind (manas). The specific quality of mind is cleverness. . . . Yoga states clearly that it is not the fact of being less clever than your neighbor that makes you stupid. Stupidity is the absence of intelligence. Stupidity can be behaving in a certain way or not learning from our mistakes. . . . Let me give you an example. Scientifically advanced nations invent many complex and terrible weapons. To do this they must be clever. Then they sell those weapons indiscriminately around the world, and the arms end up in the hands of their enemies. Is this clever or stupid? If stupid, did their stupidity consist of a sudden loss of cleverness or an absence of intelligence?
—B. K. S. Iyengar, *Light on Life*

The supreme strength of science is its objectivity. To be scientific, knowledge must accord with observable facts. However, science is also associated with a mental process: the inductive, or scientific, method. First proposed by Sir Francis Bacon, this method starts with many observations, from which the scientist attempts to abstract natural laws, a few statements of great power. Since science is inductive, observations are the only acceptable evidence for truth. But there must be an observer to make the measurements and establish the theories. The observer is the subject; the universe, the object; and the two are connected by the attempts of the one to gain knowledge of the other.

There is a similarity between the philosophies of science and yoga. Both are dualistic. Both posit a fundamental division between subject and object. When something is presented to the mind, it is probably because that thing is there. Both sets of observers then try to discover what the thing is.

Powerful as the scientific method is, it does not work unaided. The scientist, for example, perceives the falling apple. But millions of human beings, including many eminent scientists, had seen apples fall for centuries without taking the leap made by Sir Isaac Newton. That falling apple had to be presented to some faculty within. There also had to be an intense desire to know. A most powerful concentration was applied, as well as an immeasurable amount of reflection. The cleverness of the mind had to be quieted so that the calm reflection of the intelligence could perform its labors without the distraction of further perceptions. Only concentration and reflection can allow the secrets of the inner and outer worlds to be laid bare by the intelligence.

But this is where yoga and science begin to diverge. According to B. K. S. Iyengar, Patanjali has defined *yoga* as "the cessation of movements in the consciousness."* The state of reflection that awakens the intelligence, that transcends mind and its perceptions, and that produces that knowledge of the true state of the world is the end result sought. Yoga's sole purpose is nurturing the ability to reveal truths arising from within. "While I am in this condition and my perceptions are suspended, where did you come from?" says the yogi to the awakened intelligence. Maintaining that state is *dhyana* (meditation). Sutra 1:48 says, *Rtambhara tatra prajna*, or "When consciousness dwells in wisdom, a truth-bearing state of direct spiritual perception dawns."† The observer is the subject; the universe, the object; and the two are connected by the attempts of the one to gain knowledge of the other.

The scientist is very different, returning to the mind, asking it to be clever again, so that new intelligent discoveries can be elicited from new perceptions. The issue rests on what is observed by the intelligence when reflection begins and how this debate between cleverness and intelligence should be settled. To the yogi, the development of inner subjective knowledge is primary. The scientist seeks to preserve the objectivity of objects, whereas the yogi seeks to destroy this.

Mel Robin discusses this issue of what practitioners of yoga can and should observe, and how they relate to what they observe as they perform asanas.

---

* B. K. S. Iyengar, *Light on the Yoga Sutras of Patanjali* (London: Aquarian, 1993), 46.
† Ibid., 95.

From a very early age, I was attracted to the wonders of science, and until very recently, my professional life was spent in trying to understand particular aspects of the physical world, especially in the areas of light, the colors of things, and the phenomenon of color perception. At the same time, I was independently fascinated with the beauty of gymnastics and the satisfaction that came from the performance of its intricacies after years of practice. To my regret, it was many years before these two aspects of my life came together; however, it did happen for me and in hindsight, it explains my love for yoga and my fascination with understanding (from a scientific viewpoint) how the body, mind, and spirit are bound together and the many consequences that follow from this.

It was only natural that I would be attracted to Iyengar Yoga, because there are clear and frequent statements by Guruji as to the rightful place of a questioning scientific attitude toward understanding the phenomenon of this yoga. I now see that gymnastics led me to yoga; yoga led me to B. K. S. Iyengar; and Guruji has closed the circle, as I now use my training in the scientific method to explore the whys and what-ifs of yoga.

Guruji repeatedly speaks of our striving for understanding, even at the level of the *annamayakosha* of the beginner; it follows naturally from this that a beginner might ask, "How can it be that one can make conscious contact with each cell of the body? How does dropping the chin into the sternal notch at the base of the throat cause the body to relax? What is the meaning of extending the intelligence of the body to the extremities? Why is it necessary to roll the forward thigh outward in trikonasana if one hopes to increase the lateral angle of bending? Which of our senses is satisfied by the practice of yoga?"

How can you not wonder about such things and not want to go deeper in search of their rationalization? Without Guruji's questioning approach to the practice, questions such as these might never have been raised and the answers might never have appeared. Moreover, it is my experience that by asking such questions, one is motivated in ways that help keep one's yogasana practice fresh and interesting.

Of course, this attitude might well be a personal point of view, but I have come to see it as a useful adjunct to teaching beginners (Westerners, at least), and so I have become less self-conscious about talking about it to yoga teachers. My own experience has been that there is something of value in trying to understand more of how the beginner's body operates at the level of the annamayakosha, and that beginners are reassured when they are given Western medical answers to their possible questions. Thus, it is my hope that my thoughts on the more physical aspects of our practice may add to the attraction the Iyengar system otherwise holds for beginners. Again, I picture this as an adjunct to yogasana teaching that is meant to be kept on tap but not on top.

A. The Gravitational Attraction between You and the Earth

Let us consider what happens when the teacher says, "Press your feet into the floor," in a standing posture. Gravity affects us as yogasana students in several important ways, among the most obvious being to maintain balance and resist gravitational collapse. In order to understand how gravity affects us and how we might respond to this, let us first look at the inviolable law of universal gravitation first advanced by Sir Isaac Newton. Given two objects of mass (m_1 and m_2) separated by a distance (d), the gravitational force (F) attracting each of the objects to the other is given by Newton as

$$F = G \cdot m_1 \cdot m_2 \,/\, d^2$$

where G is a fixed number called the gravitational constant. When we practice standing yogasanas on the floor at the surface of the earth, then F is the gravitational force with which our feet press the floor; m_1 is our mass; m_2 is the mass of the earth; and d is the earth's radius. The magnitude of this force (F) can be measured directly by anyone, scientist or not, by simply standing on a bathroom scale and reading the dial. As G, m_2, and d are fixed quantities, the only way we can change the force with which our feet press into the floor or into the scale when in tadasana is to change our mass (m_1), for example, eat a cheesecake, slim down, or hold a sandbag. Note that in regard to the gravitational force with which the soles of our feet press the floor, there is no room in the equation for personal choice, willpower, the number of times we have been to Pune, or our years of yogic experience.

The fallacy of the following instructions, often given by teachers in beginning yogasana classes, can be induced from Newton's law:

1. Teachers often instruct students to "press your feet into the floor" in the standing postures. If you could do this on command, then you could change your weight as measured on the bathroom scale at will and instantaneously. In fact, your feet press into the floor in tadasana whether you want them to or not, and how hard they press cannot be changed as long as you stay in tadasana and neither gain nor lose weight.

2. Another common instruction is to "come up by pressing your feet into the floor" in trikonasana. Actually, your feet unavoidably press into the floor as you start the posture, remain pressing while you are in the posture, and press in as you come out of the posture; the pressure of your feet on the floor does not change unless your weight changes. The only way to increase your weight on the floor on coming up from trikonasana is to start eating more and exercising less.

3. Teachers say, "Press your forearms into the floor" in pincha mayurasana. Just as when you are standing on your feet, your weight on the floor in pincha mayurasana will not respond to your teacher's advice to press the floor harder or more heavily in this posture, because Newton's law got there first. Similarly, you cannot "press your right palm down" when attempting to lift your hips in vasisthasana; however, as explained later, you *can* press your forearms into the floor with good effect when in sirsasana i.

We have the illusion that the soles of the feet can be pressed into the floor in tadasana because we are generally not aware of the pressure on the feet resulting from the earth's gravitational pull on our mass. However, when the teacher says, "Press the feet," we quickly become aware of the pressure and so think that the teacher's instruction immediately made the pressure increase. Actually, the pressure has stayed constant, but the *awareness* of the pressure increased when the teacher gave the command.

Though you cannot change the weight that presses your feet into the floor in tadasana, you can change the distribution of your weight among the various parts of the foot touching the floor. What this means is that in tadasana you can be heavier on your heels by being lighter on the balls of your feet; you can move the weight from the inner edges of the feet to the outer edges; and you can shift the weight from one foot to the other. You can press your feet more strongly into the floor in adho mukha svanasana by shifting your weight away from your hands and toward your feet. When coming up from trikonasana, though you shift your weight between the left foot and the right and also between different parts of each foot, the phrase "pressing the feet into the floor" has no meaning. And though you simply cannot "press the forearms into the floor" in pincha mayurasana, you can lift the upper arms away from the forearms to achieve the same end, or you can be heavier on the hands and lighter on the elbows. You can also press the forearms into the floor when in sirsasana I so as to be heavier on the forearms and lighter on the head. The question of differentially pressing your weight into the floor is discussed from an experimental point of view later (section E), but all of this involves the shifting of awareness.

B. SIGNIFICANCE OF THE CENTER OF GRAVITY

When standing in tadasana, the different body parts are at different distances (d) from the center of the earth, so each body part experiences a very slightly different gravitational force; that is, each has a very slightly different weight from that which it would have in savasana where every part of the body is almost equidistant from the center of the earth. The single force (weight) that you register on the bathroom scale when in tadasana is equivalent to what you would experience if all of your mass were concentrated at one particular point in space called the center of gravity.

For a spherical object such as the earth, the center of gravity is the geometric center of the object. However, an object's center of gravity need not be within that object; for example, the center of gravity of a doughnut is within the doughnut hole rather than within the doughnut itself, and that of half a doughnut (urdhva dhanurasana) is about halfway up from the floor toward the lumbar spine. When the human body is in tadasana, the center of gravity is a few inches below the navel (at about

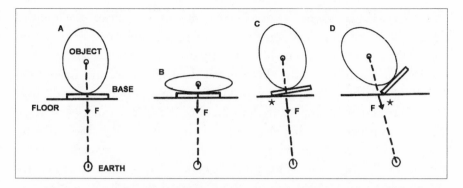

FIGURE 1: Relation of an object's center of gravity to the direction of gravitational force. *A,* The orientation of the gravitational force acting on an object resting on the floor. This object is stable toward falling sideways, as the line between centers of gravity (earth and object) passes through the base of the object. *B,* The gravitational force (*F*) may be large enough to cause the object to collapse along the line of centers. *C,* The object is tipped to the left by an external force; however, the direction of the gravitational force (*F*) still acts to tip the object back onto its base by clockwise rotation around point ★ due to the fact that the line between centers still passes through the base of the object. *D,* Here, the external force is so large that the line between centers is now *outside* of the base and the force (*F*) then rotates the object counterclockwise around the point ★ as it falls to the floor.

the height of the S2 vertebra) and halfway along the line from front to back. When we lift the arms in urdhva hastasana from tadasana, the center of gravity moves upward; similarly, when we bend the legs on going from tadasana to malasana, the center of gravity moves downward within the body. For any given posture, the position of the center of gravity is fixed with respect to that posture, regardless of the body's orientation in space. For example, the position of the body's center of gravity is the same in urdhva hastasana, supta urdhva hastasana, and adho mukha vrksasana, because in all three the arms are extended over the head, whether you are standing, lying down, or inverted. But the awareness is different in all three cases. The direction of the gravitational force between an object and the earth is always coincident with the line between their centers of gravity (fig. 1).

Often, what is sought by "pressing the feet into the floor" is a lengthening of the distance between two points in the body, one of which is constrained to the floor. The lengthening does not press the hands, feet, or forearms farther into the floor, but it does lift the center of gravity. Thus to be more accurate, we should be saying to students in tadasana, "Lift your center of gravity by lengthening the distance between your feet and your pelvis," rather than "Press your feet into the floor so as to straighten your legs." The work involved in doing the yogasanas is largely the work of lifting the body's center of gravity away from the earth's center of gravity; correspondingly, the body is most relaxed when its center of gravity is closest to the center of the earth, that is, in savasana.

It is gravity's intention to pull us flat onto the floor, bringing our center of gravity as close to the center of the earth as possible. Even when we are able to resist this action of the earth's gravitational field, as when standing or sitting, our resistance is not complete, so we tend to collapse our spine over time, especially as we grow older or become tired. This collapsed posture is not only unattractive, but it is very inefficient physiologically, as it inhibits the return of venous blood to the heart and often becomes the origin of or a reflection of negative emotions. It is one of the postural goals of our yogasana practice to counter the spinal collapse initiated by the downward pull of gravity.

C. FALLING AND BALANCE

In regard to the importance of gravity and balance, Guruji has said over the last few decades, "You have to work to obtain a perfect balance between both sides of the body. As a goldsmith weighs gold, you have to adjust your body so that it is perfectly balanced in the median plane. Balance is the gift of the Creator. The whole body is symmetrical. Yoga is symmetry. That is why yoga is a basic art." Consider for a moment how gravity affects our balance.

In outer space, where there is little or no gravity, "balancing" has little or no meaning. Since all orientations of the body are equally energetic, there is little or no force that can lead to a postural reorientation, meaning a fall. Said differently, in outer space one cannot "fall down" because the direction *down* is defined as the direction of the earth's gravitational force on our center of gravity and this force does not exist in outer space. (It is for this reason that people in the Southern Hemisphere do not fall off the earth, but instead fall toward the center of the earth, just as those in the Northern Hemisphere do.) On the other hand, balancing on the surface of a planet such as Jupiter is also impossible, as the strength of gravity is 317 times greater than that on earth; on Jupiter our body would be crushed before it could be balanced. Only here on earth have the strength of gravity and the strength of the body reached a *sattvic* state, for gravity is neither too little nor too much, balance is possible, and indeed, absolutely necessary for the yogasana practitioner.

All of the yogasanas except for savasana can be considered balancing postures if one is sufficiently unsteady. When falling out of balance in the earth's gravitational field, there are two distinct modes. In the first, one yields to gravity along the line of centers so there is no rotational torque; instead, one has a postural collapse (see fig. 1B), most often a sinking of the chest and a dropping of the body's center of gravity. It is this postural collapse that we work so hard to resist in Iyengar Yoga. In the second case, there can be an induced rotation (torque) of the body as one falls forward, backward, left, or right (see fig. 1D).

The concept of the center of gravity is most useful to yogasana students in the following way. In order to avoid falling in any yogasana posture other than savasana, the line between the earth's center of gravity and the body's center of gravity must pass through the area of the base of the body which is in contact with the earth (see figs. 1A and 1C). One remains stable in a posture only as long as the line between the two centers of gravity falls within the area of the base of the posture on the floor and the student is strong enough to avoid collapsing along the line of centers (see fig. 1B). For obvious reasons of relative strength, collapse along the line of centers will be more likely when supported on the arms than when supported on the legs.

Any momentary force experienced by the body that displaces the body's center of gravity such that the line between centers still passes through the base (see fig. 1C) may tip it but then return it to the former position, whereas if the force is strong enough to move the line of centers outside the base (see fig. 1D), then falling to the side is certain and irreversible. It follows from this that we maintain our balance in the gravitational field when the line between the centers of gravity of body and earth lies within the base of the posture; otherwise, a rotational torque that tips us to the side results, and we fall. Unlike the inanimate object which is falling in figure 1D, yogasana practitioners can react to shift the body in response to a perceived sense of falling and thereby maintain balance.

When balancing in a yogasana posture, the body is not static as is the object in figure 1, but is in constant motion as it senses the falling torque and reacts to cancel it. That is to say, when balancing, we are always undergoing a swaying motion through an angle (θ) in order to shift the body's center of gravity so as to keep the line between its center of gravity and that of the earth within the area of the base. Thus when in vrksasana-on-the-right-foot, if we sense we are falling to the right, we press the little-toe edge of the foot to the floor. This shifts the body's center of gravity to the left and balance is maintained momentarily; however, the weight is now falling to the left and will have to be countered by a response to the right. It is the endless job of consciously redistributing the weight between different parts of the base against the floor that keeps us balanced dynamically in every posture. The smaller the amplitude of this oscillating redistribution of weight, the steadier the posture, the smaller the fluctuations of the mind, and the longer our endurance for staying in the posture. "Yoga is the cessation of the fluctuations of the mind" is the definition given by Patanjali in the *Yoga Sutras*.

As can be seen in figure 2, the permissible sway angle beyond which falling is certain (θ), given a constant size of the base, is larger the lower the center of gravity; that is, it will be easier to balance if you can lower your center of gravity. Test this for yourself by noting how much easier the balance in vrksasana is while holding a sandbag in each hand at the knees (lowered center of gravity) as compared to holding the sandbags overhead (elevated center of gravity). Of course, all too often this lowering of the center of gravity has been achieved by a postural collapse. It is clear as well from the figure that if the base is enlarged while the height of the center of gravity is kept constant, then the critical sway angle (θ) is enlarged as well, so again, balancing is easier.

This lifting of the center of gravity is largest and most sustainable

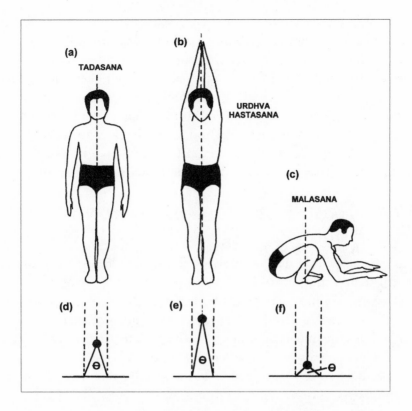

FIGURE 2: The effects on the critical angle of sway (θ) on raising or lowering the centers of gravity when moving from tadasana to urdhva hastasana or malasana, respectively.

when the bones of the body are positioned so as to bear most of the weight (gravitational stress) and the muscles are used only to keep the bones in alignment and the joints open, as with tadasana. Of course, positions in which the bones are not aligned are also possible (utkatasana, for example), but here a larger part of the gravitational stress falls on the muscles, so the posture cannot be held as long. Bones fatigue in the course of years, muscles in the course of minutes. Nonetheless, both bones and muscles are strengthened by resisting the pull of gravity, and both wither in a gravity-free environment or in an environment where there is gravity but no effort is expended to resist its pull, as when lying in bed. To experience what yogasana practice would be like in the zero gravity of outer space where bones are essentially irrelevant, try the yo-gasana postures while submerged in a swimming pool.

It is easier to balance when the center of gravity is lower and also when the base is enlarged. On the other hand, we must keep the bones in positions that support the body. For example, it is not easier to balance in adho mukha vrksasana with the hands very far apart because though this does expand the area of the base, it also opens the door to collapse along the line of centers. It is for this reason that we always work to keep the el-bows no wider than shoulder width when in sirsasana I or sarvangasana.

D. GRAVITATIONAL EFFECTS ON ANATOMY AND PHYSIOLOGY

Many scientists hold that on evolving from a quadruped to an upright bipedal stance, the human body has suffered greatly as the downward gravitational pull on our upright bodies has moved us toward flat feet, slipped intervertebral disks, hernias, various prolapsed organs, and a slumped posture, much of which must be counteracted through use of the antigravity muscles. These gravity-induced consequences can be minimized by an active physical yogasana practice that strengthens both the antigravity muscles and our postural awareness.

The body's reaction to the pull of gravity begins once we are born; from that moment on, gravity's pull is a mechanical stress to which the body must react. The body's web of connective tissue responds to gravi-tational stress by either thickening the tissue in places where the stress is intense and continuous or going beyond this to form bone where only cartilage and a vascular net existed before—all in mechanical support of the body against the pull of gravity. In fact, each of us is born with ap-proximately 300 bones, many of which are adjacent but disconnected at birth; however, once these bones are used in ways such that they experi-ence gravitational stress, the independent bones are knit into more solid structures, leading to only 206 bones in the adult body.

For the yogasana student, the physiological effects of a lack of gravity are manifold. In the zero gravity of outer space (or to a lesser extent, while confined to bed rest or limited by old age), the body's processes tend to go retrograde. Nausea can develop as the vestibular signals from the inner ears conflict with the visual signals in regard to just what is "upright"; blood and lymph pool in the chest rather than in the feet and legs; the heart weakens as its load decreases; muscles become feeble; and bone demineralizes at a rate greater than 10% per year. In zero gravity, muscles not only atrophy, but in some postural muscles, the slow-twitch fibers necessary for the long-term muscle strength needed for yogasana practice are converted into fast-twitch fibers that act more quickly and fatigue rapidly. As the bones demineralize and become brittle, serum levels of Ca^{2+} rise to dangerous levels. The immune system also seems to be adversely affected by low gravity, as is sleep quality and motor coordination. Unfortunately, many of the symptoms of living gravity-free appear in a reduced form when we are bedridden for any length of time or make the mistake of becoming old. On the other hand, these symptoms are minimized when we are physically active.

Though the skeleton and the antigravity muscles can support the body against the pull of gravity, they are not as effective in shielding the body fluids from this downward pull. In the gravitational field, these fluids tend to pool in that part of the body closest to the floor—when standing upright, in the legs; when sleeping, on the side of the body closer to the floor; when inverted, in the head and neck. In regard to yogasanas performed in the supine position, there is a more efficient filling of the right atrium of the heart when horizontal. In consequence, the volume receptors in the atrium report a high value to the hypothalamus, which in turn decreases the heart rate as compared to when the posture is performed in a standing position. It is this aspect of assuming the supine position (viparita karani, for example), which generally leads to a global relaxation of the body-mind. However, even in the standing position, there are indirect ways of using the bones for support and contraction of the muscles to elevate fluid, thereby keeping the fluid distribution more or less uniform. In contrast, without gravity, fluids move more to the head when standing and so cause stuffiness and congestion. The senses of taste and smell degrade, and each leg loses about one liter of fluid, with overall plasma volume decreasing by 20%. Once plasma volume decreases, red blood cell production shuts down and anemia sets in.

With the advent of space travel, bed-rest studies were instigated in order to simulate the physiology of extended stays in gravity-free and exercise-free environments. After twenty-one days of enforced bed rest, it was found that the male subjects had suffered a 28% decrease of the body's ability to do work (equivalent to more than thirty years of aging!) and a 25% loss of cardiac stroke volume. Moreover, their heart volumes had shrunk by 11%. Publication of these results in 1968 led to an immediate redirection of hospital practice, shifting heart patients from bed rest to exercise. Following the study, it was found that any cardiac deficits resulting from bed rest were erased by placing subjects on their feet, the cardiac recovery time being much shorter than is required for atrophied skeletal muscles to respond to weight lifting.

The effects of weightlessness due to a lack of gravitational pull on the body are of interest to us not only because they point out several important factors here on earth that we have come to ignore due to their constancy, but also because the effects of weightlessness seem to mimic closely those of old age and bed rest. Thus, space travelers are off balance when they return to earth's gravitational field and mental deterioration sets in: they suffer from motion sickness, vomiting, headache, poor concentration, and loss of appetite. All of the observations listed here parallel many of the body changes observed in the aging process and following prolonged bed rest. Clearly, a regular yogasana practice works against all of the negative effects of too little gravitational pull on the body by keeping us out of the sickbed and giving us opportunities for actively responding to gravity's pull.

E. Measuring Weight Distributions
in the Yogasanas

To quantify the concept of distributing body weight on the floor while in the yogasanas, we have made several simple measurements of the weight distribution while in various postures. This was done by placing bathroom scales (electronic and spring balance) under the various body parts otherwise in contact with the floor when in a particular yogasana and simply reading the proportion of the body weight borne by each contact. For example, one scale was placed under each foot with students in trikonasana-to-the-right (fig. 3). On average, it was found that the right foot carries 63% and the left foot carries 40% of the total body

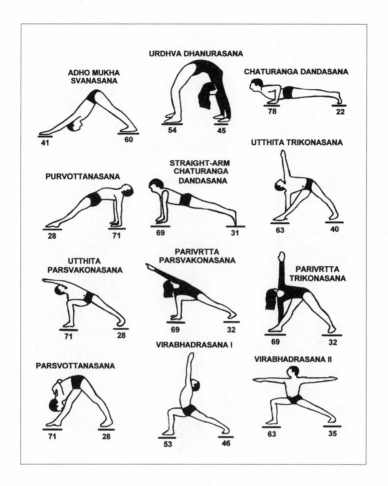

FIGURE 3: Various yogasanas in which the distribution of total body weight has been measured between the hands and the feet or between the two feet, all on the floor, as appropriate to the posture. The percentage values given for each limb contacting the floor are averages of the values found for a group of five intermediate-level Iyengar students.

weight for the intermediate practitioner; as described next, the numbers are noticeably different with beginners. Though we found that the sum of the scale readings in all postures was equal to or very close to the total weight of the student while in tadasana, this was not true in some cases, so the calculated percentages in some instances do not add up to 100%.

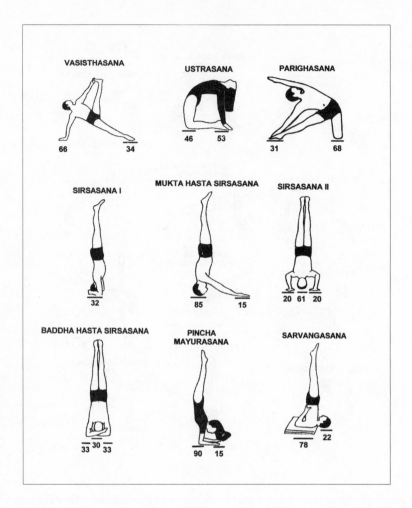

FIGURE 4: Various yogasanas in which the distribution of total body weight has been measured between some combination of the hand, the foot, the elbow, and the knee on the floor, as appropriate to the posture. The percentage values given for each limb contacting the floor are averages of the values found for a group of five intermediate-level Iyengar students.

We start with adho mukha svanasana and urdhva dhanurasana. In adho mukha svanasana, the beginner's hands/feet weight ratio is close to 50% hands/50% feet, but the more experienced students could effectively move 10% of their total body weight from hands to feet, achieving weight ratios closer to 41% hands/60% feet. The observed shift is a consequence of the experienced students being able to work the posture so as to move the pelvis upward and backward, thereby lengthening the spine and making the legs more vertical. If instead the student moves the pelvis forward to plank position (straight-arm chaturanga dandasana) from adho mukha svanasana, the weight becomes much more imbalanced, favoring the hands of course (69% hands/31% feet); this imbalance increases further (78% hands/22% feet) on moving to chaturanga dandasana, where the center of gravity is shifted even farther toward the head as the arms are bent. Plank posture done facing upward (purvottanasana) has basically the same hand-to-foot weight ratio (71% hands/28% feet) as straight-arm chaturanga dandasana and is close to that of vasisthasana (66% hand/34% foot; see fig. 4).

Note, too, that on attempting to move from chaturanga dandasana to straight-arm chaturanga dandasana, the teacher might reasonably ask the students to press their hands into the floor in order to lift the chest. However, if this were the way to lift the chest (or any other part of the body), then the percentage of the weight on the hands would increase significantly, whereas it is observed that the weight percentage on the hands when going from chaturanga dandasana to the straight-arm variation actually *decreases,* going from 78% to 69% (see fig. 3). One can take this as experimental proof that encouraging students to "press the floor" in order to lift a part of the body farther from the floor can be poor advice.

We see that the weight distribution for urdhva dhanurasana (45% hands/54% feet) is much like that of adho mukha svanasana (41% hands/60% feet), as is evident since the locations of the centers of gravity are very much the same (see fig. 3). With the body bent strongly to the right side, it is no surprise that the weight ratio in trikonasana is found to be 63% right foot/40% left foot. These figures shift to 69% right foot/32% left foot when trikonasana-to-the-right is rotated into parivrtta trikonasana, suggesting that among the intermediate students, spinal elongation-to-the-right is not as large in the rotated variation or that spinal twisting results in an unavoidable shortening of the spine. On taking parsvakonasana-to-the-right (right arm on right knee), the center of gravity is drawn farther to the right, and the weight ratio becomes

71% right foot/28% left foot. It is surprising that the left-right weight distribution in virabhadrasana I (53% front foot/46% back foot) is as close to even as it appears, given the imbalance observed in virabhadrasana II to the right (63% right foot/35% left foot). This is understandable in that the structure of the hip joint does not allow the upper body to lean to the left in virabhadrasana II performed to the right as much as it allows the upper body to backbend to the left in virabhadrasana I done to the right.

Putting beginners in sirsasana I resulted in a weight ratio of approximately 50% head/50% forearms; however, they were very unsteady in this posture, so for each of them, the scale readings constantly shifted between wide limits. Because the intermediate students are more able to lift their shoulders up and away from their elbows, taking the additional weight onto their forearms, they are able to generate a ratio of 32% head/64% forearms (see fig. 4). When placed in sirsasana II, the pressure of the hands/forearms on the floor is no longer transmitted efficiently to the shoulders and consequently the weight ratio rises to 61% head/40% hands for the intermediate students versus 32% head/64% forearms in sirsasana I. In sirsasana postures, one of the roles of the hands or forearms is to work the floor so as to shift the weight off the head and onto the hands or arms. In comparing the percentage of the total weight on the head in sirsasana I (32%), sirsasana II (61%), and mukta hasta sirsasana (85%), we see how important it is to keep those parts of the anatomy (hands or forearms) that work to keep the weight off the head as close as one can to the head and to the center line of the upper body and legs, balance permitting.

In this preliminary study, it was found that in vertical sarvangasana with blankets under the elbows and shoulders, the elbows and shoulders carry 78% of the total weight and only 22% of the weight rests on the back of the head. As with the sirsasanas already discussed, the importance in sarvangasana of keeping the point of contact with the floor close to the center line of the posture—that is, keeping the arms under the posture so as to exert the maximum sustainable lift—is apparent.

This initial and admittedly crude study involves the awkward placement of large scales between the floor and certain large body parts. With simple sensors and a cheap meter, one could sense the pressure differences between the first and fifth metacarpals (the thumb and little finger) with the hand on the floor as in adho mukha svanasana, between the first and fifth metatarsals (big toe and little toe), between inner ankle and outer ankle with the foot on the floor as in urdhva dhanurasana, and so on. Once this small step in regard to instrumentation is taken, it should be relatively simple to make quantitative measurements of relative pressure in both static and balancing postures. Such simple steps as this, and those undertaken by Dr. Krishna Raman and others in the field, will allow comparison of the relative weight distributions in a set of common postures as performed by beginners, intermediate-level students, and senior-level performers. In this way, a doorway to a fresh understanding of the anatomy of Iyengar Yogasana practice and the accompanying fluctuations of consciousness will open for whoever chooses to walk through it.

(This chapter is a condensed version of work appearing in *A Handbook for Yogasana Teachers Incorporating Modern Aspects of Neuroscience, Physiology and Anatomy,* Wheatmark Publishers, in press, 2007, used with permission.)

MEL ROBIN holds a PhD in chemical physics and worked in molecular spectroscopy research for twenty-eight years. He published four books and more than one hundred technical papers during that time. In 1988, he worked as director of student research at Science High School in Newark, New Jersey. He received the Science Mentor of the Year Award from President Clinton, the first such award ever given to a high school teacher. He then began the full-time practice and teaching of Iyengar Yoga, continually exploring how yoga and medicine might be related. His book *A Physiological Handbook for Teachers of Yogasana* is the culmination of that effort.

A Brief Analysis of Lower Limb Arterial Blood Flow in Standing Poses

DR. KRISHNA RAMAN

To the hatha yogi, the body is an exercise in concentration, its subtle inner workings an opportunity to develop the most sophisticated and deepest levels of knowledge and awareness. Dr. Krishna Raman gives an indication of the complexities of interaction of which a discriminating awareness is capable.

I started practicing yoga in school at fourteen. One of my teachers presented me with a book, and liking challenges, I attempted the poses and felt great. Being a student of karate, I was already quite flexible. I attempted the more difficult asanas, and although I could achieve them, my incorrect technique eventually caused problems. Years later, I could not cross my legs while seated in a chair. Persistent backaches and hip pain were my companions. Yet the most advanced poses remained possible. By God's grace, I met Sri B. K. S. Iyengar, and the pains of years disappeared within a week! This new approach to practicing yoga made me ponder whether there was more to it. I continued to visit the Ramamani Iyengar Memorial Yoga Institute and followed up on patients being treated there. Dr. Suresh, a highly regarded and dedicated sonologist, was a friend of mine. I became curious about the ultrasound details of yoga poses. Dr Suresh started analyzing arterial blood flow patterns while I practiced asanas. The research continues even now, and we discover more about yogic physiology.

Hatha yoga is often filled with concepts that cannot be ratified. What we think happens does not happen, while the opposite is also true. For example, our eyes may feel very comfortable while in headstand. We therefore may not appreciate that eye pressure rises to twice its resting levels no matter how well the pose is performed (with or without a bandage around the eyes). The pressure rises even if the pose is performed on the ropes.*

It is very important to be unbiased and recognize that our assumptions on the effects of yoga poses may well be incorrect. We tend to focus only on what yoga can do. Many yoga practitioners think that yoga poses lead entirely to positive effects. It is difficult to accept that negative effects could occur. As an example, we may think that standing poses increase blood supply to the legs. But they can produce minimal change and sometimes actually reduce blood flow.

Is it harmful if blood flow is reduced? The body does need to shut off its own resources at times. This helps to give "relief" from the effects of the constant hematological traffic within the body. It is important to understand the different effects on blood flow that different poses can have.

In tadasana, the force of blood flow is slightly greater than it is in dandasana. One need not execute a perfect asana to get this slight change in effect. The moment we stand up, gravity will ensure certain hemodynamic changes. Sri Iyengar once mentioned that it is possible to consciously direct blood flow to the center of the vessel—and that is what I have seen using ultrasonography (USG). He also stated that a slight change in the position of the legs in prasarita padottanasana will change the direction of flow. This was also ratified by USG (as shown later).

It is necessary to appreciate the medical importance of keeping the knees locked in standing poses. Failure to do so will weaken the supporting ligaments (medial and lateral) and the menisci will be massaged improperly. Taking utthita trikonasana as a specific example, it has been observed that the blood flow in the popliteal artery, located in the back of the knee, shows greater increases when the knees are not locked! But this does not mean that we should not engage the knees in these poses.

---

* Krishna Raman Baskaran et al., "Intra-ocular Pressure Changes and Ocular Biometry during Sirsasana (Headstand Posture) in Yoga Practitioners," *Ophthalmology* 113, no. 8 (August 2006): 1327–32.

In the end, the locking provides a greater overall blood supply than merely standing erect, since the popliteal artery is enveloped by the leg muscles and is massaged more thoroughly when the knees are locked. This indirect "touch" on the artery maintains the elasticity of the vessel, which in turn maintains healthy blood flow.

To a certain extent, the effects of locking the knees are different (1) from pose to pose, and (2) between two legs (rear and front) within the same pose. To explain the first concept, in utthita trikonasana, there is reduced peripheral resistance in the popliteal artery when the knee of the front leg is locked. However, in parivrtta trikonasana, the normal "triphasic" pattern (the normal triphasic waveform is made up of three components that correspond to different phases of arterial flow: rapid anterograde flow reaching a peak during systole, transient reversal of flow during early diastole, and slow anterograde flow during late diastole) is retained whether or not the legs are locked. There is, however, an increase in peak systolic velocity in the front leg.

To elaborate on the second concept, in parivrtta trikonasana, the blood flow in the rear leg is considerably different depending on whether the knee is locked and unlocked. This is due to a rotation of the rear leg muscles in this pose—a phenomenon entirely absent in utthita trikonasana.

It is not necessary to stretch a body part to increase the arterial flow. In utthita parsvakonasana, there is an increase in both systolic and diastolic velocities in the front leg in a suitably performed pose. But there is reduced pulsatility in the rear leg during this pose when compared to utthita trikonasana.

If we now compare the blood flow of the rear leg in parivrtta trikonasana to that in parivrtta parsvakonasana, we will notice immediate differences. In parivrtta trikonasana, the force of the stretch on the rear leg is greater than that in parivrtta parsvakonasana. Since the length of the stance is greater, we cannot exert the same force we can in parivrtta trikonasana; hence, the difference.

In the front leg of ardha chandrasana and virabhadrasana III, the flow patterns are similar because—except for the rotational component in the former pose—we stress the leg similarly. The rotation of the leg in the latter pose is evidently insufficient to produce any substantive differences.

In prasarita padottanasana, it can be very difficult to replicate identical flow patterns from one performance to the next unless we are extremely precise in the weight distribution of the body. If the pose is to feel light, then the weight should favor the inner ankles and knees. The "dead weight" must not be on the outer legs and ankles. Externally, it looks as though we bear all our weight on the lateral aspect of the legs. If this is done, the measured flow pattern in the popliteal artery changes to the same one that occurs when the leg is overstretched. The broader the stance, the greater the effort needed to prevent the weight of the body from affecting the outer legs. Hence, the need for deliberate inner leg weight bearing is recognized.

Inverted poses, unlike standing ones, are restful for the legs, yet they actually deliver a greater quantity of fresh blood to these extremities. Many yoga students feel better if they practice inverted poses after standing poses, as this relieves the fatigue sometimes caused by standing asanas. However, if the standing poses are done with "buoyancy," no difference is felt in the legs while doing inverted poses. But if they are held to the point of exhaustion and done with "heaviness," the blood flow in the legs reduces almost to zero.

It is easier to lock the quadriceps in sirsasana than in sarvangasana, because in the latter, we need to align and lift the pelvis. Against that lift, we need to press back onto the hamstring muscles. Thus, the legs must be very active in sirsasana. If beginners feel a little fatigued in the legs, it is then incorrect to advise them, and even fairly advanced practitioners, to precede their standing poses with a headstand.

Yoga poses change the vascular bed impedance of the arterial aspect of the general cardiovascular system. However, similar changes do not occur in the venous aspect because the leg veins are squeezed in standing poses, while completely collapsing in inversions. It is necessary to give standing poses to patients with varicose veins, as the veins tend to get well compacted in standing poses and not just stretched, as one would think. Being enmeshed in the musculature, the veins are impacted when muscles are held tight in standing poses. The greatest direct compression the leg veins receive is in virasana, where the venous pressure is tremendous.

It is important to be aware that standing poses are not the only way to healthy legs. We cannot and should not dismiss athletes, for their legs can also be healthy. They may face problems with aches and tears in fascia, ligaments, and muscles, but this does not preclude them from being fit. Every exercise system brings health of a particular nature to whatever part is being exercised and according to the nature of the stimulus. We must choose what we need and what we want. Taking up yoga should not make a person stop participating in noncompetitive sports. It is not just the sport per se, but rather the frequency of the sporting events, that can damage the body.

If "high-speed" athletes practice yoga regularly, their running speed might well decrease as the fast-twitch muscle fibers seen in sprinters are replaced by slow-twitch ones. They must therefore practice yoga prudently. There is a subtle tendency among yoga practitioners to "thump" other systems of exercise, and in all fairness to both systems, this is not justified. Every system of exercise gives some benefit to the body. While yoga does not involve wear and tear, a yoga student cannot engage in recreational sports as effectively as do professionals, because yoga does not build the stamina to face that kind of strain. However, yoga does offer methods of recuperation and protection against injuries.

Can we state that the yoga practitioner does not possess stamina? Or that the tennis player does not have the elasticity and quietness in the cells of a yoga practitioner? These are different kinds of exercise. It is not a good idea to compare systems. We need to consign each to their respective pedestals. That no system of exercise (however skillful one may be at it) is "superior" to any other is something we must constantly bear in mind.

Prolonged and vigorous exercise may well indicate a tendency toward longevity.★ A thirty-two-year study of 2,259 participants in the famous Dutch "eleven cities" ice-skating race demonstrated an enhanced tendency to longevity, particularly if the exercise was recreational and occasional.

Ultimately, as yoga attests, our health is in the hands of the Almighty. It is important to understand that many mighty yogis have fallen ill and then realized that the higher power can provide all. As students of yoga,

---

★ "Longevity of Men Capable of Prolonged Vigorous Physical Exercise," *British Medical Journal* 301, no. 6766 (December 22–29, 1990): 1409–11.

it is essential that we surrender whatever we have learned in yoga (and every other field) at the feet of the Almighty, who will then take us to lofty heights without ego.

⅃

Dr. Krishna Raman holds a Bachelor of Medicine and Surgery (MBBS) degree, Madras; is a Fellow of the College of Chest Physicians (FCCP), Delhi; and is a certified Iyengar teacher who has assisted extensively in the medical classes held at the Ramamani Iyengar Memorial Yoga Institute in Pune, India. He has applied his background in Western medicine to the study of yoga and has helped establish its clinical applications to the treatment of medical disorders, whether as an alternative or a supplement. He has presented case papers and given lecture-demonstrations at medical conferences and institutions in India and the United States. He has authored *A Matter of Health: Integration of Yoga and Western Medicine for Prevention and Cure* and *Yoga and Medical Science: FAQ.*

An Introduction to Ayurveda

DR. VASANT LAD

Although yoga is being increasingly validated by Western medicine, the two work on very different principles. Thanks largely to Hippocrates of Kos, the father of Western medicine, medicine is not seen as philosophy, but as an objective endeavor that rejects theories suggesting a divine origin for any ailment. Hippocrates taught that disease is caused by environmental factors such as diet and living habits. Although later theorists such as Galen introduced religious motifs, Hippocrates' idea tended to predominate.

Yoga and ayurveda are both based on the Sankhya philosophy. Their ideas on health could not be further removed from Hippocrates' theory. According to ayurveda, at the moment of creation, this "science of life" was brought to mind by Brahma, the Creator. He then taught it to Daksha, the protector of all beings, who then taught it to the Ashvin twins, the physicians to the gods, who then taught it to Indra. When sickness began to plague human beings, Bharadvaja went to Indra's court to learn the science. Atreya, one of the sages whom he instructed, taught it to his own disciples and held a competition to see who could write the best treatise to preserve the knowledge. Agnivesha won, and the *Agnivesha Samhita* became ayurveda's authoritative text. Shortly before it was lost, Charaka wrote the *Charaka Samhita,* a revised version. Charaka tells us that ayurveda is the *veda* ("knowledge") of *ayus,* which is "a combination of the body, sense organs, mind, and soul." Yoga and ayurveda affirm that an individual is a spiritualized being seeking enlightenment. *Chitta,* "the field of consciousness," records a person's experiences and seeks to understand its own condition. Yoga tells us that all ill health is a manifestation of *duhkha* (the unbalancing sorrow that ignorance of our real nature brings). Ayurveda tells us that ill health makes itself evident in our bodily existence. On one hand, we have the consciousness of health; on the other, the health of consciousness. Dr. Lad, who at one time served as the medical director of ayurvedic medicine in B. K. S. Iyengar's hometown of Pune, now tells us how chitta and ayus manifest themselves, and how they can be brought to a balanced condition through awareness and consciousness.

A*yurveda* is a Sanskrit word derived from two roots: ayur, which means "life," and veda, or "knowledge." Knowledge arranged systematically and with logic becomes science. Over time, ayurveda became the science of life. It has its root in ancient Vedic literature and encompasses our entire life: the body, the mind, and the spirit.

Purusha/Prakriti

According to ayurveda, every human being is created by the cosmos, the pure cosmic consciousness, as two energies: male energy (*purusha*) and female energy (*prakriti*). Purusha is choiceless, passive awareness, whereas prakriti is "choiceful," active consciousness. Purusha doesn't take part in creation. Prakriti is the divine creative will and does the divine dance of creation called *leela*. It is first evolved or manifested as supreme intelligence, called *mahat*. Mahat is the *buddhi* principle (individual intellect), which further manifests as self-identity or ego, called *ahamkara*. Ahamkara is influenced by three basic universal qualities: *sattva,* which is responsible for clarity of perception; *rajas,* which causes movement, sensations, feelings, and emotions; and *tamas,* which is the tendency toward inertia, darkness, and heaviness, and is responsible for periods of confusion and deep sleep.

Manifestation of Creation

The five senses are created from the essence of sattva: the ears to hear, skin to perceive touch, eyes to see, the tongue to taste, and the nose to smell. The essence of rajas is manifested as the five motor organs: the organs of speech, hands, feet, genitals, and the organs of excretion. The mind is derived from sattva, whereas *prana* (the "life force") comes from rajas. The tamasic quality is also responsible for the creation of *tanmatras* (the "subtle elements"), from which are generated the five basic elements of space, air, fire, water, and earth. It is from pure consciousness that space is manifested.

Space

Expansion of consciousness is space, and space is all-inclusive. We need space to live, and our bodily cells contain spaces. The synaptic, cellular, and visceral spaces give freedom to the tissues to perform their normal physiological functions. (A change in tissue space, however, may lead to pathological conditions.) The space between two conjunctive nerve cells aids communication, while the space in the mind encompasses love and compassion.

Air

The movement of consciousness determines the direction along which space changes position. This course of action causes subtle activities and movements within space. According to the ayurvedic perspective, this is the air principle. A cosmic magnetic field is responsible for the movement of the earth, wind, and water. Its representative in the body is biological air, which is responsible for movement of afferent and efferent, sensory and motor neuron impulses. When someone touches the skin, that tactile sensation is carried to the brain by the principle of movement, which is the sensory impulse. Then there is a reaction to the impulse, the motor response, which is carried from the brain back to the skin. This is a very important function of air. Breathing is created by the movement of the diaphragm. Intestinal movements and subtle cell movements are also governed by the air principle, as are the movements of thought, desire, and will.

Fire

Where there is movement, there is friction, which creates heat, so the third manifestation of consciousness is fire, the principle of heat. There are many different representations of fire in the body. The solar plexus is the seat of fire, and this fire principle regulates body temperature. Fire is also responsible for digestion, absorption, and assimilation. It is present in the eyes (therefore, we perceive light), and the luster in the eyes is a result of it. The fire in the brain is the gray matter, which governs understanding, comprehension, appreciation, transformation, recognition, and total understanding. In our small universe, the sun is a burning ball of consciousness, and it gives us light and heat. In the body, the representative of the sun is the biological fire: the solar plexus, which gives us heat, digestion, and liver function.

Water

Because of the heat of the fire, consciousness melts into water. According to chemistry, water is H_2O, but according to ayurveda, water is the liquefaction of consciousness. Water exists in the body in many different forms, such as plasma, cytoplasm, serum, saliva, nasal secretions, orbital secretions, and cerebrospinal fluid. We eliminate excess water in the form of urine and sweat. Water is necessary for nutrition and to maintain the water/electrolyte balance in the body. Without it, the cells cannot live.

Earth

The next manifestation of consciousness is the earth element. The heat of the fire and water causes crystallization. According to ayurveda, earth molecules are nothing but the crystallization of consciousness. In the human body, all solid structures and hard, firm, and compact tissues—including bones, cartilage, nails, hair, teeth, and skin—are derived from the earth element.

All of these five elements are present in every human cell: the membrane is earth, the vacuoles are space, the cytoplasm is water, the nucleic acid and all chemical components are fire, and the cell movement is air. According to ayurveda, humans are creations of universal consciousness. What is present in the cosmos, or the macrocosm, is present in the body, the microcosm. A human being is a miniature of nature.

MENTAL CONSTITUTION

Vedic philosophy classifies human temperaments into three categories, which correspond to the three basic universal qualities: sattvic, rajasic, and tamasic. These individual differences in psychological and moral dispositions and their reactions to sociocultural and physical environments are described in all the classic ayurvedic texts. Sattvic qualities imply essence, reality, consciousness, purity, and clarity of perception, which are responsible for goodness and happiness. All movements and activities are due to rajas, which leads to sensual enjoyment, pleasure, pain, effort, and restlessness. Tamas is darkness, inertia, heaviness, and materialistic attitudes. There is a constant interplay of these three *gunas* (qualities) in the individual consciousness, but the relative predominance of either sattva, rajas, or tamas is responsible for individual psychological disposition.

Sattvic Mental Constitutions

The people in whom sattvic qualities predominate are religious, loving, compassionate, and pure-minded. Following truth and righteousness, they have good manners, behavior, and conduct. They do not get upset or angry easily. Although they work hard mentally, they do not get mental fatigue, so they need only four to six hours of sleep each night. They seem fresh; alert; aware; and full of luster, wisdom, joy, and happiness. They are creative, humble, and respectful of their teachers. Worshipping God and humanity, they care for people, animals, and the environment and are respectful of all life and existence. They have balanced intuition and intelligence.

Rajasic Mental Constitutions

The people in whom rajasic qualities predominate are egoistic, ambitious, aggressive, proud, and competitive and have a tendency to control others. They like power, prestige, position, and they are perfectionists. Although hard-working, they lack proper planning and direction. They are ungrounded, active, and restless. Emotionally, they are angry, jealous, ambitious, and have few moments of joy due to success. They have a fear of failure, are subject to stress, and soon lose their mental energy. They require about eight hours of sleep. They are loving, calm, and patient only as long as their own interests are served. They are good, loving, friendly, and faithful only to those who are helpful to them. They are not honest to their inner consciousness. Their activities are self-centered.

Tamasic Mental Constitutions

The people in whom tamasic qualities predominate are less intelligent. They tend toward depression, laziness, and excess sleep, even during the day. A little mental work tires them easily. They like jobs with less responsibility, and they love to eat, drink, sleep, and have sex. They are greedy, possessive, attached, and irritable, and they do not care for others.

They may even harm others through their own self-interest. It is difficult for them to focus their minds during meditation.

VATA, PITTA, AND KAPHA: THE THREE DOSHAS

The structural aspect of the body is made up of five elements, but the functional aspect of the body is governed by three biological humors (*doshas*). Ether and air together constitute *vata;* fire and water, *pitta;* and water and earth, *kapha*. These doshas are the three biological components of the organism. They govern psychobiological and physiopathological changes in the body. Vata-pitta-kapha (VPK) are present in every cell, tissue, and organ. Their permutations and combinations differ in every person.

The sperm (the male seed) and the ovum (the female egg) also contain vata-pitta-kapha. Because bodily VPK change according to diet, lifestyle, and emotions, sperm is influenced by a man's diet, lifestyle, and emotions, and ova by a woman's. At the time of fertilization, when a single sperm enters a single ovum, individual constitution is determined.

According to ayurveda, there are seven body types: three mono types (vata, pitta, or kapha predominate), three dual types (vata-pitta, pitta-kapha, or kapha-vata), and one equal type (vata, pitta, and kapha in equal proportions). Every individual has a unique combination of these three doshas. To understand individuality is the foundation of healing, according to ayurveda.

Vata Qualities

Vata, pitta, and kapha are distinctly present and express differently in each human being, depending on the predominance of the different qualities (gunas). For example, vata is dry, light (related to weight), cold, mobile, active, clear, astringent, and dispersing. If a person has excess vata in his or her constitution, because of the dry quality, he or she will have dry hair, dry skin, dry colon, and a tendency toward constipation. Because of the light quality, the vata person will have a slight body frame, lean muscles, and little fat, and so will be thin and underweight. Because of the cold quality, he or she will have cold hands, cold feet, and poor circulation and will hate winter but love summer. Because of the mobile quality, vata people are very active. They like jogging and jumping and don't like sitting in one place. Vata is subtle, and this subtle quality is responsible for the emotions of fear, anxiety, insecurity, and nervousness. Vata is also clear; therefore vata people can be clairvoyant—they have clear understanding and perception. Although they understand things immediately, they forget immediately. Finally, vata is astringent, so the vata person feels a drying, choking sensation in the throat while eating. These qualities are all expressed in a vata individual to some degree.

Pitta Qualities

Pitta is a biological combination of fire and water elements. It has hot, sharp, light, liquid, sour, oily, and spreading qualities. It has a strong, fleshy smell and a sour, bitter taste. If an individual has excess pitta in the body, these qualities will be manifested in the following ways. Because of the hot quality, the pitta person has a strong appetite and warm skin; body temperature is a little higher than that of the vata person. The pitta person can perspire at fifty degrees, but the vata person cannot perspire even at a much higher temperature. This difference is very important. Pitta is hot; therefore the pitta person has a strong appetite. If hungry, he has to eat, otherwise he will become irritable and hypoglycemic.

The second quality of pitta is sharp; therefore pitta people have sharp noses, teeth, eyes, and minds, and while talking, they use sharp words. They also have very sharp memories. Because of the oily quality, they have soft, warm, oily skin; straight, oily hair; and oily, liquid feces. Because of the hot, sharp, and oily qualities, pitta people have a tendency to go gray prematurely, a sign of early maturity. Pitta girls reach puberty earlier; they can even begin menstruation at the age of ten. Pitta is light, which is the opposite of both heaviness and darkness. Because of this quality, pitta people are moderate in body frame, and they do not like bright light. They like to read before they go to bed and sometimes sleep with a book on their chest. Because of too much heat in the body, male pittas tends to lose their hair in the full bloom of youth, resulting in a receding hairline or a big, beautiful, bald head.

The next quality of pitta is a strong smell. When pitta people perspire, there is a typical sulfur smell under the arms, and socks will have a strong odor. That's why pittas love perfumes. Pitta people are lovers of knowledge and have a great capacity for organization and leadership. They are often wise and brilliant but can have controlling, dominating personalities. Pitta people also have a tendency toward comparison, competition, ambition, and aggressiveness, so they naturally criticize. If there is no one else to censure, they will criticize themselves. They are perfectionists. Pitta people tend to develop inflammatory diseases, while vata–predominant people tend to get neurological, muscular, and rheumatic problems.

Kapha Qualities

The next dosha is kapha. Subjects having more kapha in their bodies have heavy, slow, cool, oily, liquid, dense, thick, static, and cloudy qualities. Kapha is sweet and salty. Because of the heavy quality, kapha people have big bones, large muscles, and fat, with a tendency to put on weight. A kapha person may even do a water fast and still gain weight. Kapha is slow, which is reflected in a kapha person's slow metabolism and digestion. A kapha person can work without food, while it is very difficult for a pitta person to concentrate without eating. Kapha is cool so kapha people have cool, clammy skin. Although the skin is cool, the gastrointestinal tract has a high digestive fire, so they have strong appetites.

Other kapha qualities are thick, wavy hair and big, attractive eyes, as well as a slow but prolonged, steady memory. Kapha people are forgiving, loving, and compassionate. Because of the slow quality, they walk and talk slowly; they don't like jogging and jumping. They much prefer eating, sitting, and doing nothing.

Because of the cloudy quality, their minds are heavy and foggy, and after a full meal, they feel lethargic and sleepy. Unless they have a cup of coffee or strong stimulant in the morning, they cannot move. Finally, the kapha person has a sweet tooth and loves candy, cookies, and chocolate.

PRAKRITI, OR INDIVIDUAL CONSTITUTION

Individual constitution is determined at conception by the particular combination of the three doshas (vata, pitta, and kapha). Every human being is a unique entity with his or her own physical and psychological makeup. A person's psychosomatic temperament is primarily genetic in origin. The sperm and ovum carry within them the constitution of each of the parents. At the time of conjugation, the dominant factor of prakriti (vata, pitta, or kapha) in the sperm can either neutralize, weaken, or exaggerate similar attributes of prakriti in the ovum. For example, a sperm with a strong vata constitution can inhibit some of the characteristics in an ovum with a kapha constitution. The dry, light, rough, mobile qualities of vata will suppress the oily, heavy, smooth, and stable qualities of kapha. Vata and kapha are both cold, so the cold quality will be exaggerated in the prakriti of the fetus. The baby, who inherits a vata-kapha constitution, will be sensitive to the cold. If both parents are vatas, their offspring will be vata as well. The constitutions of both the parents and the baby are influenced by diet, lifestyle, environment, climate, age, and emotions.

SAMPRAPTI, OR THE DISEASE PROCESS

According to ayurveda, health is a state of balance between the body, mind, and consciousness. Within the body, ayurveda recognizes the three doshas; the seven *dhatus* (tissues) of plasma, blood, muscle, fat, bone, nerve, and reproductive organs; the three *malas* (wastes), which are feces, urine, and sweat; and *agni* (the energy of metabolism, or biological fire). Disease is a condition of disharmony in any of these factors. The root cause of imbalance, or disease, is an aggravation of VPK caused by a wide variety of internal and external factors. According to the attributes of these different etiological factors, the doshas become aggravated and start to accumulate at their respective sites. Vata tends to accumulate in the colon, pitta in the intestines, and kapha in the stomach. If the provocation continues, the accumulated dosha reaches a point at which it overflows the original site and spreads throughout the body. The aggravated dosha then enters and creates a lesion in a specific weak tissue where pathological changes are manifested in the organ or system.

Causes of Disease

Many factors affect the doshas. For instance, disease can result from unbalanced emotions. If a person has deep-seated, unresolved anger, fear, anxiety, grief, or sadness, this can upset the doshas. Ayurveda classifies seven major types of causative factors in disease: hereditary factors, congenital factors, internal factors (including misuse, overuse, or underuse of the five senses), external trauma, natural tendencies or habits, supernatural factors, and seasonal factors. The disease itself can be described by the number of doshas involved, the specific tissues affected, the quality or combination of qualities that aggravated the dosha(s), whether the disease is primary or secondary, its strength, and the length of time it has been present.

Some of the factors that cause disease are direct and easier to identify. For example, there are many recognized hereditary pathologies, which can take the form of tendencies toward a specific problem or manifest as actual abnormalities. Internal conditions, such as ulcers or a damaged liver, may be caused by the overuse of taste, such as too much hot, spicy food or alcohol. External traumas are violent actions, such as automobile accidents, gunshots, and so on. Natural tendencies, such as overeating and smoking, can be a problem, as can supernatural causes such as sunburn, lightning strikes, and the influence of planetary bodies.

Seasonal causes are usually more indirect, as are a person's tendencies to take his or her own primary dosha to an unbalanced state. There are four seasons. Summer, with its bright light and excess heat, is a pitta season. Cold, windy, and dry, autumn is the vata season. Winter's cold, windy snow and rain makes it a kapha season. Spring is both kapha—early spring—and pitta—late spring. So the four seasons have vata, pitta, and kapha qualities that can aggravate those qualities within individuals. For example, vata people have a tendency toward constipation, sciatica, arthritis, and rheumatism, which can become aggravated by the onset of autumn. Pitta people may get hives, rashes, acne, biliary disorders, diarrhea, or conjunctivitis in summer. The kapha person tends toward colds, hay fever, coughs, congestion, sneezing, and sinus disorders during spring.

Clinical Barometers of Ayurveda

Ayurveda is an ancient clinical art of diagnosing the disease process through inquiry (questioning about the past, present, and family history); observation (inspection); tactile experience (palpation); percussion; and listening to the heart, lungs, and intestines (auscultation). Ayurvedic doctrine talks much about interpreting the pulse, tongue, eyes, and nails in the clinical examination, as well as conducting separate examinations of specific functional systems.

Ayurveda describes the three basic types of pulses (vata, pitta, and kapha) and their characteristics. There are twelve radial pulses: six on the right side, three superficial and three deep, and six corresponding ones on the left. There is a relationship between the superficial and deep pulses and the internal organs. One can feel the strength, vitality, and normal physiological tone of the respective organs separately under each finger.

The art of tongue diagnosis describes characteristic patterns that can reveal the functional status of respective internal organs merely by observing the surface of the tongue. The tongue is the mirror of the viscera and reflects many pathological conditions (see fig. 1). A discoloration and/or sensitivity on a particular area of the tongue indicates a disorder in the organ corresponding to that area (see fig. 2). For example, a whitish tongue indicates a kapha disturbance and mucus accumulation; a red or yellow-green tongue indicates a pitta disturbance; and a black-to-brown coloration indicates a vata disturbance. A dehydrated tongue is symptomatic of a decrease in plasma (*rasa dhatu*), while a pale tongue indicates a decrease in red blood cells (*rakta dhatu*).

Body fluids, such as blood (*rakta*) and lymph (*rasa*), serve to carry wastes (malas) away from the tissues that produce them. The urinary system removes water (*kleda*), salt (*kshar*), and nitrogenous wastes (*dhatu malas*) and helps to maintain the normal concentration of water (*apa dhatu*) and electrolytes within body fluids. It also helps to regulate the volume of body fluid and thus maintain the balance of the three doshas and water.

Ayurvedic physicians use urine examinations as one of the diagnostic tools to understand the doshic imbalances in the body. Clinical examination is performed by observing the color of a sample. If it is blackish-brown, there is a vata disorder. A dark yellow color indicates a pitta disorder, constipation, or a low intake of water. If the urine is cloudy, there is a kapha disorder, and red urine indicates a blood disorder. Urine samples can also be tested with oil. One drop of sesame oil is placed in the sample. If the drop spreads immediately, the physical disorder is probably easy to cure. If it sinks to the middle, the illness is more difficult, and if it sinks to the bottom, the illness may be very difficult to cure. If the

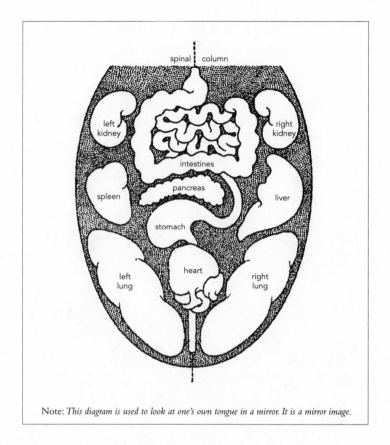

Note: *This diagram is used to look at one's own tongue in a mirror. It is a mirror image.*

FIGURE 1: LOCATION OF ORGANS ON THE TONGUE

A discoloration or sensitivity of a particular area of the tongue indicates a disorder in the organ corresponding to that area in the diagram. A whitish tongue indicates kapha derangement and mucus accumulation; a red or yellow-green tongue indicates pitta derangement, and a black-to-brown coloration indicates vata derangement. A dehydrated tongue is symptomatic of a decrease in the *rasa* or plasma dhata, while a pale tongue indicates a decrease in the *rakta* (red blood cell) dhatu.

drop spreads on the surface of the sample in wavelike movements, this indicates a vata disorder. If it spreads on the surface and multiple colors resembling a rainbow are visible, there is a pitta disorder. Finally, if it breaks up into pearl-like droplets, a kapha disorder is diagnosed.

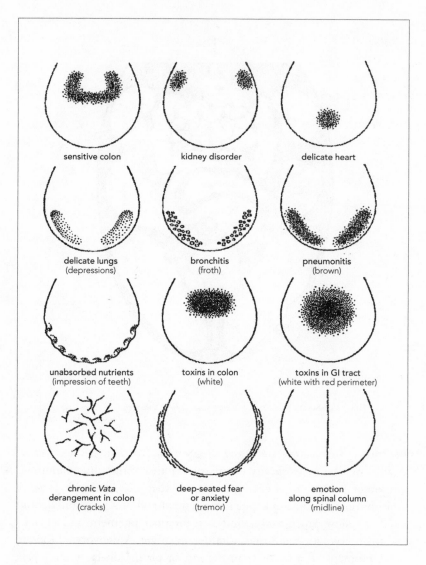

FIGURE 2: TONGUE DIAGNOSIS (JIHVA)

Normal urine has a typical smell. However, a foul odor indicates digestive toxins (*ama dosha*) in the system, while a sweet smell indicates diabetes. In the latter condition, the individual may experience goose bumps on the skin while urinating. Acidic urine that creates a burning sensation points to excess pitta. Gravel in the urine indicates stones in the urinary tract.

CHIKITSA, OR DISEASE MANAGEMENT

Ayurveda says that to restore health we must understand the exact quality, nature, and structure of the disease, disorder, or imbalance. There are four main classifications of disease management in ayurveda: *shodana* (cleansing), *shamana* (palliation), *rasayana* (rejuvenation), and *satvajaya* (mental hygiene).

Shodana

The purpose of shodana is to remove excess doshas and ama from the body. It includes *purvakarma* (initial procedures), *pradhanakarma* (the main procedures), and *pashchatkarma* (the sometimes crucial postoperative procedures of changes in diet, medication, and lifestyle). Purvakarma procedures move the aggravated doshas and ama from sites deep in the body to more peripheral locations to prepare for elimination. *Panchakarma* (five actions), which is part of pradhanakarma, then removes the doshas and ama. The five actions are *vamana* (vomiting), *virechana* (purgation), *basti* (medicinal enema), *rakta moksha* (blood cleansing), and *nasya* (nasal insufflation).

Vamana is vomiting therapy for removing excess kapha impurities from the body. Virechana removes pitta through purgation therapy. Basti removes excess vata from the body by the administration of enemas. Rakta moksha includes bloodletting by the application of leeches, withdrawing blood, or donating blood at a blood bank, as well as using certain cleansing and blood-thinning herbs. Nasya comprises the administration of certain herbal powders, medicated oils and preparations, and ghee into the nose for purification of prana, mind, and consciousness.

Ayurveda says toxins are produced when an aggravated dosha affects the biological fire (agni), which in turn affects digestion, metabolism, and assimilation. So undigested, unabsorbed, unassimilated food products remain in the body as a morbid substance. This toxic, raw, nonhomogeneous, sticky substance is ama, and it adheres to the tissues, clogs the channels, and creates poisons in the body. It enters the blood and creates toxemia, which is a root cause of disease. Since the root cause of ama is the aggravated dosha, ayurveda says that one should remove the aggravated dosha by panchakarma.

Shamana

According to ayurveda, shamana (palliation) is the balancing and pacification (as opposed to elimination) of bodily doshas. There are seven types of shamana: *dipana* (kindling the agni), *pachana* (burning toxic ama), *ksud nigraha* (fasting), *trit-nigraha* (observing thirst, or not drinking water), *vyayama* (yoga stretching), *atap seva* (lying in the sunlight), and *marut seva* (sitting meditation).

Shamana is a spiritual method of purification. People with insufficient physical or emotional strength to undergo panchakarma are good candidates for shamana. Any pitta, vata, or chronic kapha disorder that affects the immune system and the agni also makes an individual a good subject for this approach. Shamana can be done in a healthy person also, because it has both curative and preventive aspects, and prevention is better than cure.

Dipana

The first shamana method is dipana. Kindling the bodily fire is absolutely necessary in kapha and vata disorders, where the person has low gastric fire. This can be accomplished by taking certain herbs, such as *pippili,* ginger, cinnamon, black pepper, and *chitrak,* in certain proportions with honey. The fire ceremony can be performed by burning special woods; making an *agnikunda*, like a *yagyakunda* (fireplace); arranging the woods in a pyramidal, square fashion; putting camphor and cotton at the center; and kindling the fire while chanting special mantras that increase the internal fire. Concentrating on the solar plexus, the individual can also kindle the agni in the physical body, subtle body, and causal body. This kind of ceremony is very effective for kapha and vata people, but it should be done with great caution for pitta people.

Pachana

With this method, toxins are burned away using certain herbs in certain proportions. For pachana, ayurveda uses teas made from *trikatu,* chitrak, cinnamon, ginger, cumin, coriander, and fennel after meals. The process can be improved through concentration, meditation, and contemplation on improving the digestive capacity so there will be proper assimilation by and nutrition of the bodily tissue.

Ksud nigraha

Ksud nigraha is fasting, or eating a monodiet. Ayurveda suggests fasting for acute fever, indigestion, dysentery, and diarrhea. A person may only eat cooked apple with ghee, basmati rice with *mung dal* and ghee, or yogurt and rice in small quantities. For all conditions except acute indigestion, it is better not to eat anything for a couple of days, so the bodily fire will kindle and burn the internal toxins. For this, observing a fast is very important.

Trit-nigraha

Trit-nigraha, observing thirst, is very important when water (kapha) disorders are found. For example, ayurveda says to observe thirst for kidney disorders—such as edema or ascites, where there is accumulated water in the peritoneal cavity—or certain other kapha urinary disorders where too much water is retained in the system. If a person drinks too much water, it will remain in the body. Trit-nigraha means observing one's thirst and state of thirst with a possible view toward a long-term alteration in drinking habits.

Vyayama

The next important shamana is vyayama, which is exercise, or yoga. Exercise is defined here as using the muscles in a particular direction with a goal, so that you can reach the goal with effort and, in that effort, create physical stress. This stress kindles agni, like hiking in the mountains, walking, jogging, and jumping. Ayurveda says exercise has a quality that improves circulation, accelerates the heart rate, enhances the burning of calories, stimulates metabolism, regulates body temperature, and maintains body weight. Exercise makes your senses alert and attentive, and your mind sharpens and develops keen perception. These qualities are important, but again, the type of exercise required varies from person to person.

Ayurveda suggests certain exercises according to individual constitution. For example, the seat of vata in the body is the pelvic cavity, so any exercise that will help stretch the pelvic muscles is good. Therefore, the forward bend, backbend, spinal twist, cobra pose, camel pose, shoulderstand, and plow pose help to move the vata in a particular direction and calm it. Pitta is centered in the solar plexus, so fish pose, boat pose, camel pose, locust pose, and bow pose—all of which stretch those muscles—will help calm pitta. The focus of kapha is the chest, so ayurveda says that shoulderstand, plow pose, locust pose, cat pose, cow pose, and bow pose are best to improve the circulation of kapha in the pulmonary cavity.

Different kinds of exercise suit different constitutions. Jogging is not good for vata people; it is good for kaphas, but kapha people don't like jogging. Swimming is good exercise for the pitta and the vata person. Mountain climbing and hiking are good for kapha people. Proper exercise is a wonderful part of shamana.

Atap seva

Atap seva, lying in the sun, is another ancient shamana. The sun is the source of heat, light, and higher consciousness. Pitta-predominant people can lie in the sun after applying certain oils (sunblocks) to reduce their exposure to ultraviolet (UV) rays. A pitta should not lie in the sun for more than half an hour, whereas a vata can stay out for about an hour, and a kapha can stand more than an hour. If the proper care is taken, lying in the sun and meditating on the solar plexus is a wonderful shamana for kapha and vata. It improves circulation and the absorption of vitamin D, strengthens the bones, and kindles the fire in the solar plexus. The heat of a fire lit during the daytime or evening can cleanse the astral, physical, subtle, and causal bodies.

Today, extended exposure to the sun has become dangerous. The ionosphere and ozone are damaged, allowing unwanted radiation (UV rays) to reach the earth and aggravate *brajak-pitta* under the skin, which can result in skin cancer. A person with multiple moles should not lie in the sun. Lying in moonlight is also an ancient shamana for reducing pitta.

Pranayama

Lastly, there is breathing. Respiration is partly conscious and partly unconscious. One should do proper breathing through both nostrils by doing alternate-nostril pranayama. There are different types of pranayama, as well as a totally different science of breath that one can study from an experienced teacher. But if one sits quietly, inhales deeply through one nostril, holds the breath in the lower abdomen, and slowly exhales through the opposite nostril (repeating and alternating nostrils), it helps to bring balance to prana, *apana,* and *udana* (subtypes of prana). Out of that balance, one can attain the highest state of tranquillity.

Shamana as a whole brings balance to the body, mind, and consciousness and to the three bodily humors. It also cleanses the physical, subtle, and causal bodies. So by understanding the basic principles of life, one's own constitution as explained in ayurvedic literature, and the exact nature and structure of doshic aggravation, one can follow the proper guidelines of shodana and shamana.

Rasayana

Rasayana has three subcategories: restoration of tissues through herbs, minerals, and exercises; revitalization, or restoring energy to the system; and longevity, which involves slowing or stopping the aging process.

Satvajaya

The categories of satvajaya include mantra (sound); *yantra*s (physical support devices); tantra (directing energies in the body); meditation; and gems, metals, and crystals specifically for the relief of imbalances or disease.

AYURVEDA AND RELATIONSHIPS

According to ayurveda, life is a relationship and includes the relationship between you and your spouse, girlfriend, or boyfriend, and between parents and children. Equally important, however, is the relationship with yourself—the inner relationship between the three humors, which is the relationship between body, mind, and consciousness. These relationships are life, and ayurveda is a healing art that helps bring clarity in relationships. Clarity in relationships brings compassion, and compassion is love; therefore, love is clarity. Without clarity, there is no insight. The insight gained from ayurveda brings harmony, happiness, joy, and bliss to our daily lives and our relationships.

Ayurveda can definitely bring longevity. The body has its own intelligence to create balance, and ayurveda helps in the balancing process. Its definition of exercise is the goal-oriented usage of muscles in a particular direction so that you can reach the goal and attain peace. With the practice of pranayama, we can attain the highest state of tranquillity. And if we prevent potential ailments through shamana, we can succeed in healing the soul. According to ayurveda, every soul is immortal and sacred; to understand the individual, to understand oneself, is the foundation of life. Ayurveda is a total healing art. It brings a quality of consciousness such that we can get insight to deal with our inner life; our inner emotions; our inner hurt, grief, and sadness. Without this self-knowing, life has no meaning.

§

DR. VASANT LAD, a native of India, has been a practitioner and professor of ayurvedic medicine for more than thirty years. He holds a Bachelor of Ayurvedic Medicine and Surgery (BAMS) and a Master of Ayurvedic Science (MASc). His academic and practical training includes the study of allopathic (Western) medicine and surgery. He served as medical director of the Ayurveda Hospital in Pune, India, for three years, and held the position of professor of clinical medicine for twelve. He is the founder and director of the Ayurvedic Institute in Albuquerque, New Mexico. Since 1984, he has conducted one of the first full-time programs of study on ayurveda in the United States and travels widely to teach. Dr. Lad is the author of many books, including *Ayurveda: The Science of Self-Healing; The Complete Book of Ayurvedic Home Remedies; Strands of Eternity: A Compilation of Mystical Poetry and Discourses;* and *Ayurvedic Cooking for Self-Healing.*

Consecration of the Body and Rituals of Fullness

CHRISTIAN PISANO

According to Kashmiri Shaivism, when Shiva "creates" this world, he also conceals his real nature with particularity. This is his *maya* (magic). He can do this through the power of absolute freedom. As a distinct individual, Shiva loses the real and undifferentiated knowledge of his real self, thereby possessing only the differentiated knowledge of particularity. He uses this maya, or *ajnana* (ignorance), to veil himself. The first two verses of the *Shiva Sutras* say, "Awareness is the reality of everything. Bondage is having differentiated knowledge while not having undifferentiated knowledge." This bondage is to be escaped. Ignorance is not the absence of knowledge. Rather, it is the nonfullness, noncompletion, or poverty-stricken nature of knowledge. The knowledge is always present in our conscious lives, but it is limited. Self-knowledge, or real knowledge, is unlimited. It is undifferentiated and identical with consciousness. Nevertheless, every limited being must have some knowledge because it could not exist otherwise. Since knowledge is identical to consciousness, it is the essence of reality. All is absorption into the reality of God consciousness, which is the truly mystical state of being in one's own nature; in that condition, there is nowhere else to go and nothing else to do. It is replete and complete. These are the different issues presented by Christian Pisano.

Although the spontaneous brightness of childhood poured out of me, there was always the feeling of something missing. This feeling of lacking was not a "something" in itself. It was more about my condition as a so-called entity. Perhaps my being born with a clubfoot pushed me to question reality, the accepted assumption of being a body–mind. My search took the expression of yoga and India.

I first met my guru in a bookshop when I saw his book *Light on Yoga*. I didn't know at that time that he would be my teacher. I didn't know where he was or even if he was still living. It was only on my third trip to India that I excitedly found out that Guruji was alive and teaching in Pune. The play of the guru is indeed wonderful!

Being young and proud, I sent him pictures of my asanas (what a joke!), begging him to accept me as a student. He did, but it took me many years to understand what a real student is. He gave me the teaching I needed, but being eager to impress him, I regularly practiced a lot of advanced poses. The first guidance he gave me was on my legs: "You are overstretching. Work from the thigh muscle straight up, and resist with the calf muscles." But I was not an empty vessel and was too full of myself to meet the real requirement of a disciple—that of the surrendering attitude. I did not stick to the practice of basic asanas, and one morning at the end of practice, he noticed that my lower back was red. This was not a good sign. In the afternoon at the end of my practice, he asked me again to show him my back. It was still red. He then got very upset with me, saying that my body was like cotton, an overripe banana with no intelligence! He asked me to adjust someone doing a standing twist and to help turn his back. This man was very stiff, and I couldn't move him an inch. Guruji said, "Your body should become like his. Even if your body can do the pose, don't allow it! You must create tremendous resistance. If I see you practicing advanced poses again, I will no longer teach you yoga, neither in this life nor in the next!" Though he was angry with me, I could only see love in his eyes.

I then began to get fever regularly. Guruji said it was because of my overdoing. He gave me a resting sequence that I had to follow for at least a year, even during the general classes. He also showed me how to work on my clubfoot. Building this work was slow and very organic and took many years. The process continues even now.

When first I met Guruji, I knew that I was home—I could intuit that the question was the answer, for one cannot put the question of one's self if the Self is not already there. That is what the guru mirrors. He taught me in many ways relevant to my situation and frame of mind, always breaking down the identifications and personal drama I was acting out. The guru is the one who knows that you are not the body-mind. That is why his teaching goes to the core.

I offer my humble salutations to my Guruji, Mahasiddha among Siddhas, whose playground is the universe. Praise be to my Guruji, who out of compassion for my ignorance, initiated me into yoga.

The little I know about yoga I owe to my Guruji, Yogacharya Sri B. K. S. Iyengar. What follows is an expression of how his teaching resonates in me and offers an exploration of three of his now-famous statements:

> The body is my temple; asanas are my prayers.
> Each asana teaches you the art of silence.
> Each asana is free. Learn to diffuse it everywhere.

THE FIELD OF THE LORD

At the height of identification, the body serves as a proof of separation like a duke of fear to the tidal wave of existence. Without referring to memory, I cannot know what the body of separation is. The image of the body allows me to define myself as a man or a woman with certain characteristics, pleasant or unpleasant, reducing space into a simple contraction. I know nothing of this body except that it is a story that I continue to tell myself: a particular shape in a particular place, carrying out particular tasks. Although this story has an aftertaste of lack, I am very attached to it. I take great care to protect this wardrobe full of beliefs, prejudices, and preferences.

Is it really I who I see in the mirror of my projections, which seek to seal the breach of reality? Am I my twenty-year-old self or my seventy-year-old self; the youth of my body or its old age and pain? We still carry within ourselves the ever-present celebration of the lightness of our childhood dances, intoxicated and full of our own plenitude.

All feelings of life cry out for the sinking of the sense of separation, where we may glimpse the body as a breath of air, a morning mist announcing the nascent light of day, a divine veil.

> This entire world is the shadow of His essential parts.
> And those who exist through the veil of His life,
> Are not just part of him, they are His very Self.★

★ Rumi Koraïchi Rachid, *Le miroir infini* (Paris: Éditions Alternatives, 2001).

The body is called *sharira, kshetra, pinda, rupa, purpura puri, anga, murti,* and *deha.* So many expressions signifying that it is no more than a pointer, the signifier of the breath, the caress of the absolute. The body is no more than a representation, an object, and cannot be regarded as the subject. The body's ephemeral nature is beyond all doubt. As the *Isha Upanishad* says, "The body has its end in ashes."

The Sanskrit term *sharira* has a far-wider meaning than the Western concept of the body. It refers to different condensations and coagulations. The contemplation of the total transience, of the utter lack of substance of this body, is the ultimate oblation. The body is the vibrating place of tides called envelopes (*koshas*), which are different waves (*urmis*) of crystallization and conditionings. The exploration of the subtle to the most subtle of Shiva's semen (*Shiva bija: spanda-sharira; shakta-sharira; puryastaka-sharira; prana-sharira; sthula-sharira*) becomes the ritual of consecration of the body.

The ritual of consecration is the actualization of fullness in the limited and conditioned body. The means can never achieve the *anupaya,* which is beyond and is the source of activities. "No discipline or practice can be possible with regard to the highest reality or Shiva, which is also one's essential nature. Nothing can be added to or removed from the highest reality; of what avail can practice be here?"★

That which is described in these rituals must not be taken in the literal sense of the mundane liturgy where one accomplishes certain actions to achieve some goal. The flavor, the primal emotion (*rasa*), the upsurge at the heart of these rituals is that of fullness. "That is whole; this is whole; from the whole, the whole becomes manifest. From the whole when the whole is negated, what remains is again the whole."†

Downstream, this upsurge imposes crude, fragmentary, and volitional activities on the body. The mundane ritual, which is born of the sense of lack (*raga tattva*), wants to change or obtain a body-mind more in agreement with its idiosyncrasies, thus becoming a slave of the syndrome of

---

★ Lilian Silburn, *Les voies de la mystique ou l'accès au sans-accès* (Paris: Éditons Les Deux Océans, 1993).

† Swami Chinmayananda, *Discourses on Isavsya Upanishad* (Bombay: Bombay Central Chinmaya Trust, 1980).

"more and less." One sets oneself into a practice of reform, change, and intentions. Whatever the movement, be it accumulation or renunciation, both are manifesting the farce of separation. It is inescapable that this very movement in its crudest expression of hegemonic and colonialist practices recognizes itself (*pratyabhijna*) upstream as being the upsurge from the heart of fullness.

There is no seeker, but a search, which becomes exhausted with itself. There is no practitioner, but merely a practice of making offerings like drawing patterns in water, lost in the texture of its depths. The sharira and its different envelopes become the vantage point for the exploration of the states of consciousness. This process, called *karana,* is where the body and its attributes are used as means of contemplation to reveal itself, free from any superimposition. "The varieties of karana are meant to subordinate and ultimately assimilate all objective phenomena to the consciousness of the essential Self."*

There is always a certain contraction tied to the image of the body, to its gluey definition. The karana intends to resorb the grasping of the body. The observation of bodily processes allows the structure to rest within its natural conditioning.

> There are two categories of conditioning: the necessary and the unnecessary. The unnecessary has it roots in ignorance and a sense of separation. When this is relinquished, the necessary conditionings only hold up the body. It is purely biological.†

THE POSTURAL FIELD (KSHETRASANA) AND POSTURAL CONTEMPLATION (ASANASAMAVESHA)

Like an ancient epic poem recounting the deeds of heroes, the asanas are a celebration of the absolute in all its forms and flavors. The different groups of asanas testify to a circumambulation (*parikrama*) that follows a rhythm in their execution and pedagogical aspect:

---

* Jaideva Singh, *Shiva Sutras: The Yoga of Supreme Identity* (Delhi: Motilal Barnasidass, 1979).

† Svami Venkatesananda, *The Supreme Yoga* (Fremantle, Calif.: Children Yoga Trust, 1976).

Although thirty spokes meet at the hub,
it is the empty space at the center
Which makes the cart move.★

Asana is not a psychophysical posture, but the power of the supreme *shakti* as conscious light, not limited by space and time or the activities of the body: "The nature of the I is celebrated as conscious light resting within herself. It is designated 'rest' because all waiting is destroyed and there reigns liberty, activity and sovereignty."†

One of the etymologies of the word *asana* is "to be seated." This sitting is essentially establishing all the envelopes of the sharira within their source. For Shankaracharya, the posture is that where attention flows spontaneously. In the *Shiva Sutras,* it is said,

> Taking his seat in the middle breath (udana) in between the passages of Prana and Apana, holding firmly on the jnanashakti, the stable posture that the yogi acquires is the real asana.‡

What then is this asana if it is not the pulse of the *spanda*, which takes myriad forms? Thus the postures become a mirror of this pulse, of this sensation (*sparsha*) also called tingling (*pipilika*). It expresses itself in every form, which is why the postures recreate it by means of the different groups, the infinity of all its structures, be they geometric, geographic, mineral, vegetable, animal, human, heroic, demonic, or divine. Touch is the most radiant act of consecration in the asana.

RITUALS OF POSTURAL ACTION (KRIYAVASTHA)

All traditional arts demand an apprenticeship. The great musicians can allow themselves to improvise and forget technique because they have been absorbing it over many years of intense practice. In the *Vastu Sutra Upanishad* (the upanishad of the architects, sculptors, and builders of temples), it is said that there are six essential disciplines within this art. These

---

★ *Lao-Tseu philosophes Taoïstes* (Paris: Éditions Galimard, 1987).
† Lilian Silburn, *Sivasutra et Vimarsini de Ksemaraja* (Paris: Collège de France, Publications de l'Institut de Civilisation Indienne, Éditions de Boccard, 1980).
‡ Ibid.

can be applied equally to the art of asana: knowledge of stone (*shailam*), which in our context becomes the body; composition of diagrams (postures) and knowledge of the vital points (*marman*); cutting stone (*shailabedhana*); arranging component parts (*angaprayoga*); the emotional attitude evoked by the composition (*nyasabhavana*); and intuition of the unity underpinning the composition (*sambandha prabodhana*).

The first contact with the body reveals its inertia. At first, asanas will simply be creating movement and mobility wherein there is a reorganization of the body. It is a return to sensation, to a nonverbal perception wherein the body is no longer thought or named. The asanas become an opportunity to observe how the body is constantly agitated, restricted, or contracted. This stage is called *chikitsa krama* (gradual purification).

The language of posture refers to three rhythms, which are described as emanation (*shrishti*), maintenance (*sthiti*), and resorption (*samhara*). The *Vaijayanti Kosha* defines *shrishti* as the natural state (*svabhava*); *sthiti* as the act of maintaining or continuing (*maryada*); and *samhara* as that of ending or dissolving (*pralaya*).

Entering into the posture, holding it, and releasing it refer to the currents of the spanda. These three rhythms find their whole meaning in the sense of direction. Everything that is perceived, including the universe itself, is regarded as the field of consciousness. The universe, as yantra or mandala, spreads out in all eight directions: east (*purva*), west (*pashchima*), south (*dakshina*), north (*uttara*), northeast (*isha*), southeast (*agneye*), northwest (*vayau*), and southwest (*nairakta*). When these directions are applied to the mandala of the body, the anterior side of the body is the east and the posterior side the west, the north being the head and the south being the feet.

> According to the space-directions, the guardians of the quarters are worshipped. (Aditya in the east, Yama in the south, Varuna in the west, Soma in the north and Agni in the center.)★

The sense of direction in an asana is the basis of the alignment. By alignment, we are referring to the concept of *samatva* (equanimity).

★ Alice Boner, Sadasiva Sarma, and Bettina Bäumer, *Vastu Sutra Upanishad, The Essence of Form in Sacred Art* (Delhi: Motilal Barnasidass, 1982).

Initially, one uses the external means of movement and action. Movement can be vertical, horizontal, spiral, and lateral in expansions and contractions. These actions are applied to different parts of the body in the various postures. Thus the body becomes the object (*grahya*) of a dynamic concentration resting on the different parts (angas) of the organism. Mobility will become action, which is intelligence in motion, unfolding different and opposite senses of direction, some parts being stable and others mobile. Precision in adopting the posture and the refinement of the shape itself thus reveal its exterior texture.

The median line (*brahmakila* or *brahmadanda*), like the center (*bindu*), is the support of all the postures. Alignment or median line is only another name for cosmic order (dharma or *rita*).

> All limbs have to be set along lines.
> The middle line is the support. . . .
> The hole is the center (marman) and is to be contemplated as Brahma.★

Thus the source of the asanas is the *shantarasa*. *Samasthiti* is therefore "the even posture," where all the fluctuations of opposites reabsorb in the center.

Every posture has its source in samasthiti, which is the actualization of shantarasa. If samasthiti is present, the wave of resorption (*shavasana*) is also there. The different attitudes (*bhava*) open up to the taste of unity (*samarasatva*).

ATTENTION AND FEELING (VIJNANA RASA)

In the initial phase (*kriyavastha*), dynamic concentration is fragmentary, dividing the body into parts, using movement and action. Now concentration must give way to attention (*vijnana*) which is no longer focused, but diffuses into a unifying whole. An image of warm oil that spreads out is used. In this phase, sensation is even more predominant, and one observes the body's texture during the course of the asana. The phases of

---

★ Alice Boner, Sadasiva Rath Sarma, Bettina Bäumer, *Vastusutra Upanishad, The Essence of Form in Sacred Art* (Delhi: Motilal Barnasidass, 1982).

adjustment and action are minimized. Alignment in the earlier kriya phase insisted on the outer form of the asana, without being concerned by the final or achieved form, and more on the harmonic and aesthetic arrangement of the various limbs in the space. In the vijnana phase, this convention is obsolete. It remains present, rather like musicians who tune their instruments before playing but do not spend all their time just tuning them, or like birds gliding, using rising or falling currents of air, occasionally adjusting, but not beating their wings unceasingly.

Here the postures take on the character of mudra, symbolic gestures of three energies: there is energy of will (*iccha shakti*); energy of knowledge (*jnana shakti*); and energy of activity (*kriya shakti*), where contemplative moods gain the upper hand. The external manifestation is just a pretext for the recognition that the object (*grihya*) is bathed in the light of the subject (*grahaka*) without separation. Technically one undoes more than one does. This phase is also called *shakti krama* (the succession of the energies).

The Sky of Consciousness (Chidakasha)

Here, even attention dies and evaporates into the space of consciousness (*chidakasha*). Postures become mandalas (from the root *manda,* meaning "essence"). All the dynamism of doing, of actions, is extinguished and the asana becomes the reflection of its source. The nonvolitional aspect of the posture becomes a unifying obviousness. The asana is nothing but the space of consciousness. This nondoing completely burns up the object itself to make us recognize what we are through the discriminative emptying of all that we are not.

In the outer aim, any object whatsoever can be used: the blue of the sky, a sound, the sun, the moon, a flowing river, water, and so on. The outer aim gathers the diversity of phenomena (*vikalpa*) toward an undifferentiated perception. In postural practice, the outer aim relies on the various parts of the body, their interaction, and their unity.

The internal aim relies on the various parts of the internal geography, organic and subtle. Initially, the various organs will be the centers of attention. The organic aim will open into a bridge of space (*adhara*), a place of contemplation where the *panchavyomana* (five firmaments) unfold.

Here one becomes sensitive to the currents that flow in these spaces, the *panchavayu* (*apana, samana, prana, udana,* and *vyana*). Thus the internal aim creates intimacy with the marrow of life and reveals how it is robed in different colors and different contractions to become the so-called compact mass that is the body. When these two aims reach maturity, they die into the median aim (*madhya lakshya*), where all notions of body-mind disappear. This stage is called *adyatmika krama* (plunging into the self).

INVOCATION, FILTRATION, RESONANCE, OR THE RHYTHMS OF SILENCE (VINYASA KRAMA)

The ritual of consecrating the body goes through *nyasa*. In the traditional nyasa, the fingers are used to consecrate the different parts of the body. It is interesting to note the etymology of the Sanskrit word *hasta* (hand), "that which blossoms outward" (*hasati vikasati*). The base of the thumbs (*angushtha*) becomes the dwelling place for the waters of Brahma, symbolizing the creative force—the hypnotic power of the mind, which, like a colored lens, projects our own expectations on reality. "When a pickpocket meets a saint, all he sees in him are his pockets."

The index finger (*tarjani*) is the one that warns, that reprimands but also points out. It discriminates. The ring finger (*anamika*) does not have a name; it is unnamable because Shiva used it to decapitate Brahma. It signifies the nonconceptual, the no-mind. The little finger (*kanishtha*), called the smallest or weakest, represents the dual nature (vikalpa) of the thought process. The greater or middle finger (*madhyama*) becomes the representation of the unifying vibration of consciousness where the characteristics of the other fingers no longer exist.

In the postural ritual that we are considering, the asana becomes the offering of space (*akasha*) in different parts of the body or limbs: the anatomical, physiological, respiratory, and sensory functions participate in the nyasa of impregnation. According to the *Dhatupatha,* the root of *krama* is *kram,* which means "to take a step." Krama indicates a time sequence, a cycle, the succession of days, nights, months, the cycle of seasons, years, and the course of the sun. The intuition of a rhythm (emanation, maintenance, and resorption) in the relative sequence of events brings us back to their silence, to their absolute transparency. The actual vinyasa in postural practice is the codification of the bodily attitudes, as well as the groups of postures and the precise positioning of the various parts of the body, which begin to interact to produce certain effects. The vinyasa krama encompasses a diversity of definitions:

- The starting position; the attitude for entering into, staying in, and coming out of the posture according to a rhythm synchronized with the breath
- The gradual linking of asanas according to a sequence in a flow synchronized with the breath
- The gradual preparation of asanas, not yet mastered, spread over several months
- Precision in establishing and unfolding the asanas
- Unfolding variations for intensifying the postures or modifications brought to a posture
- The resorption phase and the postures that spread a feeling of calm (*prashant*)

It is in the series that postures reveal their melody and can reflect their different energetic coloration and tones. A series is an invocation that generates clarification and an intuitive resonance of the absolute. The texture, the flavor of a posture would be different according to the place within the sequence, but this has nothing to do with counterposture because asanas are not postures. Asana mirrors totality, unfolding quietude (*shanti rasa*) of the body, breath, and mind. Thus each asana is self-sufficient and has no need for an "opposite action." Rather, the notion of equalization of energy (*pratikriyasana* or *samashaktikriya*) is used to avoid certain undesirable effects or to reinforce certain desirable ones. For instance, one would not end practice with sirsasana or a backward extension, even if this were followed by savasana unless one were a master in the art of resorption.

The attitude is the acceptance of the energetic flow of the asanas in their anatomical, physiological, neurological, sensory, and mental effects. There is, therefore, a vinyasa krama of initiation into asanas. Thus the introductory vinyasa krama of the inverted poses would start with setubandha sarvangasana (cross bolsters), viparita karani, ardha halasana, halasana, and sarvangasana. When these asanas have been introduced, having themselves been introduced by prior asanas, then sirsasana may be undertaken. Once sirsasana has been introduced, the vinyasa krama of the energy would be sirsasana, sarvangasana, halasana, setubandha sarvangasana, viparita karani.

The various energetic colorations of the asanas or groups of asanas are fundamental to the art of sequencing. Certain asanas are warming, whereas others are cooling. They can be stimulating and enlivening, or calming and relaxing, simple or complex. In an elementary vinyasa krama, one begins with standing postures (*utthishtha sthiti*), the seated postures (*upavishtha sthiti*), the forward extensions (*pashchima pratana sthiti*), lateral extensions (*parivritta sthiti*), and inverted postures (*viparita sthiti*). When these groups have created a degree of mobility, the backward extensions (*purva sthiti*) are introduced, followed by the abdominal postures (*udara akunchana sthiti*). A sample of a supine posture (*supta sthiti*) is given during savasana. In regard to the vinyasa of energy, one never performs sirsasana, backward extensions, or sun salutations after sarvangasana. Sarvangasana is included in the group of asanas of resorption and must be followed by postures that spread and deepen the wave of resorption.

Vinyasa krama has an infinite number of aspects. The crudest is that where one moves from one posture to another in a continuous flow. The link between the postures is surya namaskar. Here the movement is peripheral, and one cannot truly understand the notions explained earlier about alignment and maturation from staying in the asanas, because in this approach the practitioner moves quickly from one asana to the next. This method is ideal for children and young people who need a vigorous practice and challenge, for experienced practitioners who have a tendency toward inertia or dullness, or in cold weather. But it is selective and is therefore not suitable for everyone. The danger in the overuse of vinyasa would be to unleash the mind of a monkey driven mad by the sting of a scorpion and locked in a room without windows. In this approach, one could easily become obsessed with achieving the final posture at any cost.

In the same register, *vishamanyasa* is the mix of postures that seem to oppose each other and have no links. *Viloma vishamanyasa* is the practice of a group of postures linked by a posture in an opposite direction, such as backward extensions interrupted by paschimottanasana. "The sculptors (silpakaras) apply a softening mixture."★ The sculptor does not begin to use his chisel until he has already applied four substances to make the stone malleable. This quotation introduces one of the most interesting aspects of the vinyasa krama, which is that of intimacy (*parichaya*) or welcome (*svagatam*). Here the achievement of a final posture in its external form has no significance. A gradual approach is used to welcome the essence of the postures as they unfold by a passive observation of neurophysiological processes.

The svagatam vinyasa krama proceeds from the simplest to the most complex forms, where one may integrate resistance as it grows and flirt with the more achieved aspect of the asana. By *achieved,* we mean the fully extended sensation and tone of a posture, without moving into the so-called final posture. Fundamentally, there is no final pose. For example in halasana, the feet, instead of being on the ground, could be raised up. There is, in fact, a gradual approach for each posture. This vinyasa krama, called "framing" (*samputana kriya*), unfolds two processes: revitalizing and pacifying. One could adopt some preparatory vinyasa krama that would not only lead to the desired posture with a degree of maturity regarding observation, but also allow a release from various parasitical movements such as agitation, panic, and fear that impede breathing or create pressure in the throat, eyes, ears, tongue, and brain.

Sirsasana can be framed in its upward phase by uttanasana, adho mukha svanasana, prasarita padottanasana, janu sirsasana, paschimottanasana, adho mukha virasana, and sirsasana. The asanas are then repeated in the downward phase in the opposite direction. The same asana could be framed in a more dynamic postural environment such as adho mukha vrksasana and pincha mayurasana.

A sequence only acquires its true value when it is accompanied by yoga practice adapted to the needs of the individual (*viniyoga*), where it is in harmony with the internal and external environments and is not merely imposed. The constitution (deha), place (*desha*), gender (*linga*), time (*kala*), age (*vayas*), abilities (shakti), aspirations (*marga*), and occupations (*vritti*) of the practitioner must be taken into account, while

---

★ Alice Boner, Sadasiva Rath Sarma, Bettina Bäumer, *Vastusutra Upanishad, The Essence of Form in Sacred Art* (Delhi: Motilal Barnasidass, 1982).

respecting the seasons (*ashrama*) of existence, the different stages of life, and each person's predilections, which can alter according to circumstances. If a person suffers from hypertension or if a woman is experiencing menopausal hot flashes, the postural programs naturally need to be adjusted. During the menstrual cycle, certain asanas such as the inverted postures must absolutely not be practiced, and one must give greater emphasis to other asanas. Seasons and changes in the seasons also have their importance. One must not practice the same way in winter as in the middle of a hot summer. Various techniques are adapted to meet the needs of the practitioner's age. *Shrishthi*, which relates to youth, uses a dynamic practice emphasizing agility, rapidity, suppleness, and strength. Sthiti, which relates to adulthood, emphasizes organic and pranic action. *Antya*, which relates to older people, makes maintenance and good condition of the circulatory and respiratory systems high priorities and concentrates on the movement of natural resorption.

One can also adapt the practice to meet the needs of the moment and the maturity of the practitioner. Chikitsa krama is the practice known as "purification" and is intended to clean and detoxify the body. Shakti krama targets those who use the postures from the perspective of churning, for example, through the advanced postures. Adhyatmika krama is the practice of offering and oblation, where the postures are a surrendering of the sharira and its various envelopes into the source.

Respect of the individual structure leads to an emptying out of its personal history to reflect its latent abilities at a given moment, rather like a plant that has not reached ideal conditions, yet is at one with its environment and makes the best of it. The body is no longer stifled by a personal commentary that restricts it within an image. This unity with its own ground enables the structure to breathe freely.

Supports of Contemplation, Junctions, and Gates into Infinity (Adhara and Sandhi)

Adhara, from the root *dhr,* literally means "that which retains," or "that which contains but also supports." The word *laksha* (an object of contemplation) is also used. Goraknath describes sixteen adhara, or supports, for contemplation:

1. *Padangushthadhara* (the base of the big toes). The root of the big toes and the spaces between them and the second toes have great importance in postural stability. The big toes must "see." It is said that there exists a connection between the big toes and the optic nerves.
2. *Muladhara* (the perineum). The site of contemplation for the paths of *ida, pingala,* and *sushumna.*
3. *Gudadhara* (the rectum). The site of contemplation for apana prana. Numerous postures help to vitalize apana prana in this part of the body, which regulates the excretory functions. Certain asanas—such as samasthiti, sirsasana, sarvangasana, urdhva dhanurasana, ustrasana, and paschimottanasana—are imperative to learn the upward suction of the rectum (*vikasa-samkocana* or *ashvini mudra,* known as the "horse's gesture" because it is reminiscent of a horse's stance while urinating).
4. *Medhradhara* (the lingam, situated at the root of the penis, though some say the penis itself). This is the site of contemplation of prana, which rises with the syllable SVA, hence its alternative appellation of *svadhishthana* (pleasant). Here the life force (*pranashakti*) becomes semen (*bindu, virya, retas*). Certain postures induce a saturation of the body by the life force (*bindu stambhana*) instead of its usual loss (*bindu ksharana*).
5. *Uddiyanadhara* (spot situated above the navel). It controls the vitality of the *jathara agni* (digestive fire), helping to cleanse the intestines as well as the urinary and excretory systems.
6. *Nabhyadhara* (situated at the root of the navel, a spot also known as *kandasthana,* or the bulb root of the *nadis* network). "In the lower region of Manipura turned towards the south and towards the north is the zone of the anus. At its center, the bulb of the navel resembles the lotus flower and so it is said, is the receptacle of all the nadis."* This adhara is the site of contemplation of *pranava* (AUM) in its subtle, still-unified form. It is only in *hridayadhara* that it becomes

---

* Lilian Silburn, *La Kundalini, l'Énergie des Profondeurs* (Paris: Les Deux Océans, 1983).

distinct, although still in a continuous manner. Then it bursts into an infinite number of sounds at the level of the vocal cords.

7. *Hridayadhara* (the heart). The site of contemplation for the union of prana and apana.

8. *Kanthadhara* (the throat). The site of contemplation of the throat by the *jalandharabandha,* among others.

9. *Gantikadhara* (the root of the palate). The site of contemplation of the *amrita kala,* the nectar that flows from the *chandra mandala* to pour into the *sahasrara.*

10. *Taludhara* (the roof of the palate). The site of contemplation of the *kechari mudra* (unlimited consciousness).

11. *Jivadhara* (the root of the tongue). The site of contemplation of the emanation and resorption of speech, called "the one that is spread" (*vaikhari*). "Keeping the tongue in the center of the wide-open mouth one should fix the mind there. Uttering the letter 'h' mentally, one will be dissolved in peace."★

12. *Bhrihu-madyadhara* (point between the eyebrows). The site of contemplation of the lunar disk.

13. *Nasadhara* (the tip of the nose). The site of contemplation of the gates of the breath and the *tattva akasha.*

14. *Kapatadhara* (the roof of the nose). The site of contemplation of the respiratory passages and the nose's stability during inhalations. On the wave of exhalation, one can notice a natural descent in the eyes and also the bridge of the nose. (They tend to be pushed back upward in aggressive or nonrhythmic inhalation.)

15. *Lalatadhara* (point in the center of the forehead). The site of contemplation and resorption of the frontal brain.

16. *Bradharandradhara* (the center of the skull). This is also the area called "the bee's cave" (*bhramaraguna*) at the apex of the spinal column and in the lower parts of the sahasrara site of contemplation of space (akasha).

In postural practice, one extends the notion of adhara to the whole body, meaning all parts whether anatomical or physiological. Different

---

★ Swami Lakshman Joo, *Vijnana Bhairava, The Practice of Centering Awareness* (Varanasi, India: Indica Books, 2002).

parts of the body thus become fulcrums for contemplation and absorption (*samavesha*). These fulcrums are a way of dissolving the tensions, or grips, of the body, allowing the vital functions to spread out to their full organic extent, thus pouring out their effervescence, the sap of life. This effervescence dissolves the limits of the body, spreading it out into the universe. These adharas are the buds of life, recognized as divinities (*devata*) in their energetic aspect.

The practitioner will observe how certain zones evolve within the asana itself, but also how they maintain their stability from one asana to another. This junction is called sandhi. Sandhi is the meeting point, the connection, the union. *Sandhana* is a synonym that in Kashmiri Shaivism signifies awareness and the fundamental unity of reality. In grammar, *sandhi* means the junctions between words and between sounds. They are the liaisons that transform themselves when they meet. But *sandhi* also means the joints of the body that during postures become a storage place of infinite space or synapses, helping the diffusion of infinity between the limbs and thus avoiding compression. Sandhi applies also to the spaces around each breath. Sandhi reveals the center. Intuition of sandhi and its unfolding are essential to the practice of asana.

There are some gross sandhi connected with outer conjunctions. For example, the position and opening of the armpits in virabhadrasana II will help the understanding of their positioning in parsvakonasana. Some sandhi are more subtle, affected by the conjunctions of the organs of action and perception by the breath. Certain postures will educate the various diaphragms, and they become pranic junctions. Essentially, all postures become contemplations of the incomprehensible, the unknowable. These junctions, or doors of space, permit the practitioner to experience the asana subjectively and no longer overobjectify it by exteriority. It is rather like two strangers who meet with a glance that intuitively reveals all, without the need for introduction.

EMANATION, MAINTENANCE, AND POSTURAL RESORPTION (TRIKALA)

The intuition of what we are has no need of a time process or progression. According to Abhinavagupta, it is instantaneous, like a flash of lightning. However, its actualization and diffusion, in the order suggested by the *Shiva Sutra,* "to implement within the body the resorption of the fragmentary activities," takes time. This is why kala is an important element in asana. In early apprenticeship, duration does not matter; it becomes significant later. To establish oneself in the duration of a posture is to no longer occupy the body verbally, but to relate with its sensations in the moment. This feeling is always new and leaves one free within the forever-renewed freshness of the sensation.

Staying in an asana permits it to evolve. Abhinavagupta speaks of the two faces of energy: the one of fire, or igniting—the face of effervescence (*kshobhita*), and the other of earth—the face of noneffervescence (*akshobhita*). In the igniting aspect, the practitioner unfolds in his body itself the process of opening; of awakening (*unmesha*) organic effervescence; of unfolding various orbits from the most gross to the most subtle, including all the tattvas, the five gross elements (*panchamahabhuta*), the five subtle elements (*panchatanmatra*), the five organs of action (*panchakarmendriya*), and the five organs of perception (*panchajnanendriya*). The duration permits the practitioner to immerse himself in a particular attitude that provokes a virile shudder of the energy (virya) through a particular breath and permits him to become saturated with the flavor, with the energetic coloration of the posture and its resonance.

Steadiness, heaviness, hardness, capacity to germinate, fragrance, strength, association, fixing, and holding are qualities linked to the earth (*prithvi*). Coolness, fluidity, dampness, oozing, flowing, lubrication, softness, salivation, and bubbling are qualities linked to water (*jala*). Terrible brightness, heat, burning, resplendence, affliction, redness, swiftness, intensity, and what rises are qualities linked to fire (*agni*). Lack of control, sense of touch, speech organs, independence of movement, rapidity of movement, power, defecation, activity, agitation, and subtle movements of the breath are qualities linked to air (*vayu*). Sound, vastness, expanse, freedom, the unsupported, invincibility, shapelessness, indestructibility, the inanimate, immutability, and mutability are qualities linked to space (akasha). Then begins the process of involution, or withdrawal (*nimesha*), that is described as the practice of fainting, engulfing, and linking to the earthly character of energy. All the different categories from the grossest to the most subtle are resorbed in their source, a process also called purification of the elements (*tattvashuddi* or *bhutashuddhi*). In purification, it is implied that one loses consciousness of the objective world in the dissolutions of all psychophysical references and grips. This is the art of dying, which is at the heart of the fundamental practices in yoga. Time in asana allows the sharira and its envelopes to pause, so it can be surrendered in quietude (*vishranti*).

From Support to Supportlessness and the Caress of Spontaneity (Sagunasana, Nirgunasana, and Sahajasana)

The sensitivity of the body can be extended to the universe. Whatever is perceived becomes the direct extension of that intuition. Perhaps that is why the postures unfold archetypal energies that can at first seem strange to us but are brought together by a unifying intuitive perception (*sattarka*): postures of the tree, the dog, the triangle, the half-moon, the warrior, the ferocious one, the eagle, the horse's head, the cow's head, the crocodile, the fish, the fetus, the cobra, the royal pigeon, the scorpion, the bow, the archer, the bridge, and so on. "Those who know, cut down at its roots the dreadful tree of division (bedha) with the axe of intuitive reasoning (sattarka) sharpened to the finest edge; for us it is a certainty."[*]

The universe itself becomes an extension of this sensitivity. All is nothing but support. Each situation becomes the support of the inexpressible, the indescribable, of an astonishment that precedes all known, all definition.

Regarding the asana, the introduction of support may be an aid for the awakening sensation as the prolongation of awareness, or it may at least serve as a pointer. The support can direct the practitioner toward the "magnificent form of the supreme firmament." This is how my Guruji himself introduced props in his own practice and teaching. In the preliminary phase, the props allow practitioners to unfold space while increasing the degree of mobility and also to acquaint themselves with certain

---

[*] Lilian Silburn, *Abhinavagupta, La lumière sur les Tantras* (Paris: Collège de France, Publications de l'Institut de Civilisation Indienne, Éditions de Boccard, 1998).

asanas that would be too difficult to practice without support. The props engender understanding of the correct gesture (mudra) and attitude (*bhava*) of the asana. They allow prolonged timing in the asanas, thus permitting deeper penetration of certain areas of the body not yet explored. It then becomes easier to incorporate certain breathing patterns and see how the various colorings of the breath (*pancha prana*) unfold themselves in different constellations of the body. The props can be regarded as an outer loom leading to the very heart of the posture in a purely subjective way.

There should therefore always be a balance between using an external prop and using the body itself as a prop. In the final analysis, the body-mind is only an external prop.

> As for the Yoga depending on props, the dependence on specific spheres, such as the hands, feet, etc. of the body is salambayoga. As for the propless Yoga, contemplation in which all names and forms are far distant and the Atman is a mere witness of all desires and other movements of the inner senses, free from dependence on them is Niralambayoga.*

Perhaps when there is no longer a focus on any of the envelopes (*annamayakosha, pranamayakosha, manomayakosha, vijnanamayakosha, anandamayakosha*), when these are resting in their source, it could be possible to intuit what Guruji practices and teaches—that the body itself is no more than an evanescent web of space.

> Either sitting on a seat or lying on a bed one should meditate on the body as being supportless. When the mind becomes empty and supportless, within a moment one is liberated from mental dispositions."†

---

* A. A. Ramanathan, *The Vaisnava Upanishads* (Adyar, India: Adyar Library and Research Centre, 2002).

† Swami Lakshman Joo, *Vijnana Bhairava, The Practice of Centring Awareness* (Varanasi, India: Indica Books, 2002).

CHRISTIAN PISANO is a long-term student and advanced teacher of Sri B. K. S. Iyengar. He has studied Iyengar Yoga for more than twenty years. While in his early twenties, he lived for several years in Pune, India, so he could study directly with his guru. His philosophical inclinations are those of the nondual approaches, especially that of the Trika system known as Kashmiri Shaivism.

PART TWO

"Light on Life"

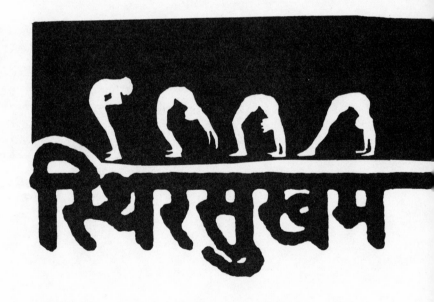

स्थिरसुखम्

"Asana is perfect firmness of body, steadiness of intelligence, and benevolence of spirit."
—B. K. S. IYENGAR, *Light on the Yoga Sutras of Patanjali*, II:46.

Light on Asana

BOBBY CLENNELL

> As a well cut diamond has many facets, each reflecting a different color
> of light, so also does the word *yoga*, each facet reflecting a different shade
> of meaning and revealing different aspects of the entire range of human
> endeavour to win inner peace and happiness.
> —B. K. S. IYENGAR, *Light on Yoga*

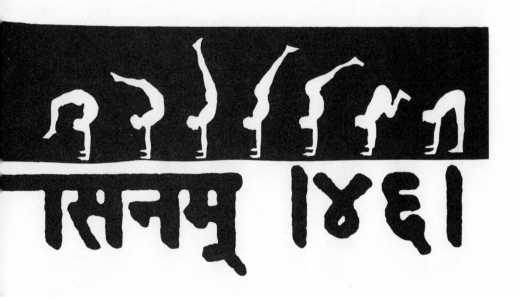

Dear Guruji, thank you.

With love and gratitude from Lindsey, Bobby, and Jake Clennell.

S

BOBBY CLENNELL has practiced yoga since 1975 and taught since 1977. She has studied with B. K. S. Iyengar and the Iyengar family in India more than fifteen times. She has written and illustrated three yoga manuals: *Props and Ailments,* detailing the therapeutic applications of Iyengar Yoga props; *Iyengar Yoga Glossary,* an introduction to the unique "language" of Iyengar Yoga; and *A Cosmic Body Map,* a key to the Vedic gods, their location and function within the body, and their mythological significance. She is experienced in using yoga for therapeutic purposes, including fertility and prenatal needs. Her newest book, *The Woman's Yoga Book: Asana and Pranayama for All Phases of the Menstrual Cycle,* was published in 2007.

Spirit of Community

Anne O'Brien

> Peace in words, thoughts and deeds, whether awake or dreaming, is a
> sign of goodwill and love towards all.
> —B. K. S. Iyengar, *Light on the Yoga Sutras of Patanjali*

Health and medicine go hand in hand, for the second is a conscious attempt to restore the first. Bioethics, medical ethics, and biomedical ethics
help us to negotiate the interface between medicine, humans, and the
sense of well-being. Practitioners and administrators often struggle to
elucidate general principles for health care, where a *principle* is a rule, or
general truth, basic to others. Modern Western health practices struggle
to form and apply such general precepts as "respect the wishes of all
competent persons"; "do not kill, impose cruel or harsh treatments, or
do harm to others"; "seek to benefit others"; "seek to produce a net balance of benefit over harm"; "ensure access to medical care for all"; "keep
promises and contracts"; "disclose all necessary information"; and "respect privacy and protect confidential information." Some of these
guidelines are taken as primary and fundamental, others as secondary
and derivative. Unfortunately, different schools of thought have different
priorities and produce different rules. Nevertheless, the four generally
accepted foundational principles are autonomy, nonmaleficence, benef-
icence, and justice.

There are immediate problems, of course, because justice can be understood in many different ways. To an egalitarian, equality of access is
important, whereas to a Marxist, the question of need is critical. Liber-
tarian theories emphasize rights, while utilitarian theories ask that efforts be made to maximize public and/or private benefits. Furthermore,
since the ideals set by any given theory of justice can only rarely be realized, the Western philosophical tradition carefully distinguishes between "formal" and "material" justice. The former deals with pure
theory (for example, all premature babies are entitled to incubators), but

the latter grapples with what happens "on the ground" (What should be done when there are seven babies and only six incubators?).

The earlier list of principles arises from the view of Immanuel Kant (1724–1804) that since all rational beings have the capacity to act in a consistent moral manner, they should be allowed to do so. This defines autonomy. It combines with individualism to determine that, in medicine, all patients are their own primary decision makers. The net result is the doctrine of informed consent. Doctor and patient must both agree to any proposed treatment, because consent can only exist when two or more people in full conscience agree that something should be done. This is consonant with the Western emphasis on individuals and their right to define their own vision of suffering and the best way to alleviate it.

This is a very far cry from the Confucian approach. Confucius taught that a person's body is a gift from his or her parents. The primary duty is therefore to take good care of it and not abuse it. To fail in that duty is to contravene the mandate of heaven; it is unrighteous behavior, possibly deserving of punishment. The family is the center of attention. Collective autonomy and social determination replace the Western emphasis on the individual, because it is only through this basic unit of familial reference that a harmonious universe and the greater good of the community can be realized.

The fundamentals of the Indian approach are stated in the *Charaka* and *Sushruta Samhitas*. The *Charaka* says that physicians should be celibate, vegetarian, truthful, and nonviolent (carry no arms). They should be committed to helping their patients, relieve them from harm, never abandon or injure them, and never be the cause of anyone's death. The *Sushruta* says that doctors' duties include ritualistic responsibilities. They are the *arthavan*s who perform important religious functions within a domestic setting, aiding patients in their houses by assuaging their various crises.

The important difference vis-à-vis the Western approach is the role given to dharma. Every idea and entity have their own distinct characteristics. That is their dharma. The dharma of fire is burning. For as long as an entity burns, it can be called fire. When that burning property is lost, it has lost its essential nature and is no longer fire. From this standpoint, health cannot really be promoted until its true nature, or dharma, is understood. And that requires an understanding of existence itself.

The cosmogony of health and well-being adopted by yoga states that *purusha* (spirit) and *prakriti* (nature) both emerge from *brahman* (the absolute all). Purusha dharma is the practical—since it is experiential, it is also scientific—attempt to grasp the true nature of spirit. It is divided into *jivatma dharma,* the science of the individual soul, and *paramatma dharma,* the science of the universal soul. On the other hand, prakriti dharma is the science—or true experiencing—of nature. This again has two parts. *Achetana prakriti dharma* investigates the true nature of inanimate entities, or those devoid of consciousness; *sachetana prakriti dharma* investigates living, conscious entities.

The dharma of human beings is that they are composed of consciousness. Knowing that we have a physical body and acknowledging that it has needs that can be gratified do not define the limits of human consciousness. This implies that stressing individuality and sensory gratification through inanimate objects merely promotes suffering, because it can only perpetuate the illusion of separateness that produces individuation. Coming to such a realization should be part of the dharma of being fully human. One subset of sachetana prakriti dharma is *tiryak dharma,* the dharma that relates to transverse creatures (animals). The other subset is *atiryak dharma,* which is the dharma of vertical creatures (humans). It is an essential characteristic of the latter that they should at least strive for the lofty ideals their physical construction implies.

The first step in the search for health and well-being—that is, enlightenment—is coming into the light of the knowledge of the true self. It includes eliminating suffering to make humans "fully human" and guiding them to a life that extends beyond the merely physical. True health thus demands an extension of the being to the heights of divinity. Humans should be invested and seek to invest themselves with love, serenity, and due humility in the face of the divine. Furthermore, dharma insists that life cannot be lived "separately." Health is not, and cannot be, an individual affair. It is a community—indeed, a cosmic—affair. Individuation is the root cause of all suffering. A community, even a yoga community, sickens when its individual members do not extend the bonds of unity to one another through the exercise of divine awareness and purusha dharma. The community sickens when its members fail to alleviate their mutual suffering through a benevolent "knowing" of the truth that stands behind each other's existence. Dharma insists that human-heartedness, benevolence, and compassion be a full part of wellness, for that is the way that suffering ends and the absolute is restored.

True health is powerfully radiative, seeking to transcend the boundaries of self and to encompass all. As Anne O'Brien now describes, when seekers grow in health through practice, their benevolence also grows as they seek to unite with others, to become at one with other seekers—and through that with all.

What a wonderful experience of fellowship to be a part of this book. With each author I work with, each interview undertaken, the expansiveness and diversity of yoga resounds. Yet so does the intimacy and familiarity of the yoga community. It is deeply satisfying to feel the interconnectedness of teachers and practitioners from around the world sharing the same human condition, following the yogic path.

The "sound wave" that is yoga resonates through this family of contributors. It is a wave that echoes and reverberates through all yoga practitioners everywhere. Some yogis are deep in the wave, living yoga intensely; yoga is their being; they are part of the "orchestra." Others hear the sound softly or even faintly; perhaps it is daily background music, a weekly concert, or an occasional crescendo experience. All yogis are connected to this vital yogic pulse, individually and in community, this practice that invites us to live humbly and harmoniously with courage and clarity.

The sound wave of yoga has been here from before the first AUM to today. Sometimes the practice is quiet in the world; other times (as now), it is a strong sound and the vibration is powerful. Who struck the first yogic note, plucked the first string? The One, the Spirit, Vedic scholars, Patanjali? Does it matter? For us in this era, B. K. S. Iyengar is the master musician and conductor who has struck the note that powerfully reverberates. And how complex and rich that note is! The practice that was honed from the intense individual practice of one man going deeply inside himself created an energy that cannot be contained in one being. It must be shared. His gift to the world of *Light on Yoga* awakened the individual and collective consciousness to the richness of this tradition.

Yoga is replete with paradoxes; the deeply personal, individual practice of yoga is at the same time a group exploration. Yoga classes, intensives, and retreats are not full just because students want to practice asanas or meditate or breathe. This fundamentally solitary human journey is enlivened and enriched by company. We learn from and help our fellow learners, sharing in others' joys as they accomplish a pose or gain insight. Coming together to practice, to learn, to inquire, and to discover is contagious. Individuals practice, play, and tune the instrument of their bodies and harmonize together. If, as Patanjali said, one of the aims of yoga is ultimately to discover that one's inner voice is the voice of all beings, how better to discover that unity than in community?

In my life, it seems that I have had hidden yoga ushers guiding me to people and experiences that have expanded my fellowship of practice:

- To live in London, find Edward Clark, practice with his company, and experience a taste of beauty
- To study sirsasana sequences with Dona Holleman in my own town
- To meet a man in yoga class who would become my husband
- To appreciate an amazing group of people who call themselves my students
- To have a friend in Rodney Yee
- To meet others from all corners of the globe and share the common language of yoga
- To be in the presence of a teacher from whom all of us in the room feel the magic
- To know Kofi and appreciate his intellectual depth and deep dedication to his guru
- To teach in community with wonderful teachers

We all have these magical experiences—the connection is yoga, yoga in company with others.

As seekers on the path, we always have more to learn, to share, to compose. As I reread *Light on Life,* how affirming it is to hear Mr. Iyengar proclaim that even he is still learning. He remains fully immersed in *svadhyaya,* finding new depths in his instrument, and in sharing those finely tuned discoveries with his worldwide community. I am inspired by Mr. Iyengar's dedication and curiosity, and I hope that I may retain that essence of humility, that place of unknowingness in my practice where I, too, may remain open to new music and continue to offer and share what

I learn. Thank you, Mr. Iyengar, for continuing to strike the note, increase the volume, tune the techniques of the practice of yoga, and give us the tools to continue to compose symphonies.

᳚

ANNE O'BRIEN has practiced yoga for many years and has taught since 1990. She has enjoyed the great fortune to live in several countries and feed her curiosity about life and yoga. Anne has studied in the United States, England, Mexico, and India with master teachers in several yogic traditions and continues to draw on the richness of study and discoveries on her mat to enrich her practice and teaching. Her yoga path has included working at *Yoga Journal,* establishing and directing a yoga teacher–training school, leading retreats, and assisting in the compilation and editing of this book. Her yoga and life are deeply enriched by her family, her students, and her community.

Sri B. K. S. Iyengar

My "Grand" Uncle

KAUSTHUB DESIKACHAR

We once again hear about B. K. S. Iyengar from a family member—someone who has known him his whole life.

My earliest recollection of Sri B. K. S. Iyengar takes me back to an important milestone in the history of our family. The year was 1985. My grandmother had just died, and we were waiting for the entire family to come together before completing the necessary rituals, which traditionally are spread out over a minimum period of thirteen days.

When Sri Iyengar arrived at our home, the first person he met was my grandfather, his brother-in-law. Few words were spoken. The moment of greeting was shaded by sadness. My grandfather had lost his pillar of support, his wife of more than five decades. Sri Iyengar had lost his sister and the person who had helped him make his first connection to the world of yoga. She was important, in a very special way, to both men. Their silent exchange of mutual consolation remains fresh in my memory to this day.

Over the next week, as we participated in the funeral rituals, although our grief was great, the mood of our family became somewhat lighter. As the days passed, I watched Sri Iyengar cheer those around him, even as he dealt with his own sadness. Everyone respected him and recognized that he was a giant in the world of yoga, yet no one felt intimidated in his presence. He was unpretentious and gracious.

Before Sri Iyengar took his leave to return to his home, my father invited me and my two siblings to take our granduncle's blessings. I remember vividly Sri Iyengar's words to me: "Be a good boy and make your father proud, just like he is making his father proud." I said that I would, and then I ran off to play with my friends. This is one of my first significant memories of Sri Iyengar, and it is still precious to me today.

In the following year, my father began teaching a children's yoga class at the Krishnamacharya Yoga Mandiram (KYM). I joined as a student when I was about ten or eleven and practiced with the other children of the KYM teachers. At the age of thirteen, I became one of the class's teachers.

To inspire us to learn the postures, the KYM hosted an annual film presentation that we still put on for the children's yoga class. Every year in the summer, we show the children an old 1938 film featuring my grandfather, a young Sri Iyengar, and my grandmother practicing yoga. Back in 1986–87, when I saw this video, it was a momentous occasion. At the time, video technology was in its infancy in India and extremely expensive, so we were thrilled to have the opportunity to watch a video. We told all of our friends and quickly became the coolest kids in school.

However, the hype about "video" was short-lived and long forgotten when we actually watched what was on the film. We were astounded. Although this was a silent film, it spoke clearly and openly to our hearts. Every student wanted to be Krishnamacharya or Iyengar, and in the following weeks, months, and years, these two men continued to serve as our inspiration. Viewing this film was a turning point in our yoga education.

In 1989, my grandfather passed away. It was one of the most significant moments in the life of our family, as not only was he a grandfather, but also a teacher to my father, my uncle, my granduncle (Sri Iyengar), and so many other people who had passed through the doors of our home and into his heart. My grandfather was one of the greatest yoga teachers and healers of modern times.

My father was calm and quiet, but I knew that he was hurting over the loss of his father and his teacher of three decades. His face lit up when Sri Iyengar arrived, and their mutual sadness somehow seemed to bring strength to my father. No words were said, but in the silence, volumes were spoken. I was still a boy at the time—only fourteen—but old enough to remember and recall things. Maybe at the time, though, I was not old enough to understand the depth of human emotion connected with the loss of a teacher and father.

Before he left, I remember hearing Sri Iyengar tell my father and mother to count on him for support whenever they needed it, and he has proved that he meant these words many times over in the years since my grandfather's death.

There are clearly differences in the way yoga is taught by Mr. Iyengar and the way it was taught by my grandfather and today by my father, but the bond of family remains strong and deeply respectful. It is also clear from Sri Iyengar's own commentary that as a young boy, he experienced difficult moments with his teacher. Yet I have seen that he holds his teacher in the highest regard—in the same way his own students regard him.

On a visit to Pune a few years ago, my father asked me to take along a group of long-time students to visit Sri Iyengar on the occasion of his eighty-fifth birthday celebrations. We had received a personal invitation as family members, but my father thought it was important for my students to visit and seek the blessings of Sri Iyengar. When we called to ask him if this would be acceptable, he readily agreed.

Before we left for Pune, I told my students that it was possible that Mr. Iyengar would meet us along with his own students, and they must not expect anything more. When we arrived, however, we were in for a surprise. Sri Iyengar invited us to his center, and we spent nearly three hours together while he patiently answered all of our questions. Every one of my students was overwhelmed by his generosity.

And this was not all. When the time for the evening public lecture drew near, Sri Iyengar's students started to arrive. We were happy to wait with them until the evening programs would begin, but Sri Iyengar invited us to his home, arranged a special snack of saffron milk and other local delicacies for us, and introduced us to his family and students. This was totally unexpected, and we cherish the memory of this event.

More surprises awaited us on this trip. When the evening lecture began, Mr. Iyengar insisted on honoring my father and introducing him as the ambassador of Krishnamacharya's teaching. The warmth and sincerity with which he spoke about my father, who is also my teacher, touched me deeply. I realized then why my father always said that Sri Iyengar was his "favorite uncle." While Sri Iyengar's technical expertise is what impresses most at first, it is his openheartedness that always comes to my mind when I think of him.

In the few instances that I have had the opportunity to contact Mr. Iyengar directly and request small favors, he has always responded positively and with the greatest promptness. In the last two years, I wrote to him twice—once to request an essay to be included in a biography of my grandfather that I was writing, titled *The Yoga of the Yogi*. My second request was related to a tribute to my father that the KYM was publishing to commemorate the thirtieth anniversary of the founding of the Krishnamacharya Yoga Mandiram. On both occasions, I heard back from Sri Iyengar almost immediately. That a man of his stature took the time to read my simple letters and respond so quickly is a mark of his humanity, which to me, personally, is the mark of true greatness in any person.

Mr. Iyengar's work in the field of asana is phenomenal, and it is probably the reason why so many in the West are now practicing yoga. I myself have many students who have come to me after beginning their yoga journey through Iyengar Yoga.

Yet while a great deal is known about Sri Iyengar's work in the field of yoga, especially asanas, I urge people to move beyond technique and look at him as a human being as well: as a teacher, a devoted father, a caring husband, a friend to many, and a champion of yoga.

This is why I have chosen to share some of my personal memories of Sri Iyengar. Much is said and known about his work in yoga, but there may not be many who can share simple, everyday stories about Sri Iyengar, a giant in the world of yoga, who continues to inspire practitioners around the world.

I am proud that he is my "grand" uncle.

CHENNAI, INDIA
NOVEMBER 2006

§

KAUSTHUB DESIKACHAR is the son of T. K. V. Desikachar and the grandson of B. K. S. Iyengar's guru, Krishnamacharya. He lives and studies with his father and is world renowned in his own right as a yoga teacher and yoga therapy consultant. Among his varied writings, he authored *The Yoga of the Yogi,* a book on the life and teaching of his grandfather, and co-authored *The Viniyoga of Yoga: Applying Yoga for Healthy Living* and *The Vedic Chant Companion* with his father.

Yoga in Daily Life

DONA HOLLEMAN

> Peace and harmony are wonderful words. Harmony is the language of
> the heart and not that of the head. Being the language of the heart, it is
> very difficult to express the experience of inner quietness. Yoga is the
> means to attain it.
> —B. K. S. IYENGAR, *Astadala Yoga Mala*

> Happy is the man who knows how to distinguish the real from the un-
> real, the eternal from the transient and the good from the pleasant by his
> discrimination and wisdom. Twice blessed is he who knows true love
> and can love all God's creatures. He who works selflessly for the welfare
> of others with love in his heart is thrice blessed.
> —B. K. S. IYENGAR, *Light on Yoga*

> Yoga on the mat is all very well. But as Dona Holleman describes, we
> should take it off the mat sometimes.

Cisco is standing between the trees, the sun through the leaves making mottled patterns on his coat. When I approach, he looks up and
then comes toward me with a soft nicker. Standing before me, he lowers
his head so I can caress him on his forehead, and I reflect for the
umpteenth time with wonder how far we have traveled together. Cisco
is a rescue horse, and without my forty-five years of yoga, I do not know
if we could have arrived where we are now, standing next to each other,
content to be in each other's company.

Yoga is an age-old philosophy, but like all philosophies, it remains
sterile unless applied in daily life and not confined merely to memoriz-
ing words and concepts. As many know, the word *yoga* means "union."
There are as many interpretations of this word *union* as there are yoga
practitioners. At this moment, reflecting on the struggle of the last three

years with Cisco, of the peace at the end—my heart overflowing with love for this massive, gentle creature, who taught me that yoga has to be applied in a 360-degree circle, including everything, even old, abused horses—I am in union with all of life, with all living beings, with the matrix of life.

Yoga has traveled through many centuries and brought forth many great teachers. In our times, we have witnessed Babaji, Yogananda, Aurobindo, Krishnamacharya, Pattabhi Jois, T. K. V. Desikachar, B. K. S. Iyengar, and many others. It has been my good fortune, together with thousands of others, to have been a student of B. K. S. Iyengar. It was my double good fortune to be one of the first to travel to India in the early sixties, witnessing the birth of "Iyengar Yoga." It has also been of great fascination to see how all of the thousands of students of Krishnamacharya, most notably Pattabhi Jois, B. K. S. Iyengar, and Desikachar, bring out different aspects of this teacher, thus enriching the original teachings.

B. K. S. Iyengar, with his great interest in the physical-therapeutic aspect of yoga, has undoubtedly brought this practice of yoga to a new dimension and has contributed to enriching the legacy of thousands of years of yoga. As such, he has helped many people to overcome their physical problems and alleviate their suffering.

Suffering is not confined to human beings, however. Actually, it is often human beings who inflict suffering on their relatives, the animals, in a very "unyogic" way. Meeting Cisco was a highlight in my life, and the chance of my life to apply all that I learned from B. K. S. Iyengar and yoga philosophy. Working with Cisco required physical control; discipline combined with suppleness; the ability to let go at the right moment; and above all, the facing of one's fears, doubts, and "unskillfulness"—just as in our daily yoga practice. But there is a difference between making one's own body a perfect instrument of skillfulness and one's own mind clear and confident, and having to do the same thing with a five-hundred-kilo flight-animal that has been abused and wants nothing more in life than to run as far away as possible from anything human. Here *karuna* (compassion) has to bloom fully, or the struggle to "win" is in vain. To move with control and gentleness, and at the same time with determination; to not allow confusion to enter into the game;

to make all movement a tai chi dance, a *vipashyana,* a meditation, a perfect asana, in order to not set off the flight response—this was an extremely rewarding yogic exercise and one that would probably have been much harder to accomplish if I had not practiced yoga for so long. Thus, I am greatly in debt to my teacher, B. K. S. Iyengar, who taught me all those things and much more.

Each yoga student has to find his or her own niche to carry the flame forward. Each yoga practitioner is different and will speak to a different audience. It takes integrity and courage to find one's niche and to carry the teaching of one's teacher forward on one's destined path. One thing I have learned in my dealings with Cisco and my other rescue animals is that without love and compassion, any practice—yogic or otherwise—is a practice in vain isolation.

☙

DONA HOLLEMAN is one of the leading pioneer women yoga teachers in the world, with more than forty-five years of study and experience. Born in a Japanese concentration camp in Thailand during the Second World War and raised in Indonesia in the early fifties, Dona became interested in Asian philosophies, especially Buddhism and Taoism. In the mid-fifties, she became a student of Jiddu Krishnamurti, and also began practicing yoga. Dona remains convinced that yoga is the most complete form of exercise for interacting with the forces of life. It was through Krishnamurti that she met B. K. S. Iyengar. Dona spent two years in India (1964 and 1969) studying with Mr. Iyengar and founded the B. K. S. Iyengar Yoga Work Group in the Netherlands. She has taught many teachers who have gone on to earn international reputations. In the early seventies, Dona moved to Italy and became an intimate friend of Vanda Scaravelli, a concert pianist and student of B. K. S. Iyengar. Dona spent many years studying the piano with her in Florence, discovering the correlation between music, yoga, dance, and religion. She started the B. K. S. Iyengar School in Florence, and taught there for the next twenty-five years. She currently teaches at the Epona Yoga Studio in Soiano del Lago in the Lake Garda area. She is the author of several books, including the best-selling *Dancing the Body of Light.*

Kriya Yoga

Transformation through Practice—
A Western Perspective

GARY KRAFTSOW

> The whole educative thrust of yoga is to make things go right in our lives. But we all know that an apple that appears perfect on the outside can have been eaten away by an invisible worm on the inside. Yoga is not about appearances. It is about finding and eradicating the worm, so that the whole apple, from skin inward, can be perfect and a healthy one. . . . It is natural for worms to eat apples. In yoga we simply do not want to be the apple that is rotted from inside.
> —B. K. S. Iyengar, *Light on Life*

Gary Kraftsow now tells us how we can remove the worm from the apple.

> *Tapah svadhyaya ishvara pranidhanani kriya yogah*
> *Samadhi bhavanarthah klesha tanukaranarthas ca*★

The classical yoga tradition developed in the context of the spiritual traditions of India. Thus, yoga evolved as a means of recognizing and ultimately eliminating the root causes of suffering that have plagued humanity, as the ancients said, since beginningless time. These causes are as prevalent today as they have ever been.

★ *The Yoga Sutras of Patanjali*, II:1–2.

According to this view, suffering is largely the result of a fundamental misapprehension concerning the nature of who we are and what is going on in this life—a misapprehension that lies at the root of and distorts our perception. We are confused at a very basic level about our own identity; we are unaware of this confusion; and as a result, we develop all kinds of false identifications. According to the yoga tradition, it is this misapprehension, and the subsequent identification with the "me," that is the field in which all the other seeds of human suffering grow: greed, anger, fear, and delusion, for example.

Thus, the fundamental goals of yoga are to reduce and ultimately to eliminate these seeds of suffering by making the mind quiet and clear and by helping us to achieve our full potential as human beings. It is toward these goals that the science of kriya yoga, as presented by Patanjali in his *Yoga Sutras*, leads us.

This science rests on the recognition that, as human beings, we are constantly involved in activity and that our activity can either reinforce our conditioning or be the ground for positive change. As such, kriya yoga practice is linked directly to our daily activities and to the transformation of our relationship to those activities, as well as to the conscious and sustained application of certain practices oriented toward self-development.

In relation to this fundamental human condition, the image of a seed is appropriate. A seed sprouts, shoots up, and becomes a plant or a tree. In the same way, say the ancients, emotions such as anger, frustration, sadness, jealousy, envy, fear, loneliness, anxiety, and depression exist within us as seeds waiting to sprout. In other words, we act continuously. Most of our daily activity follows conditioned patterns that we have acquired since childhood. In new situations, we rely on old patterns of behavior and activity. Thus, our actions serve to reinforce our patterns. For example, consider the way we move our bodies. If we had a short video sequence of ourselves walking down the street—today, last week, last month, last year, two years ago, five years ago, even ten years ago—so that we could digitally view our walking sequence over time, we would see that certain patterns condition the way we walk. Whenever we walk, we reinforce those patterns. And this phenomenon of patterning is true at every level of our systems—from the way we move our bodies, breathe, communicate, and emote to the way we relate to food, sex, people, and the world around us.

The classical teaching of Patanjali on the purpose of kriya yoga can be expressed poetically as follows: to reduce the seeds of suffering and to awaken the higher potentials of our minds. In keeping with this purpose, personal practice is said to have two fundamental orientations: the reduction and ultimate elimination of undesirable or negative characteristics, dysfunctional patterns, and impurities from our systems; and the awakening of our inherent potential, discriminative awareness, or the wisdom-mind.

The yoga teachings are grounded in the recognition of this reality and the suffering that results. But they also acknowledge the existence of these within each expanded consciousness—that is, once we get in touch with our own suffering. In fact, the ancients suggested that the first wisdom is the recognition of suffering, and from that recognition arises the desire to end suffering; it is exactly at this point that the kriya yoga teachings become meaningful.

KRIYA YOGA: A THREEFOLD APPROACH TO PRACTICE

Kriya yoga can be understood as a threefold practice (*sadhana*), or a threefold approach to practice. The three elements of kriya yoga are *tapas, svadhyaya,* and *Ishvara pranidhana.* Traditionally, these refer to specific activities, but they may also be understood in the context of an overall relationship to action. We will now present the teachings of kriya yoga as they apply to our day-to-day experience, giving examples to illustrate each point.

Tapas: The Purifying Heat

The purifying heat of tapas concerns mastery of the body and senses (*kaya indriya siddhih tapasah*).

Tapas comes from the Sanskrit root *tap,* which means "to cook." The heat of the cooking process purifies and transforms. The word *tapas* is also linked to the idea of deprivation. In order to deprive ourselves of something that we are habituated to, we must resist acting in our habit-ual patterns. This resistance creates a kind of internal heat that purifies, strengthens, and transforms us. Concepts and practices of intentional self-deprivation can be found in all of the ascetic traditions of the world. The word *tapas* is, in fact, often translated "austerities."

In classical religious traditions, we can find many differing forms of ascetic practices, from fasting to self-flagellation. The most common form of tapas is fasting. Throughout the year there are certain times dur-ing which partial or complete fasts were prescribed. The more extreme means of tapas were reserved for monks or ascetics.

An example of extreme tapas was demonstrated in the life of Saint Francis of Assisi, who renounced his wealth and lived like a beggar. He went without shoes, dressed in rough clothes, and begged for food. In medieval times, this extreme form of ascetic practice represented a view that the soul was imprisoned in the body and that the mortification of the flesh was a means to free the soul. At the end of his short life, Saint Francis confessed to his disciples that he had "abused this donkey," refer-ring to his body, and exhorted them to avoid such extreme asceticism.

The story of the life of Buddha explains that he, too, practiced this type of extreme asceticism until he discovered the middle way. It is said that on hearing a simple fisherman playing a stringed instrument, he rec-ognized that too loose a string would not sing, that too tight a string would break. And it was at this point that he renounced the path of ex-treme tapas.

The practices prescribed by yoga are not about self-abuse. They are intentional means of purifying and strengthening our systems. They may be understood to be any discipline designed to reduce physical, emo-tional, or mental impurities. In this context, tapas refers to a process of "getting rid" of something that is not desirable in our system (*klehsas*)—ranging from chronic subliminal muscular contraction, to toxicity in the colon, to deep-rooted emotional and behavioral patterns.

According to the ancients, without tapas, there can be no real success in yoga. The various means and methods of tapas used in yoga practice include asana, pranayama, and meditation, as well as other actions—such as dietary restrictions, fasting, refraining from idle gossip, or other forms of selective renunciation—that serve to break our habits. Controlling breath, limiting speech, and restricting diet are said to be the three most important areas for tapas. And it is to these ends that we are taught to eat less, speak less, and work on our breathing.

When we do asana practice, we bring our attention to our normally unconscious movement patterns. Through asana, we are able to develop more useful movement patterns, as well as purify and strengthen our systems. But if we are doing asana the same way all the time and it has become a mechanical practice, it would be tapas to stop doing that practice and go for a hike instead.

When we fast, we purify our bodies; we gain an appreciation of the nourishment that we usually take for granted. We also have the opportunity to recognize how much we rely on food for our sense of emotional well-being and even as a source of entertainment. When we avoid idle gossip, we save energy, and our minds may become more focused. When we control our breathing, we interrupt an automatic process that is going on at every moment. This is a very deep and profound method of tapas that is immediately accessible to any practitioner. Though many in our society have well-developed asana practices, few have deep pranayama practices.

There are things we desire that are harmful for us. There are also things we desire that are beneficial, or at least not harmful. It is easy to understand how it can be useful to give up things we are attracted to that are harmful. This is a form of tapas. For example, we may be attracted to practicing certain asanas because we are apparently able to do them well, even though they are harmful to our structure. Recognizing this, tapas would be either to eliminate them from our practice all together or to modify them in such a way that they are no longer harmful to our structure—even if that means they do not appear to be as picture-perfect. Another example would be giving up a habit like smoking cigarettes or drinking coffee that we may enjoy but that may cause unnecessary stress to our system.

On the other hand, tapas may sometimes involve giving up something we like that is not harmful to us at all. This form of disciplined renunciation—in which we give up something that we like—is known as *tyaga*. It should be done carefully in order to avoid any harm to the body or the mind. The ancients suggested that this form of selective renunciation will accelerate our progress in personal practice.

We all know how we can be slaves to our habits and addictions. Consider New Year's resolutions. Many of us are lucky if they survive the month of January. Before we know it, the strength of our habits takes over, and we find ourselves acting out the same behavior that we intended to stop. The various methods of tapas are a means to strengthen ourselves so that we are able to break the cycle of habitual and addictive behavior and, as it were, come out of slavery. They challenge us to wake up out of the momentum of our daily lives, to pay attention, and to look at life in a new way.

In applying the concept of tapas not to specific actions, but to our entire relationship to action, we might look at the quality of the attention we bring to any given moment. In our daily activities, we are rarely 100 percent focused on what we are doing. Often, tensions and other preoccupations divide our attention. Tapas requires that we cut through distractions and bring our full attention to the present moment. To do this, we must break patterns, and that requires energy. The means and methods of personal practice are designed to help us build sufficient energy to break free of our conditioned responses.

If tapas remains only at the level of the body, its beneficial effects will not be lasting. If done as a kind of penance without deep self-reflection, it may not help us make deep changes and may even harm us. One of my acquaintances, after making many mistakes in his marriage, decided to radically restrict his diet as a kind of penance. Though the diet was actually beneficial for his health, it became a mechanical process that didn't impact his behavior. Not long after, he repeated similar mistakes in his relationship and finally ended up divorced. I have worked with many students who originally went to a gym or who practiced extreme forms of asana with the intention of improving their condition and who ended up in surgery. In both of these cases, though effort was present, something was missing—in the first case, tapas without self-reflection was ineffective; in the second, it was harmful. So taking a lesson from Saint Francis and the Buddha, we can say that our tapas should not be adverse to our physical health or our mental composure (*chitta prasadanam*).

Svadhyaya: The Reflecting Mirror

Svadhyayat Ista Devata Samprayogah
(Return to Oneself, Discover the Divine)
—*The Yoga Sutras of Patanjali*, II:44.

The second element of kriya yoga is svadhyaya. It is a beautiful word. Its verbal root is *i,* which means "to go" or "to move." *Adhi* is a verbal prefix meaning "toward." *Adhyaya* then is a verbal derivative meaning "to move toward." *Sva* is a reflexive pronoun meaning "self" or "one's own." *Svadhyaya* then means—literally and etymologically—"to move toward one's self," "to return to oneself," "to come back to who we are" by some means. If we can understand tapas as purifying or refining our systems, then svadhyaya is self-reflection, coming deeper into a self-understanding and a self-awareness.

Tapas makes us fit for svadhyaya. Tapas cleans the vessel; svadhyaya looks at the vessel. There is a mutual relationship. After svadhyaya, we clean the vessel some more and then look at it again.

This suggests that we find a means to discover who, in essence, we are. It means to reflect deeply on our actions, to use all of our actions not only to achieve something external, but as a mirror to see ourselves more deeply in terms of what we are doing and how we are motivated. It means piercing through the veil of our self-image. It means inquiring into the nature of our being through deep inner reflection. This implies looking honestly at our behavior, our motivations, and all of the strategies we use to maintain our self-image.

Classically, *adhyayanam* is a technical term that involves chanting texts and mantras that have been learned exactly from a teacher and that are about *moksha. Svadhyayanam* refers specifically to chanting texts and mantras that are part of one's lineage—in other words, that have been passed down by one's ancestors.

In a more general sense, svadhyaya suggests that the study of sacred or inspirational texts can result in insight into the human condition. Such classical texts include the *Yoga Sutras* and the *Bhagavad Gita,* the Bible, the Talmud, various writings of the saints, or any spiritual or inspiring text—again, not abstractly or academically, but as a means of understanding ourselves more deeply. It also means chanting, using a mantra, or singing hymns. It means receiving *darshana* (teachings from a particular text) from the guru or going to hear a sermon.

All these activities are seen as mirrors that reflect back to us our true nature. The ritual of confession in the Roman Catholic faith is an example of a different kind of svadhyaya process. In confession, we reflect on our past actions and expose ourselves to ourselves before God. In this ritual, the priest serves primarily as a medium through which the confession is transmitted and the prescribed penance and absolution is received. In both the Jewish and Islamic faiths, to take two different examples, repenting and seeking forgiveness are integral parts of the process of purification and illumination. And in yet another form of svadhyaya, the Tibetan Buddhists contemplate the "great thoughts that turn the mind" from the worldly toward the spiritual life.

In all of these contexts, spiritually inspiring teachings are tools to help us understand ourselves and, through that understanding, to change our attitudes and behavior. When we are practicing with this self-reflective quality, we will deepen our self-understanding.

This teaching is not meant only for those dedicated to the spiritual life. It has great practical meaning for all of us who recognize that there is room for improvement in our lives. In this context, svadhyaya represents a process through which, at any given moment, we can assess where we are in relation to many things. In this sense, it is like tuning our inner navigator. Am I at the right place at the right moment? Where am I now, and where am I going? What is my direction, and what are my aspirations? What are my responsibilities? What are my priorities? We often find ourselves on cruise control, acting habitually, and being so swept up in the momentum of our daily responsibilities that we fail to take the time to check where we are or where we are headed. As our lives are in motion, svadhyaya at this level is an ongoing process. Where I am today is different from where I will be tomorrow.

If, in this process, we find that we are not where we want to be, we must find a means to develop new attitudes and new behaviors. The mantras and textual studies offered by the classical traditions function as references from which we can measure where we are. If we come back to the image of the inner navigator, then the mantras and texts are like the polestar, which shows us true north. Since most of us live in a society with a predominantly secular orientation, it is difficult for us to use these ancient texts as mirrors in which we can see ourselves. In this case, other means are recommended.

Svadhyaya is also the ability to look in the mirror of how people are responding to us and let that be an opportunity to understand something about the way we are operating. For example, one of the greatest opportunities we have to see ourselves is in the mirror of relationships. It is difficult to hide aspects of our personality from our mates, our parents, and/or our children. Even with intimate friends, our pretenses are not likely to endure long. And while we are quite able to play the game of avoidance, if not self-deception, in the mirror of our relationships, it is difficult to hide—that is, if we are willing to look, to avoid deflecting messages that would be valuable for us to hear, and to avoid playing the victim or becoming self-righteous. Thus, svadhyaya suggests that we can use all of our activities as mirrors to see something about ourselves—a way of coming deeper into self-understanding—for we can use the feedback from all of our interpersonal interactions and reactions. However, svadhyaya is also suggestive of a mirror to remind us of our higher potential.

Classical means of svadhyaya include using a mantra, reading a text, or sitting with a spiritual master (guru). The ancients used the word *darshanam,* which means "something like a mirror," to describe the teaching contained in a particular group of sacred texts. They used the same word to describe what happens when we sit with a spiritual master. We take darshanam from the guru. The idea is that when we study a sacred text or sit with a spiritual master, we see ourselves reflected back. We see all of our neuroses, our small-mindedness, our pettiness mirrored completely back at us. At the same time, we see beyond our current state to something like the divine potential. And that, too, is who we are.

Svadhyaya is ultimately a means to reach that higher potential, a way into the interior where our "true selves" reside. But in the process, svadhyaya implies doing some reflection on how we are operating, how we are behaving. We can use many things as mirrors for that purpose. Though mantras, texts, and spiritual masters were classically suggested, we can use our wives, husbands, lovers, friends, yoga students, or yoga teachers.

Everybody. Everything. All of our activity can be an opportunity to see more deeply who we are, how we are operating, and how we can refine ourselves, how we can become more clear and more appropriate in our behavior. This is very important. Thus, we see that svadhyaya leads back into tapas on the one hand and toward Ishvara pranidhana on the other, for each of these elements of kriya yoga, while independent, is interdependent and mutually supportive in practice. We cannot truly consider tapas separate from svadhyaya. An intelligent practice of tapas must include svadhyaya. For example, if we do an intensive asana without being adequately self-reflective, we may end up destabilizing our hips, creating vulnerability in our lower back, and ruining our knees. Instead, if we consider that the asana practice itself is a mirror, helping us understand more about who we are, we are much more likely to avoid injury.

This is a tricky point, because many of us are drawn to styles of asana practice that reinforce our existing tendencies. For example, if we are the fast-paced, hyperactive type, we might be drawn toward a very active practice—one that makes us sweat and generates lots of heat—whereas what we may really need is a more soothing and calming practice. If, instead, we are the slow-moving, sluggish type, we might be drawn to a gentle practice that is very relaxing, whereas what we may really need is a more active and stimulating practice.

This is tapas without svadhyaya. Not only will this approach reinforce our patterns, it can lead to injury and, ultimately, to illness at some level. So when we are practicing, we must look carefully at who we are and what is actually happening. In the tapas, there must be svadhyaya so that we learn more about ourselves. With svadhyaya, we have a kind of constant feedback mechanism, feeling what is actually happening in our system. In short, tapas accompanied by svadhyaya ensures that tapas is not an abusive, mindless application of technology, but a transformational activity.

As we go deeper and deeper into this process of self-investigation and self-discovery, as we go deeper into our selves, according to the ancients, we will slowly discover or uncover the divine. The ancients say that svadhyaya develops tapas, that tapas develops svadhyaya, and that together they help us awaken to the spiritual dimension of life. One great teacher has described this process with the image of a drop of water dissolving into the ocean. At first, we wonder whether we are the drop of water. But eventually we discover that we are not the drop, but the water, and that we have always only been the water, never the drop.

Ishvara Pranidhana: The Refuge

Ishvara Pranidhanat Samadhi Siddhih
(Open Your Heart, Master Your Mind)
—The Yoga Sutras of Patanjali, II:45.

The third element of kriya yoga is Ishvara pranidhana. Although *Ishvara* is the Sanskrit equivalent of the word *God,* it is not personalized. The ancient teachers of yoga were not offering a theological testament on the godhead, but rather a deep psychological analysis of the transformational potential of opening the human mind and heart to the divine. In the *Yoga Sutras,* Ishvara is described as a being without suffering or the seeds of suffering, and not as the Creator God of traditional religious doctrine. In fact, it is for this reason that the traditional religious schools of Hinduism rejected yoga philosophically, though they appropriated its practices. In this context, Ishvara represents that living symbol of the divine that is in our hearts. For the Christian, it could be Jesus; for the Muslim, it could be Allah; for the Hindu, it could be Krishna; for the Buddhist, it could be Buddha; and for the atheist, it would represent whatever is the highest value in his or her heart.

Pranidhana is a technical term usually translated as "surrender." It consists of the root *dha* (to sustain), plus the verbal prefixes *pra* (in all directions) and *ni* (deeply or intensely). The implication of this word is the profound recognition of that which sustains us and gives meaning to every dimension of our lives. It is a kind of faith—in the sense of the "place" where we put or give our hearts. It implies an element of self-sacrifice—the sacrifice of our own self-importance.

In a traditional religious context, Ishvara pranidhana means the recognition of God as the source of one's being. For the mystic, it means that God is there at every moment, all that is seen is God, and God is all that is seen. God is always present, in everyone, in everything, and in every situation. For the devotee, it means standing in awe before the mystery and in gratitude for the gift of life, dedicating that life to God. This recognition is celebrated by the religious through communal and personal songs of praise, as well as through blessings, prayers, rituals, rites, and offerings.

Consider, for example, the ritual of Communion at the pinnacle of the Roman Catholic Mass. In this ritual, the individuals of the congregation are communing, merging, with the mystical body of Christ through the sacrament of bread and wine. Consider the completion stage practices at the pinnacle of the tantric Buddhists deity yoga. In this ritual, the individuals of the *sangha* (congregation) merge and become one with the deity.

These rituals, however, are for the faithful. In our contemporary and secular society, fewer and fewer of us are able to confidently embrace the spiritual heritage of our ancestors, even though many of us long to experience this quality in our lives. But we must ultimately be authentic and true to ourselves. We cannot fake at this level. Unfortunately for many of us, the rituals of our ancestors have lost their meaning. We are constantly exposed to faiths and religions distinctly different from the ones of our childhood. Science and technology are rapidly and radically changing the way we live. It is as if we are entering a collective identity crisis. And in the midst of this crisis, we are longing to find our way back to faith.

This is the greatness of kriya yoga, which from ancient times has echoed a nonsectarian path that will lead us beyond suffering and in the direction of realization. Stripped of all sectarian religious images, we have seen that *tapas* can be understood as "being present" and *svadhyaya* as "being reflective." In this contest, Ishvara pranidhaha can be understood in relation to attitudes of openness, availability, humility, and gratitude. There is an implicit knowing that we are not in control of everything and cannot know what is ahead. In this sense, there is a surrendering of control and an openness to receive whatever life brings. This attitude is antidotal to the pervasive fixation around "me and mine" that dominates most all of us most of the time. It implies an open attitude toward our own mistakes and a sincerity in relation to repentance. Ultimately, it is faith, deep in our hearts, in our potential to become free from suffering and to achieve our destiny as human beings. The ancients said that when this quality is in our hearts, all our action is done as an offering, without regard to personal gain.

I remember a woman asking me to help her with the idea of surrender. She told me that her husband was a marine and would never go for the idea of surrender. After considering the implications of what she was saying, I asked if he could relate to it better as "dedication to the mission."

Another woman, who had been a yoga teacher for five years, came to see me. She was a professional psychotherapist and an avid trekker—very bright and very tough. She had also been doing mindfulness meditation, a popular form of Buddhist meditation, for ten years so she could sit and control her breath. However, at a certain point in one of her private sessions with me, she realized that, in her words, "something was missing"—something in her heart. It was the Ishvara element: the sweetness of devotion. I discovered that she used to go to church as a child, so I taught her a chant—an Italian chant composed by Saint Francis of Assisi, not a Vedic chant—that praises the beauty of nature and gratefully acknowledges it as a gift of God's immense love. That filled her heart and made her practice more meaningful.

How sweet it is to feel how, in my heart
Now, humbly, love is being born
How sweet it is to know that I am no longer alone
But am part of an immense life
How generous the splendor that surrounds me
Gift of Him and His immense Love.★

What we can see from this is that Ishvara pranidhana is fundamentally about a relationship to something higher than or beyond ourselves. It may be a higher force, as in the context of traditional religious traditions, or it may be in relation to human values, such as kindness and compassion. In either case, it will manifest in our lives as the ability to let go of the tyranny of our self-importance—whether it reveals itself as pride and arrogance, or self-pity and low self-esteem. It will awaken in us attitudes such as gratitude and appreciation. As a result, we will be able to simply wake up in the morning and say, "Ah, I'm alive another day." We will feel grateful in our heart for the gift of this life. We will take the time to look and appreciate the beauty around us. In our relationships, we will be-

---

★ *Dolce Sentire*, Saint Francis of Assisi. Original translation by Gary Kraftsow.

come open to receiving each other with respect and appreciation. And if we make this the spirit and foundation of our practice, then surely, as the Buddhists say, we will have "attained the stream" that will lead us to the river, that will return us to the ocean from whence we came.

GARY KRAFTSOW began his study of yoga in India with T. K. V. Desikachar in 1974. He founded the Maui School of Yoga Therapy in 1983 and received a Viniyoga special diploma from Viniyoga International in Paris soon after. Since then, he has become a renowned speaker and teacher of the Viniyoga methodology, and in 1999, he founded the American Viniyoga Institute. His work on yoga for chronic low back pain and generalized anxiety was funded by the National Institutes of Health. He is the author of *Yoga for Wellness* and *Yoga for Transformation*.

The Union of Body, Mind, and Spirit

JOHN LEEBOLD

In *Yoga Sutra* II:46, Sage Patanjali describes an asana as something that is both steady (*sthira*) and comfortable (*sukha*). But since nothing about the body can be known without the agency of the mind, this does not tell us exactly what it is that should *be* steady and comfortable. Is it the body? Is it the mind? Both? Neither? Guidance on this point comes from the following sutra (II:47), where we are told the effects that the pose should have on the mind. When the body has assumed a suitable posture, it should present possibilities for pleasure and freedom to the mind. These possibilities encourage the mind to understand not only that a release from the totality of bondage imposed by the material world is possible, but that due acquaintance with the infinite should be made immediately. However, the mind can only direct itself toward such an end if all the effort needed to maintain the pose has disappeared. In other words, the practitioner should be exhibiting such a high degree of skill that maintaining the asana is completely effortless. Patanjali confirms that, done this way, asana is a medium for the exploration of consciousness and tells us that the correct posture will free us from all possible oscillations; we will no longer be tossed about by the opposites and dualities so characteristic of this humdrum existence. The essential lesson of asana, therefore, is that no matter what position is adopted, the body should provide an undisturbed and undisturbable physical matrix or framework for the exploration of consciousness. If *samadhi* (enlightenment) is to be experienced, then an asana capable of allowing for it is essential.

This immediately raises the issue of what "health" actually is. Yoga's view is that if the body is anything at all, it is the embodiment of the soul. As such, it is not intended to be an object for enjoyment, but for liberation. The *Upanishads* say, *Nayamatma balahinenalabhyah,* or "The soul cannot be realized by those who are weak or unstable." Therefore, complete stability is essential, and asana is the recommended tool for creating the structural and biomechanical stability that will allow the goal to be attained. John Leebold now compares yoga's search for structural stability with an alternative approach current in the West.

Sri B. K. S. Iyengar first ignited my interest in yoga when I read *Light on Yoga*. We met in Pune in the seventies, at which point I began a journey that combined osteopathy with yoga. I returned regularly to Pune for further studies, being anxious to assimilate Guruji's vast biomechanical knowledge. Since then, like many of his students, I have endeavored to combine yoga with my professional life and interests. I have found that my chosen profession of osteopathy integrates very well with yoga, even though yoga has many other dimensions that transcend the strictly therapeutic.

It was Guruji's insistence on a firm foundation in the asanas, particularly the standing ones, that first prompted my inquiry into how these poses related to the biomechanical and physiological effects I had studied in what osteopaths call "manual medicine." Yoga and osteopathy share many common dicta, and when performed well, yoga asanas definitely correct mechanical dysfunctions.

But yoga brings benefits that are broader and more profound then the merely physical. A practitioner of yoga must, by necessity, be his or her own doctor, philosopher, and scientist. With the guidance of a sound teacher who has trodden the path—or a master such as Guruji— the yogi can learn how to achieve and maintain good health and sound physical and spiritual well-being by balancing nature's forces both inside and out.

The science of osteopathy dates back to the United States' post–Civil War days, when it was introduced in 1874 by Dr. Andrew Taylor Still, a frontier doctor, after years of arduous studies in and concerns over conventional medicine. The first osteopathic school opened in Kirksville, Missouri, in 1892. From the outset, the science included not only anatomy and physiology, but also a philosophy of the integration and restoration of the harmonious functioning of the body, mind, and spirit. Using that philosophy, together with a clinical diagnosis and treatment, osteopaths seek to restore the inherent biomechanics of the body and its systems.

Compared to osteopathy, *yoga vidya* (the body of yogic knowledge) dates to the Vedic period more than five thousand years ago. Patanjali is credited with the systematization now known as "classical yoga," and its philosophy, science, and art have been passed down through many lineages. In the modern era, Acharya Sri B. K. S. Iyengar has participated in this tradition of handing down ancient wisdom by redefining, synthesizing, and clarifying the practice of asana and pranayama, as well as by demonstrating their beneficial effects on body and mind. It has become increasingly evident that his teachings correlate soundly with modern science; yet at the same time, the subject has been kept accessible to all. To come to Iyengar Yoga is to undertake a journey. It is not a cult or a religion; rather it is religiousness itself. In essence, it is a yogic passage.

Osteopathy teaches its practitioners that its point of reference is the Maker. Dr. Still was a devoutly religious man and pointed to what he called the "master mechanic." He taught that osteopathic principles are as old as the cranium itself, predating even human evolution. By definition, osteopathy applies itself to the bony faculties of the body. But it deals with much more than that, for it is a science of structural and functional interdependence. It is the reciprocal relationship between optimum stability and movement and those internal forces that propel us in life. As a practice, osteopathy teaches that disease is chiefly due to a loss of structural integrity and that that integrity can be regained by manipulation of the parts that contribute to the affected structure. Dr. William Garner Sutherland, one of Still's closest disciples, later recognized, for example, that the cranial anatomy has beveled bones that resemble the gills of fish, indicating that a primary respiratory mechanism is the driving force of life and that it is accompanied by a normal fluctuating ebb and flow of the cerebrospinal or cranial fluids. This rhythm creates an inner dynamic balance of life, manifesting itself through membranes that, quite literally, hold us together. Osteopaths engage with these tension membranes by subtle tactile contact, thereby seeking to assist the inherent forces and rectify the dysfunctions of the body.

By his dedicated practice, Guruji has also clarified a way to balance these inner forces. The practice of asana and pranayama calms the mind and restores the body. We learn that the inherent breath and biophysical forces have an intelligence; they are self-regulating. Therefore, we have the potential to rebalance and harmonize ourselves. He teaches us that we cannot reach higher levels of meditative awareness unless and until we learn the fundamentals of asana and pranayama and learn to educate our senses of perception so they can go beyond the gross physical body and contemplate our inner state. Guruji gives us the tools and the method to grow from a connection to our inner spirit, but not without the constant purging of awareness that must take place during practice. This is a spiritual *kriya,* a transformation achieved by constantly clearing and rebalancing ourselves. His teaching is direct and unambiguous, for he has a firsthand knowledge of the process that has been gleaned from thousands of hours of repeated practice, investigating and feeling in asana and pranayama the stretches, tensions, expansions, and contractions, as well as varying pressures, pains, liberations, and freedoms. It is a science of the pragmatic and the paradoxical. None can match his penetration of the subject from the little toe to the stratosphere nor his application of the philosophical and psychological practicalities of the vast subject of yoga.

Osteopathy, as practiced in the United States today, includes pharmaceuticals, general medicine, and surgery in addition to the traditional manual therapeutics from which the modern science sprang. In the rest of the world, osteopaths are better known for their manual skills—their expertise in the structural and functional corrections they make to neuromuscular joint and connective tissue and the related blood, lymph, and endocrine/humoral elements. But although these treatments are effective, osteopathy fails on the level where yoga so brilliantly excels: the education of individuals to participate in their own healing process. Although this shortcoming is addressed by osteopaths, among others, through many of the new-wave exercise regimes, few (if any) have the sound biomechanical foundations or discipline of Iyengar Yoga, which, in my view, is able to reinforce osteopathic corrections. Through its balancing actions taken in the panoply of postures, this yoga provides the means to develop substantive improvements and long-term stability.

Guruji's medical classes have become legendary, particularly since he often treats difficult cases abandoned by the traditional medical establishment. Over the years, he has developed asana sequences to deal with many and varied ailments. But importantly, all of these have the common element of looking at the alignment not just of the body, but of the whole individual—of body, mind, and spirit. This has always been Guruji's ethos. The varied sequences always include that uniquely yogic element of looking at the total individual. They ask the individual for a committed involvement in self-help that is understood in the very broadest of contexts, that of both the physical and the spiritual self. That self, or *atman,* which can occasionally be glimpsed, is the inner light that keeps us on the path to becoming whole in the truest health. It is a seeker of harmony and peace, inside and out. *Yoga* means "to yoke," to join the parts to the whole. This means the *inner* life. We seek for union with the self, for that harmony inside and out that is essentially union with the universe. Therapy in whatever form it takes is remedial, and this is certainly important. But what is even more critical is prevention, and as Patanjali so presciently noted, we must, through yoga, seek to prevent those pains that are yet to come. But how do we prevent these "yet-to-come" pains?

In that light, teaching us how to systematically unite body, mind, and spiritual awareness is Guruji's biggest achievement. Furthermore, it is an achievement forged in the great fire of his *sadhana*—his practice of uninterrupted, long, and sustained refinement. We all do our personal best, and we all have a natural drive to improve ourselves, even when we fail. Do our best. Improve. It is our challenge to carry on his torch of *tapas,* that fire that burns brightly in him even after nearly ninety years of life and seventy years of continuous teaching. We offer our thanks, our love, and our best wishes to a master who has given us a road to follow.

John Leebold, from Sydney, Australia, has been a student of B. K. S. Iyengar's since 1973, making his first visit to the Institute in Pune in 1978, following travels through Europe and Southeast Asia. He opened the Western Australian School of Yoga in 1986 and has taught extensively within Australia, New Zealand, Bali, Indonesia, the United States, and the United Kingdom. He is a practicing registered osteopath.

Namaskaram

SHIVA REA

According to the Sankhya philosophy at least three things are needed to make a universe like this one: subjects to do the perceiving, objects to be perceived, and some method for connecting the two. Every object has to have its fund of "objectness" telling it how to behave. This is called its *bhuta,* or gross element. It also has to have its "perception potential," which determines how it is going to be perceived. This is called its *tanmatra,* or subtle element. Bhutas and tanmatras then associate with each other to create both nature and the impression it gives.

All material objects are classified according to the effects they have on consciousness. Since there are five senses, then the universe must be created by bringing together five principles known as earth, water, fire, air, and space or ether, the substance that spreads out so all creation—material and nonmaterial—can be supported. Through the earth principle we come to know the cohesiveness and inertia of things; through the water principle their variety. Through the fire principle we appreciate their immediacy; through the air principle their mutual interactions; and through the ether principle their penetrability into consciousness and space.

The bhuta, or gross element, associated with the earth principle is *prithvi*, earth, the attempt by an object to convince all potential subjects of its reality. The bhuta of the water principle is *ap*, water, each object's ability to convince perceivers of its specific characteristics. The bhuta of the fire principle is *tejas*, fire, the projectivity each object must have if it is going to be perceived. The bhuta associated with the air principle is *vayu*, air, the web of relations each object forms with others. Finally, the bhuta of the ether principle is *akasha*, the ethereal substratum permeating both our inner and outer spaces.

The tanmatra, or subtle element, of the earth principle is *gandha*, smell, how real to each of us a given object seems. The tanmatra of the water principle is *rasa*, taste, our perception of each object's individuality.

The tanmatra of the fire principle is *rupa*, form, the perceived structure of things. The tanmatra of the air principle is *sparsha*, touch, our impression of how one thing relates to all others. And the tanmatra of the ether principle is *shabda*, sound, representing its penetrability into consciousness.

Perhaps the most nebulous and untranslatable of the five tanmatras is rasa, which can also be thought of as human feelings and emotions. Could it perhaps better be thought of as whatever is being tasted and/or enjoyed? But as Shiva Rea points out, there really is no proper English equivalent.

Perform each asana as a mantra and each pose as a meditation then the light will dawn from the center of your being.
—SRI B. K. S. IYENGAR, *Iyengar: His Life and Works*

S ri B. K. S. Iyengar has been like the sun to so many practitioners around the world—shining the light of his own devotion and awareness from his own being to illuminate the universal path of yoga. His legacy has not only made yoga accessible to all regardless of needs and limitations, but has offered a path of conscious embodiment at the heart of yoga. Sri B. K. S. Iyengar's teachings bring us through the gateway of our physical bodies, using breath as the bridge, to access to the intelligence and awareness that resides within our cells for self-realization and wisdom in action.

As a student of yoga, Kashmiri Shaivism, and classical Indian dance forms, I am interested in all the ways we can transform a mundane relationship to our body, to the earth body, and to the universal body to realize the unified field of consciousness pervading creation. It is the aim of yoga—like dance and music—to go beyond the long struggles with technique and performance to rasa, that state of embodied communion with what is within us. Abhinavagupta describes rasa as the self tasting the self, the juice of life, its essential essence. Rasa is the transformational state (for both doer and observer) where the thinking mind quiets and pure feeling pulses through the body. This feeling of rasa—of connection to our deeper selves and the universal self—can arise during any of life's activities. It is a heightened state of communion between us and what surrounds us. We feel rasa not with the thinking mind but with the feeling mind of our heart-intelligence, which is called *bhava*. We must first become aware of our bhava or true feeling state. In this fast-paced world, a lack of connection is common with the ever-changing rhythms of technology challenging our nervous system to be constantly pulled externally. Sometimes the very diligence of yoga practice, or a cold application of *vairagya*, nonattachment—deliberately avoiding feeling in order to still the fluctuations of the mind—can dry the soil of our natural inner connection. We need to tune in to our inner bhava and harmonize with the environment around us for rasa to emerge.

I believe that all human beings on this planet have consciously or unconsciously experienced rasa. There is one yoga practice that we have participated in that has allowed us to have the experience of *bhava-rasa*, regardless of background, karma, or dharma. In spontaneous awe all beings—the truck driver, teacher, farmer, politician, child—have at some time in their lives lifted their faces to the radiant, transformative power and beauty of the sun. This mighty star touches us intimately from some 96 million miles away. Eyes closed or open, this visceral, inherent response in which a human being enters—even if for moments—is instinctual meditation. It is the moment that blends us all, humans, animals, ocean life, plants, into a natural intuitive yogic consciousness. This "thoughtless" communion with the microcosm and macrocosm, this unconscious act of devotion, is a universal experience of yoga. This is *surya namaskar*—sun salutation, arising from the natural bhava of the sun.

Surya namaskar is that special sequence of asanas that is the yogi and yogini's prayer to the sun. It tunes into the flow of life, the seasons and the heavens, the natural circadian rhythms. It is a progressive sequence that unfolds with an inherent harmony and cellular intelligence like the opening of a water lily's petals or the series of ocean waves breaking on the shore. The words have a reverential connection to the life force of the universe; this is clearly lost in the translation from the Sanskrit *namaskar* to the slightly stiff "salutation." This archaic greeting word is rarely used in everyday English and brings to mind the rigid Roman greeting or the formal military salute, imbued as it is with acknowledgments of power and submission. This is completely lacking in the all-encompassing and compassionate feeling of the consummate greeting of *namaste* or *namaskaram* that permeates life in the Hindu/yogic world of India.

As with so many Sanskrit words, namaskar is imbued with so much bhava. With *salutation* as its equivalent translation, the vital inner link to both the universal and the deep roots of yoga is lost. The roots of namaskar as *nama* is literally "not me," implying an inner bowing that awakens our receptive awareness to feel, to connect, to open, to receive, and absorb this miracle of life. At the same time, we reflect outwards our own personal divinity back to the universe and to all beings regardless of race, sex, or creed. We place our hands in the universal symbol of prayer, connecting palms and all fingertips to symbolize unity and oneness with the divine. We magnify the healing energy within ourselves and manifest it outward into the universe. With that one act we realize that we are all created equal; that we are all connected with one another and with the ultimate source of spiritual energy in the universe.

This "lost-in-translationness" seeps over into our practice of the sequence itself, where sun salutations, as the consummate hatha yoga fitness can be done without namasakar. As B. K. S. Iyengar's teachings illustrate, when movement is done mechanically, the power of yoga dissolves. We lose the rasa of our innate spiritual connectivity to the radiant sun. Allowing surya namaskar to arise from our natural connection to the source of life, the outer sun, we awaken the feeling-mind of bhava-rasa to stimulate our body-mind-heart connection. As B. K. S. Iyengar has offered, "To live in the moment is spirituality. To live in the movement is divinity."* By aligning the outer world (environment and physical body) and the inner world (energy, breath, emotions, consciousness), we can transform our practice into a vibrating connection to our life force. If we stay true to the original spirit of namaskar, we can traverse mundane mind and enter the sacred light that existed at the beginning of the universe and that brought all into being. In our postmodern secular society we have lost the grounding power of daily ritual. The idea of Ishvara pranidhana, or surrendering to a higher source, of being willing to become part of a bigger picture, initiates a sacred shift of perspective that is urgently needed in these times of ecological peril. The act of surrender-

---

* B. K. S. Iyengar, *Iyengar: His Life and Works* (Toronto: Timeless Books, 1987).

ing is a potent method of dissolving the endless agitations of the mind and shifting our perspective from individual selfishness to universal interconnectedness. If yoga is ultimately about connecting to the bigger "dance" of life, then surya namaskar, in its true origin as a meditatively moving prayer, is a very potent method of awakening transformative bhava-rasa in one's body, life, and the world. And as the great yogic artist Sri B. K. S. Iyengar fully embodies: "Yoga is like music: the rhythm of the body, the melody of the mind, and the harmony of the soul create the symphony of life."★

SHIVA REA is a leading teacher of prana vinyasa flow yoga and yoga trance dance worldwide. Her studies in the Krishnamacharya lineage, tantra, ayurveda, *bhakti, kalaripayattu*, world dance, yogic art, and somatic movement infuse her approach to living yoga and embodying its flow. She is known for bringing the roots of yoga alive for modern practitioners in creative, dynamic, and life-transforming ways. She leads retreats and pilgrimages all over the world and is active in movements promoting the environment, yoga, and the arts.

★ Iyengar, *Iyengar: His Life and Works*.

A Tribute to the Fire of
B. K. S. Iyengar

John Friend

It is possible to sit over a page and read the words time and time again. The sentences are all there, the words read correctly and make sense, but something is missing. There is no real understanding of what is being read. This is an objective kind of knowledge lying on the page . . . and then suddenly, a transformation takes place. The words fall into place and understanding dawns. This is subjective and experiential. It is then that the light of knowledge arises and an inner journey is undertaken that not only bestirs life, but brings understanding.

The physical sun that hangs in the sky is called Surya, the son of Dyaus (the sky). Surya is a dark red man with three eyes, four golden arms, and golden hair. He is called the Divine Vivifier. He rides a golden chariot that is sometimes yoked to seven mares and sometimes to one mare with seven heads. The seven represent the days of the week and also the seven gateways to the body—two nostrils, two eyes, two ears, and a mouth. Surya stirs lifeless things and awakens them into life. He is the eye of the Vedic gods, including Agni (fire); Varuna (ocean); and Mitra (friendship, honesty, and right dealing). Surya has command over waters and wind. He is the overlord of all, the moving and the unmoving alike. He is the god of wisdom and of knowledge. It is Surya who stimulates and guides us to understanding. Surya is enlivening and enlightening.

Even though knowledge and understanding can sometimes seem far away, the sun always shines deep within us and is always ready to guide us away from *avidya* (ignorance) by lighting up our darkness. When *brahman* (the absolute all) first sought to manifest all existence, *purusha* (spirit) appeared at exactly the same moment as *prakriti* (nature, or that which was to be created). One does not exist without the other. Together, purusha and prakriti created everything, eternal and noneternal. In the same way, the sun cannot be separated from its light. Surya is the Illuminator. It is written in verse 5 of the *Isha Upanishad: Tad ejati tannaijati, tadantarasya sarvasya,* or "It moves and it does not move; it is far and it is near; it is within all of this and it is outside all of this." When sunlight appears to travel as a beam of light, is anything really moving? Perhaps all that happens when night appears to fall is that we are invited to rest in a quietude that is always present and is beyond light and dark, for the sun and its light are ever one.

But the sun is not just an illuminator. It is nothing without its *tapas* (fiery heat). Its earnest drive is to shine its light on everyone and to emanate its enlivening and enlightening heat to all. John Friend can tell us something about this ceaseless striving of the heat of the sun to announce its existence and to proclaim the possibilities it holds for us up there in the sky and in the depths of our beings through the fire of the teacher that now stands before us.

The first time I met Mr. Iyengar, in the summer of 1987, he was sitting on the lawn of the Harvard University campus, the venue for the first North American Iyengar Yoga Conference. I had just flown into Boston from Santa Barbara, where I had been studying with Pattabhi Jois and a small group of his senior students at the White Lotus Foundation. Seeing Mr. Iyengar sitting casually with only a couple of students around him, I respectfully approached him to have his *darshan* (the blessings received from being in his presence). As he sat very quietly and wholly relaxed on the grass, he appeared diminutive and gentle. After everything that I had heard and read about him, I was expecting him to appear like a great military general, radiating dignity and power. Instead, he looked almost childlike in his extremely loose and fluid posture, as if his body was flowing with gravity.

With my hands in *anjali* mudra, I slowly approached to greet him and introduce myself: "Namaste, Mr. Iyengar. It is an honor to meet you, sir. My name is John Friend, and I am a yoga teacher from Texas."

Instantly Mr. Iyengar extended his long arm to shake my hand, which surprised me since many Indian teachers will simply fold their hands in front of their hearts in greeting. In turn, I respectfully extended my hand to shake the master's with an intentional soft-heartedness. With mercurial quickness, his superbly dexterous, intelligent hand completely enveloped my smaller one. In the flash of a moment, he utterly seized my hand and squeezed with tremendous might. My mind stopped in his crushing handshake. After living in Texas for almost ten years, I was used to this type of ritual, because it is part of the Texas ethos for men to shake hands very firmly to show their strength. Yet the absolute confidence and power of his grip conveyed much more than just physical strength. I felt the brightness of Mr. Iyengar's mind, the ultra-intelligence of his body, and the fire of his heart. It was evident that I had just shaken the hand of a master.

Those of us who have been touched directly by B. K. S. Iyengar have received a profound initiation by a rare man whose soul burns with the brightest aspiration for the ultimate freedom. I have never met anyone more intensely fiery than Mr. Iyengar. Outside the classroom, you will sometimes find him soft, jovial, and gentle. Yet anytime the subject of yoga is brought up, especially during practice in the classroom, he often becomes an uncompromising ball of fire that ignites anyone in range of his passionate flames. Comparing Mr. Iyengar's fire and passion for yoga to other teachers' fire is like comparing the sun to a candle flame. When instructing students to give their full effort in a pose, his eyes often spark and his words are hot like lightning. There have been times in the classroom when he has stood over me while I performed a pose such as urdhva mukha svanasana. He can give an imperative command like, "Take your head back!" with such fiery force that every cell of my body is infused with a screaming urgency. Once at the Iyengar Institute in Pune in 1989, under Mr. Iyengar's fiery authority, I took my head so far back in this pose that I saw the baseboard on the wall behind me. I've never bent that deep in that particular pose again. Once you have been touched directly by the fire of B. K. S. Iyengar, you vibrate at a different frequency. You are never the same again.

Mr. Iyengar's fire is fueled by the most intense aspiration to live this moment fully in order to disentangle his spirit (purusha) from his material constitution (prakriti). The possibility of not being completely present in whatever action he performs does not enter his awareness. He acts with the conviction that to experience the ultimate freedom, the yogi must give everything he has to every moment. This inner fire of longing for the ultimate freedom consumes him. Spacing out, being unfocused, not giving enough effort, or not having enough desire for the ultimate are not traits that could ever be used to describe him. There is no tolerance of laxity, indolence, or any effort less than 100 percent with Mr. Iyengar.

Once Mr. Iyengar was giving a presentation at a conference and asked a student to set up her sticky mat on the stage to perform headstand in front of the audience. The student hurriedly folded her mat and got into the pose as efficiently as she could. Within seconds of her being upside down in the full pose, Mr. Iyengar roared, "Come down!" The student instantly came down onto her knees and looked up sheepishly at the master, who was glaring with his huge, classical frown. He then turned to the audience and proceeded to make a few comments on the benefit of mental focus in yoga practice. With a swift kick of his foot, Mr. Iyengar moved the student's yoga mat to the side, exposing a metal ventilation grill on the stage floor exactly under the place where the mat had been. With one hand nonchalantly on his hip, he boomed, "No presence of mind—at all!"

To be taught directly by Mr. Iyengar is like being tempered by fire. You can always recognize his senior students because they engage every part of their muscles to the core of their bones. The master's lightening touch is clearly evident in the pupil's vibrant poses. Most students today have no idea of the degree of muscular engagement it takes to fully perform asanas as Mr. Iyengar teaches them. He is the king of "old school" yoga, from a time when the foundation of hatha yoga was intense discipline and hard work. Times have changed in the yoga world over the years. The mainstream has taken to it, so the vast majority of yogis now practice it on a more superficial level. They attend class once or twice a week simply as a form of recreation and, in many cases, a time to socialize. I sometimes think that if Mr. Iyengar had begun his career in America in the twenty-first century, he would have been derailed by numerous lawsuits filed from students shocked by the intensity of his fire!

The public practice of hatha yoga has changed since the first time Mr. Iyengar visited the United States fifty years ago. Tens of millions of people now practice it throughout the world, which is many times more than the number just fifteen years ago. Consequently, yoga has become big business in the United States today, with large yoga studios in most metropolitan areas and many practitioners choosing yoga teaching as their full-time profession. Yoga teachers present their classes in ways that will be enjoyable and attractive to the public. So it is rare to find one who is not personable, kind, physically fit, and attractive. People in the West, particularly in America, have become hypersensitive to words and actions that might be perceived as offensive to anyone's ethnicity, religion, gender, physical attributes, sexual orientation, or political view. Therefore, most teachers who want to make a career of yoga present their classes with a pleasant neutrality that reduces the risk of losing these sensitive students. Satisfying the superficial desires of their students is the primary objective of most teachers, so those students are catered to in order to sustain the popularity of the classes. Most teachers and students, especially of Iyengar Yoga, would say that discipline is an important element within a yoga class. However, the degree of discipline in the average yoga class is relatively nonexistent compared to the enforcement of the one-pointed focus that I witnessed in class with Mr. Iyengar.

Throughout that first Iyengar Yoga conference at Harvard, I repeatedly witnessed his brilliance and an intense fire for the yoga that I had never seen before in anyone. The conference was structured with small yoga classes taught by certified Iyengar Yoga teachers throughout the campus in a variety of conference rooms and classrooms. All of the tables and chairs were moved out of the rooms or to the side, so all the students could lay out their yoga mats on the floor. Each participant filled out a questionnaire during registration and was assigned a particular "track," depending on his or her level of yoga experience, level of status in the Iyengar Yoga community, and physical abilities. Although I exaggerated my credentials, I was still assigned a moderate-level track!

During one of the afternoons, I decided to audit an advanced-level class focusing on inversions. Sitting against the wall at the back of the room, I watched the senior instructor guide a group of about thirty advanced-track students into headstand. All of the students were organized into rows and columns in the middle of the room and facing the tall windows on one side. The senior instructor proceeded to give a litany of detailed anatomical instructions from how to press the forearms down on the floor to the action of the shoulder blades, tailbone, and legs. The students were up for about five minutes before some of them started to

come slowly down out of the pose due to fatigue. After another five minutes, more than half the students had come out of the pose and were sitting watching the rest of the class continue to be guided in the postural
details of headstand. At about the fifteen-minute mark, there were only
about a half a dozen students still holding the pose; several of them were
sweating through their clothes and shaking with fatigue but still not re-
linquishing the pose. One advanced student in the middle of the room,
Richard Freeman, was still performing an apparently effortless headstand
with very erect and graceful posture.

I was admiring the beauty and poise of Richard's asana, when suddenly the double doors to the classroom burst wide open and an entourage of senior instructors quickly fanned into room as if it were a
police raid. In the wake of this stream of authority walked Mr. Iyengar
dressed in a fine, white cloth that wrapped around his waist and draped
to his ankles, and a white kurta that hung down to his knees. As soon as
some of the students still performing headstand realized that Mr. Iyengar
and his entourage had entered the room, they promptly came down out
of their pose, leaving only four students, including Richard, still upside
down.

Mr. Iyengar walked directly to one of the upside-down students and
barked an alignment correction to her. The student attempted to adjust
her posture to his command, but her adjustment was not to his satisfaction, and he repeated his instruction with greater fire behind his words.
He then took hold of her feet with one hand while adjusting the front
of her thighs with the other and intensifying his verbal commands. After
such a long time in the pose, the student's stamina was spent and her legs
and hips were quivering. She struggled to follow Mr. Iyengar's guidance,
but she didn't have the strength to maintain the integrity of her alignment. Recognizing her waning reserve, he gave the back of her heels a
dismissive little push and told her to come down. He then swiftly turned
his head to look at another student who was still in headstand fifteen feet
away. After a flash of his laser perception, Mr. Iyengar turned to face his
entourage with his hands on his hips and began listing half a dozen mis-
alignments of the student's pose. It was like watching Sherlock Holmes
presenting his "elementary" findings after ascertaining a tremendous
amount of informational minutia from a moment's glance at a subject.

When he was finished with his report, Mr. Iyengar turned to Richard Freeman. I was curious to hear what he would find misaligned in Richard's pose, since it looked perfect to me. Surprisingly, there was a deafening silence. No one seemed to breathe as the master began to slowly circumambulate around Richard's pose, which resembled a stone sculpture in its steadiness. With every quarter turn, Mr. Iyengar's facial muscles seemed to flicker more and his thick white eyebrows jumped up and down as the anticipation in the room mounted. I thought that perhaps he was waiting for Richard to tire so that a postural weakness would then show itself. After a long silence, Mr. Iyengar finally commanded Richard to make some esoteric action with his intercostals to affect the alignment of his rib cage. I didn't understand the command, but Richard made some almost imperceptible adjustment around his floating ribs, and Mr. Iyengar let out a deep grunt of approval.

Now Richard slowly came out of his headstand. He stood up to face Mr. Iyengar, who began to quiz him about his yoga experience. To each question, Richard answered eloquently and with aplomb. At one point in the interview, Mr. Iyengar asked him, "In what subject did you earn your college degree?"

"Philosophy," Richard replied with his typical urbane flair.

"As I suspected, you have sand for brains," Mr. Iyengar jabbed.

To this playful insult, Richard began chuckling, which then ignited a paroxysm of laughter in Mr. Iyengar.

"There will not be another yoga master like Iyengar for three hundred years!" This prophecy was bellowed to an audience of hundreds of Iyengar Yoga teachers assembled in the University of Michigan gymnasium bleachers at Ann Arbor, Michigan, in 1993 by Mr. Iyengar himself. Like a lion surveying his pride, he stood regally on the gym floor with his hands on his hips, one foot a little in front of the other, and his chin slightly raised as he addressed the public gathering at the national Iyengar Yoga conference. When I first heard him make this statement that afternoon I thought it was one of his typical hyperbolic, arrogant, wild self-proclamations. Since then, however, I have wondered if it wasn't an understatement. I am not sure the world will ever see such a fiery, passionate, and intensely bright teacher of hatha yoga again for a very long time.

॰

JOHN FRIEND is the founder of Anusara Yoga. He studied intensively in the Iyengar Yoga system from 1986 to 1996 and had the opportunity to study directly with B. K. S. Iyengar on many occasions during those years. He also served on the Board of Directors of the Iyengar Yoga National Association of the United States (IYNAUS) from 1991 to 1995.

Embodying Emotion and Myth with B. K. S. Iyengar

Richard Freeman

Having stated that the ultimate aim of yoga is mastery over the many depths and levels of the mind, Patanjali also tells us how that mastery can be attained. He gives us two methods: *abhyasa* (practice) and *vairagya* (detachment). Since yoga is an essentially practical discipline, these techniques are fundamental. Nearly everything else rides on them.

Abhyasa, or practice, is not simply about asana. It is a request that we positively cultivate a lifestyle, a mode of speech, a set of actions, a body of thought, and the spiritual practices (possibly including our time spent on the mat) that head us in the appropriate direction. Vairagya, or detachment, asks us to gradually expunge from ourselves any and all mental habits and conditionings that might feed our terrible tendency toward backsliding. One element of this pair cannot exist without the other. Abhyasa and vairagya are often described as the two wings that make the bird of effort in yoga soar. Abhyasa is persistent effort, while vairagya is putting aside, for example, the fear of failure along with all those other things that might turn into an obstacle or distraction.

A lot of the success in applying these two techniques depends on us improving our sense of discrimination. We must constantly seek to improve our discernment regarding what words, what actions, and what thoughts we should and should not indulge in. Abhyasa can take us to a state of stability and tranquillity; vairagya ensures that that state is never lost. Abhyasa can take us closer and closer to a direct engagement with the essential core of our being; vairagya helps the process by releasing us from the false identities and perceptions that gather around and can cloud or obscure the true self. As B. K. S. Iyengar puts it, "The two balance each other like day and night," with vairagya being the practice that releases us from those desires and passions that hinder us in the pursuit of the elusive primordial soul. Richard Freeman is now kind enough to give us further insights into this practice.

Much of what I have learned from Mr. Iyengar has been at a safe distance: by watching how he moves and how he readjusts, by listening to how he talks and makes listeners think for themselves, by the marvelous effect he has on others. I consider him to be like a storm with wind, lightning, and thunder—beautiful and almost too elemental for the survival of my ordinary, inattentive self. I look on many things in nature, such as the ocean, the rivers, and mountains, with the same sense of awe, thrill, and dread of self-destruction. This dread is a visceral, instinctive reaction to dissolution. I liken it to the *abhinivesha* of the *Yoga Sutras*. It is a visceral fear of yoga, of dissolution, of death, of love, of life. It is not a result of thinking. I am not to be reasoned out of it. My hair stands on end. I am enchanted, even obsessed with that which will stun my mind and stop my breath. It is like the heightened, electrical feeling in the skin, in the eyes and ears, in the nose, when there is a tornado coming. One can read on and on about it in books, hear others talk about it, even become expert in it, but direct contact is something else—raw, dangerous, vital, perhaps ecstatic.

Then there were the direct, immediate, and sometimes unexpected immersions with Mr. Iyengar, such as the time we saw him across a large hall at the Bangalore airport. He came straight over from at least a hundred feet away, grinning, chin up with ecstatic self-confidence, striding with the enthusiasm of youth. It was like being caught in a sunbeam. From him, friendly, pointed questions and from me, gushing, awkward answers. As I gave mostly inadequate explanations about where I had been and what I was up to, he kept up the small talk while patting me on my shoulders and kidney area. I was being trained and realigned with an intelligence that no longer left out feeling and emotion. Then we went our separate ways. He was off with a flourish, like Surya in his chariot, with emotion, grandeur, and myth radiating like beams from his body. I was left once again with the feeling of the living body as the world. Currents of sensation mixed with music; emotion and stories came together in strong mudras deep inside and were silent.

Mr. Iyengar gives not only precise lines of mechanical connection and the wiring and tubes that make up an awakened body in an open mind. He gives the juice that flows through them. It is an eternally repeating myth—that of Shiva catching the Ganga on his head, bringing rivers of primordial feeling and clarity to earth, which is the body. Mythology is made real in our own bodies. In the body, we find not only all the places of pilgrimage, sacred places in which to weep with relief, but all of the gods and goddesses who make them live. To be most honest, the demons, the shadows of the gods, are there too to make the stories we live rich and true. Shadows are now to be brought into the full service of yoga. No more pious hypocrisy. No more dry, theoretical escape into narcissistic self-love. No more dead stupor of *tamasic* meditation. The gods have reawakened. Mythology is understood with waves of ecstatic emotion, in between the cells, in between the thoughts and the techniques. They say that the age of mythology is gone and the age of the gods, too. But thanks to Mr. Iyengar, the human body and the worlds that extend out from it are now repopulated with variety, beauty, story, and emotion. Saved from the dry, disembodied abstractions that claimed selfhood and closed our senses and our imaginations, we can relax into the body as it is: the feeling in the skin, the pressure in the finger, the sound in the space, the pattern in the pattern, the story in the story. He is like a thunderstorm that leaves the air fresh and clear.

RICHARD FREEMAN has been a student of yoga since 1968. He spent nearly nine years in Asia studying various traditions, which he incorporates into the Ashtanga Yoga practice taught by his principal teacher, K. Pattabhi Jois of Mysore, India. His background includes Zen and Vipassana Buddhist practice; *bhakti* and traditional hatha yoga in India; Sufism in Iran; and starting in 1974, an in-depth study of Iyengar Yoga. He is still an avid student of both Western and Eastern philosophy, as well as Sanskrit. His ability to juxtapose various viewpoints, without losing the depth and integrity of each, has helped Richard develop a unique, metaphorical teaching style. He lives with his family in Boulder, Colorado, where he is the director of the Yoga Workshop.

The Perfect Fit: Adaptive Iyengar Therapeutic Yoga and Managing Multiple Sclerosis

Eric Small

A theory on the origin of disease is impossible without a partner theory on the origin of life. In an age without microscopes, many believed in the spontaneous generation of life. How else to explain the sudden appearance of maggots that erupted from nowhere to smother a piece of meat? Based on the widespread acceptance of this theory, the Dutch scientist Jan Baptist van Helmont, 1580–1644, gave the following as a recipe for mice:

> If a dirty undergarment is squeezed into the mouth of a vessel containing wheat, within a few days (say 21), a ferment drained from the garments and transferred by the smell of the grain, encrusts the wheat itself with its own skin and turns it into mice. . . . And, what is more remarkable, the mice from corn and undergarments are neither weanlings or sucklings nor premature but they jump out fully formed.★

Diseases could thus be caused by external agencies such as lint, which could "foster contagion." It was the discovery of microorganisms that paved the way for the acceptance of the germ theory of disease, which declares that when an individual contracts a disease, a self-propagating— and external—microorganism is often the cause.

Yoga has a very different theory of disease because it has a very different theory of the origin of life. Its premise is the apparent distinction between subject and object. If, for example, I am an unskilled dancer and

---

★ Earl D. Hanson, trans., *Understanding Evolution* (Oxford: Oxford University Press, 1981), 319.

invite someone to dance with me, I am dependent on the other person to teach me the steps. So at that first level, I am constantly directed by my partner. As I gain competence, things move to a second stage, where our dancing becomes more fluid and I can respond more effectively to my partner and the music. I have some input into the dance. Eventually, a third stage is reached in which our partnership is so complete that we two are one, and all sense of identity and separateness is gone.

The first three sutras in the *Sankhya Sutras* of Kapila explain yoga's view of disease and freedom from disease. They imply that human affairs can be divided into two categories: *laukika* (worldly) and *alaukika* (otherworldly). This establishes three levels of reality. In the first, we are directed by mundane affairs. In the second, we infuse a more spiritualized awareness into our existence. In the third, we realize the true nature of things and act with complete selflessness. Alternatively, there are three types of vision. The first is to see only the physical world and its constituent *bhutas* (elements). The second is to internalize and use reasoning, meditation, and concentration to appreciate that the world really is not what it seems. The third is to become a vehicle of *anugraha* (grace).

These sutras also establish the ground for yoga and ayurveda. They outline the *tritapa* (threefold suffering) that a material existence inevitably brings. These are the *adhibhautika* (externally caused sufferings); the *adhyatmika* (internally caused sufferings); and the *adhidaivika* (supernaturally caused sufferings brought on by earthquakes, floods, and the like). External sufferings (adhibhautika) are caused by other humans, other creatures, or inanimate objects; those that are internal (adhyatmika) have a twofold origin: the body and the mind. Bodily sufferings are due to energetic disturbances in the bhutas—the elements and humors recognized by yoga and ayurveda. Mental sufferings come from desire, anger, fear, and other emotions and the constant oscillations around and among them.

Regarding adhidaivika, we must remember that simply existing is suffering. Yoga argues what Eric Small now affirms—that developing awareness and consciousness immediately gives us greater understanding and tolerance. That self-same effort in awareness, along with the understanding that it brings, helps to alleviate suffering. It allows us to transform the very nature of suffering, no matter what its cause. Recognition of our indwelling nature changes our sense of who we are and our place in the universe, and it institutes a new sense of being that immediately makes our afflictions easier to bear. Thus, our sufferings become the genesis of our heightened understanding and transformation. Our suffering diminishes, our joy increases, and our gratitude to existing becomes limitless.

Who would have known more than thirty years ago that when B. K. S. Iyengar showed me his book *Light on Yoga*, my life's path would become a dynamic process of change. After opening the book, he quickly pointed out a series of asanas and pranayamas and said to me, "Do this and this and this." That started the process that would help me and affect thousands of others dealing with the day-to-day effects of multiple sclerosis (MS).

Why is Iyengar therapeutic yoga a perfect fit with a diagnosis of multiple sclerosis, which has no known source and—at this time—no known cure? One answer is that the sequences of the asanas are based on a solid knowledge of the workings of the physical body, the psychological body, and the emotional body, as well as the need for spiritual balance. A major factor in using therapeutics with multiple sclerosis is the wide range of symptoms that are presented to the teacher. No one teaching formula applies to everyone. The challenge to the instructor is to design a sequence that is readily available to the student. It is most important that the sequence be clear and concise so that it can be performed at home. It is the home practice that becomes so important in managing MS.

The instructor must have experience and training. That is why Guruji insists that his teachers have at least five to eight years of training and be certified at an appropriate level in order to facilitate effective and positive results.

What are some of the results that have occurred using therapeutic yoga? First, there is a reduction of the chronic fatigue caused by MS. A study produced by the University of Oregon at Portland showed that fatigue could be reduced or brought to a manageable level. A proper sequence made up of supported standings, supported inversions, supported forward bends and twists, supported backbends, and pranayama accomplished this.

Second, one of the major emotional symptoms presented by the MS student is depression, which responds well to Iyengar therapeutics. The sequences are based on supported inversions and backbends to open the heart and chest, supported forward bends and twists to calm the nervous system, and pranayama with no breath retention.

A third important result deals with range of motion. Because of the deterioration of the nerves' protective covering caused by the body's

autoimmune reaction to the disease, signals to the muscles are interrupted or misdirected, causing loss of function. At this time, no long-
lasting treatment has proven effective in stopping the body from
attacking itself. Iyengar therapeutic yoga does not restore muscle function, but it does dramatically increase range of motion. Props such as
chairs, bolsters, and belts are used to relieve cramping, contractions, and
stiffness in the limbs. Thus, as range of motion increases, so does circulation, digestion, elimination, strength, and muscle tone.

Finally, many chronic medical conditions affect more than the physical body. There is also an effect on the student's personal environment.
Isolation from the general population and from family and friends is a
dramatic effect of MS. We take the ability to move for granted, almost as
if it were a given right. When MS limits that ability, we begin to remove
ourselves from full participation in life. Providing a class or group of
"MSers" with a positive, healthy activity that is going to improve quality
of life has an amazing effect on the students and the instructor. We have
seen, over the span of twenty-five years, students picking up their lives
and managing their symptoms. The reentry into family and professional
life is most rewarding and sustaining.

Mr. Iyengar has always stressed that in teaching the science and art of
yoga, it is not only the technique of teaching, but also the passion of why
you teach that is important. Adaptive Iyengar Yoga is not used to "cure"
MS. It is taught as a tool to manage the disease, to increase the student's
ability to regain a sense of empowerment, and to begin the journey toward self-discovery.

As students improve in their ability to rejoin life, there is an opening
of their awareness to their personal spiritual nature. A balance begins between their physical condition, their ability to cope with their symptoms
in a positive manner, and their renewed belief in themselves. In 2006, the
Southern California chapter of the National Multiple Sclerosis Society
created the Eric Small Optimal Living with MS Program at the University of California–Los Angeles (UCLA), Casa Colina Rehabilitation
Center, University of Southern California, and Rancho Los Amigos. This
program focuses on teaching clients how to utilize various methodologies to become more independent and self-sustaining. Adaptive Iyengar
Yoga is an important factor in the training of physical and occupational

therapists in these programs. Mr. Iyengar has been a source of inspiration and encouragement. There are not enough words to express the gratitude and love we have shared over these many years.

ERIC SMALL was diagnosed with MS at the age of twenty-two and soon after became a serious student of hatha yoga, which began to help him with the effects of the illness. He has been teaching yoga since the mid-1960s, first teaching at the University of California–Berkeley. He then taught for the Los Angeles Unified School District, Beverly Hills Adult Education, and at the Iyengar Yoga Institute (Los Angeles). He has also served on the teaching staff of Iyengar Yoga conventions. He frequently travels throughout the United States, conducting yoga workshops and seminars for both MS and non-MS students and instructors. He has received countless awards and commendations: in 1999, the Hope for MS Award; in 2001, induction into the National MS Society Volunteer Hall of Fame; and in 2002, the Dorothy Corwin Spirit of Life Award for Outstanding Volunteer Service to MS patients. Together with Dr. Loren Fishman, Eric wrote a book, *Yoga and MS,* that contains illustrations and descriptions of the various uses of Adaptive Iyengar Yoga.

Attention and Love

RODNEY YEE

Yoga seeks to develop the attention for a reason: to instigate the development of that wisdom that makes our lives fruitful. Directing our attention develops a particular kind of contact with the world, a contact that ultimately produces wisdom. According to *Yoga Sutra* II:27, this growth of wisdom shows itself in seven ways: (1) by making it possible for us to know everything that should be known; (2) by enabling us to discard everything that should be discarded; (3) by giving us the wherewithal to attain everything that should be attained; (4) by helping us to appreciate what should be done so that we can do it; (5) by helping us to realize that peace of mind really exists and inspiring us to strive for it; (6) by making us realize that we can and should be our own source of fuller comprehension; and (7) by illuminating that light, that soul, that dwells within.

Yet, as Rodney Yee points out, these are not the only consequences that developing a focused attention brings to us.

Once in a while, the energies of the universe come together in a person to produce a genius. Among these people, there are a precious few who have the fortitude and virtue to channel that genius toward service to humanity. B. K. S. Iyengar is such a man.

In 1984, Manouso Manos told our class at the Iyengar Yoga Institute in San Francisco that the most a teacher can do is inspire the student. Though thousands of miles away, throughout the last twenty-six years, B. K. S. Iyengar has inspired and compelled me to hone my attention a little more every day.

Krishnamurti equates attention with love. If attention is love, then B. K. S. Iyengar is full of the divine energy embodying that idea. More than anyone I have ever known, Iyengar, through passion and complete absorption, has remapped the yoga asanas and pranayama. He has done this through tireless attention and devotion to the art of yoga. He has painstakingly moved from the gross body to the most subtle bodies, far deeper than most of us can comprehend. But like a great artist, Iyengar has not only done the research in and with his own soul and body, he has made it accessible and tangible for the common person. Through precise work and alignment, he demands that the student wake up. It is like toiling with advanced mathematics—a casual curiosity or cursory study is not enough. I remember reading Iyengar's detailed descriptions of triangle pose that went on for three pages in the smallest, single-spaced type. That description was written in the early 1970s, so one can only imagine the level of detail and insight that would be in his present-day dissertation.

The physical alignment is key to allow for symmetry, balance, and proper flow of prana. But it is the *dharana* (mental concentration) that begins to grow when studying with Mr. Iyengar that leads to yogic breakthroughs. His presence demands concentration. Being in his classroom is the essence of the often-quoted idea from Ram Dass, "Be here now." If students can get past their own fear and be truly present as this giant of a man looms in the room, they will be astounded by the journey on which Mr. Iyengar ably guides each practitioner.

Many people have called him a physical yogi, but I feel he is one of the few yoga teachers who has woven the body, mind, and spirit into their undeniable tapestry of beauty. In his work, the body, mind, and spirit all join into the infinite center. As one's concentration is honed through his precise system, the magic begins. Like a great conductor orchestrating an entire symphony, Mr. Iyengar begins to reveal the relationship of the infinite number of interrelated parts that encompass a yoga practice, a yoga life. The relationship between infinite vibrations is his composition, and direct contact to the soul is his music.

We hope to honor you, Mr. Iyengar, in the way that you have honored us, with great care and attention, with love and respect, and with devotion and service. Peace, peace, peace.

RODNEY YEE has been curious about the mind and body for as long as he can remember. He was a gymnast, a ballet dancer, and a philosophy and physical therapy major. Following the thread of curiosity about mind and body, he took his first yoga class in 1980 and knew from the start that it would be a lifelong passion. Now that his mind and body are going through midlife, he is much more curious about the spirit. His spirit is fed by his wife, Colleen, and his four children. Life is abundant and chaotic and keeps Rodney returning to asana, pranayama, and meditation. Teaching is still a main vehicle for Rodney to understand union. He has created dozens of DVDs and has written two books— *Yoga: The Poetry of the Body* and *Moving Toward Balance*—both with Nina Zolotow. He teaches workshops and retreats worldwide and leads national teacher-training intensives.

The Manual for Life

Chuck Miller

> ... a good book is better than a bad teacher.
> —B. K. S. Iyengar

Chuck Miller was interviewed by Anne O'Brien in September 2006.

CHUCK MILLER: Many people ask me how I got into yoga. My best friend and I used to sit in full lotus in fourth grade, and even before that, I used to sleep cross-legged. Around the time I was sixteen, I started reading authors like Hermann Hesse, Carlos Castaneda, Suzuki Roshi, and other Zen authors. I picked up a copy of *Be Here Now* by Ram Dass. It had just come out in 1971, and I loved it. There was something about the journey, the exploration, that really intrigued me. Growing up in suburban America, I was disillusioned with what was going on in the world. I was looking for something else. Going to church was just empty for me. I would sit there and wonder, *What is this guy talking about and how is it relevant?* Suddenly, this stuff was exciting to me. The shamanistic, the Eastern approach, was a completely different perspective on spirituality; it was not just following religion or dogma. In the book by Ram Dass, there was a little yoga routine in the back. I thought it was pretty cool, so I started practicing with that and looking for other books. I found Richard Hittleman. There was not a lot available in 1971 in Rutland, Vermont!

One day in 1974, I was in a bookstore and I picked up a copy of *Light on Yoga.* A girl I had never seen before just looked over and said, "That's the book." I took it as a sign from above and bought the book. I went home that night and read the introduction, fifty-five pages, and it blew my mind. It changed my life. I felt like I had my hand on the operating manual for the human being. I was really into the mental part of it, but the more subtle practices of the pranayama, as well as the physical practices, really intrigued me too. I started working with *Light on Yoga,* but I had the old version of the book, where all the pictures were at the back and the instructions were elsewhere. So I just began looking at the pictures and trying to copy what B. K. S. was doing. I remember one night coming home and seeing his pictures of dropbacks, and I thought, *Wow, that looks cool.* I landed on my head the first time; got my hands to the floor before my head the second time; and the third time managed to keep my head from hitting the ground! I then started reading the instructions more and was appreciative to have such a conscientious guide, a great teacher available to me in my little town in Vermont. It was fantastic, and it became a very important book for me. I actually sewed a special pocket in my knapsack, and it was with me all the time for nine years. I was carrying it with me when I landed here in Point Reyes, California, in 1980, when my car broke down and I found Pattabhi Jois.

Ashtanga was a great tool for me, and I am very happy that I had the training from *Light on Yoga* before I came to Ashtanga. The first day I came to Pattabhi's class, he asked me who I was and if I was a new yoga student. When I told him I had actually been practicing for years, he asked who my teacher was. I showed him my book, and he laughed, "How can you learn from a book? Oh, you are an Iyengar student. Today you watch." He probably thought I wouldn't come back, but I did and loved it. I found that it was great to have an actual teacher. I practiced it diligently for years. But *Light on Yoga* continued to help me in my Ashtanga practice. We were not getting a lot of instruction in Ashtanga; it was more the practice of doing. *Light on Yoga* helped bring intelligence to the practice.

ANNE O'BRIEN: You and Maty [Ezraty] were innovators in blending the two practices of Iyengar and Ashtanga Yoga at Yoga Works. Could you elaborate on that?

CM: When I met Maty in 1987, I swore I wouldn't move to L.A., but that didn't get me very far! I moved to L.A.; we were running Yoga Works in Santa Monica together and began to look for ways to augment the teachings. We started inviting workshop leaders: Richard Freeman, John Schumacher, Ramanand Patel, Aadil Palkhivala, Dona Holleman,

Judith Hanson Lasater, and others—some of the best in the world. We invited them because we wanted to study with them and share them with our students. Their knowledge and that of other senior Iyengar teachers continued to augment our Ashtanga knowledge.

In 1990, we went to the Yoga 90 Iyengar Yoga event in San Diego, and I met Mr. Iyengar for the first time. It was an interesting experience. The Iyengar community was surprised to see us there, to say the least, and placed us in a beginning class! We were in class, and I was working with one of Mr. Iyengar's teachers—Victor Oppenheimer, I think—in twisting triangle when Mr. Iyengar and his entourage walked in. He came right over to see what was going on and worked with me in twisting triangle on the one side for about five minutes. It was intense, as you can imagine. But I was really prepared to work with Iyengar after having been with Pattabhi. There is a similar intensity. It was a great experience, and I learned a lot—on the right side! I then needed to go home and work for about two years to find the similar intelligence on the left side.

AOB: You were recently in India with Mr. Iyengar. How was that experience compared with your first?

CM: We were invited by one of our Iyengar teachers to come to Pune. We had some trepidation, wondering how we would be welcomed as Ashtanga teachers, but we had a wonderful experience. A nice surprise was to work with Prashant; I found him to be an excellent teacher. I felt blessed to have been there with Mr. Iyengar and all the other teachers and students. Early in the morning, I would practice in the same room with Mr. Iyengar. One morning, he left early during the practice. As I finished my practice, I was sitting there quietly meditating before I went into savasana. I was really, in my mind, just feeling the privilege to have been there in that room to study with him. I was feeling that gratitude and was thankful that he has been able to teach yoga the way he has taught it and to share with all of us what he has learned to make the practice what it is—a safer practice. At the end of my meditation, he was lying in front of me in savasana.

We felt, too, that a corner had been turned in both the Iyengar and Ashtanga communities, a coming together perhaps, or appreciation of both practices. We could feel the similarity between Pattabhi and Iyengar.

It comes from the same place. And there continues to be a richness in blending the two traditions.

CHUCK MILLER has been practicing yoga earnestly since 1971 and began studying Ashtanga Yoga with Sri K. Pattabhi Jois in 1980. These studies have included numerous extended and familial encounters in America, and seven trips to Mysore, India, over nearly two years. Chuck enjoys teaching with a focus on the holistic nature of Ashtanga Yoga, teaching it as both a philosophical system and one with a strong practical method at its core. He is known for his gentle but deliberate hands-on adjustments, which are both reassuring and challenging. Teaching since 1988, Chuck was director of Ashtanga Yoga and a co-owner with Maty Ezraty of the original Yoga Works in Santa Monica, California, for more than sixteen years.

Om Namah Shivaya
B. K. S. Iyengar

Sri Dharma Mittra

The purpose of the asanas, especially as systematized by Guruji, is to maximize the health of the individual. According to the *Upanishads*, neither the development of the spirit nor the attainment of the primary ends of life can be achieved without this.

> *Shariramadyam khalu dharma sadhanam*
> *Dharmartha kama mokshanam arogyam mulamuttamam*

> The primary duty of the body is indeed to be the instrument
> for enacting dharma, or duty.
> Health is the key to performing duty, earning wealth, or using
> life for enjoyment or for emancipation.
> —UPANISHADS

Sri Dharma Mittra is also famed for assisting others to pursue the aims and purposes of life.

I bow to you who brought much light and inspiration to my asana practice. Since the late 1960s, I've been sneaking into your masterpiece *Light on Yoga* for references. This is especially true when I was making the Yoga Chart of 908 Postures in 1984. For me, it is like a "yoga bible," and I often refer students to it. Concerning "alignment," you're the best.

Mr. Iyengar, I see you as an embodiment of Lord Shiva for the way you teach and of Lord Rama for your elegance, love, and the way you dress.

We have shared many students over the years in our love of these teachings. When things come from experience, they can truly be trusted.

OM OM RAM RAM,

DHARMA MITTRA

❦

Sri Dharma Mittra, born in Brazil in the late 1930s, began practicing yoga in 1958. He went to New York to study with Swami Kailashananda. He is the founder and director of the Dharma Mittra Yoga Center in New York City and is perhaps best known for his creation of the 1984 *Master Yoga Chart of 908 Postures*, which has sold 100,000 copies. A vital septuagenarian, Dharma teaches weekly classes (still constantly demonstrating poses) and holds his Life of a Yogi teacher-training courses and workshops worldwide. His book *Asanas: 608 Yoga Poses*, a compendium of photographs from his groundbreaking yoga chart, is a major inspiration to today's yogis. His DVD set of *Maha Sadhana Levels I & II* demonstrates his legacy in teaching over the past forty years.

The Voice Within

JOAN RODGERS

Our essential humanity as purveyors of action rests in the use of three instruments (*karana*) with which we are endowed. These are the *trikarana* of thought, word, and deed—or mind, voice, and body. The ideal life is one in which all three have been purified (*trikarana shuddhi*) and complete harmony exists between them. Life is then guided by ideals.

Gayatri is a Sanskrit word meaning a "song" or "hymn." It is also the name of a meter of Vedic poetry consisting of twenty-four syllables arranged as three lines of eight. Any hymn composed in this meter is then a gayatri. There is, however, one particular mantra that is so revered that it is called "the Gayatri." It is attributed to the sage Vishvamitra and is itself regarded as a goddess, being a representation of *parabrahman* (the supreme essence). It is a divine awakening of the mind and the soul, and chanting it is regarded as a way to attain the highest levels of existence. It is a way to unite with *brahman*.

Gayatri has three aspects, and all three are present in all of us. As Gayatri, she is mistress of the senses. As Savitri, she rules over prana and signifies truth. As Sarasvati, she is the ruler of *vak* (speech). Therefore, when taken together, the three names of Gayatri represent *trikarana suddhi*—purity in thought, word, and deed—with the chanting of "the Gayatri" being a way to attain realization. Joan Rodgers now sings to us about the purity of voice.

I have been practicing yoga for about fifteen years and am so grateful for Iyengar Yoga. The precision of the practice has afforded me a deeper understanding of myself. Practicing yoga helps me to find inner strength and has certainly enhanced my operatic career. It gives me focus, helps me focus, makes me learn to focus. It strengthens and relaxes the body, something a singer definitely needs.

Practicing yoga and meditation before a concert clears my mind and allows my performance to flow freely. It makes all the difference. I will do sun salutations and some forward bends—especially forward bends. I find these so useful to release energy and to bring calm. Any poses I can do that seem to open the sacroiliac area help me.

Mr. Iyengar is an enabler of the practice. He has enabled us to release something inside ourselves. At the same time, he has enabled us to find ourselves or find something inside ourselves that perhaps we didn't even know we had. Thank you, Mr. Iyengar, for enabling us.

§

JOAN RODGERS, a renowned British soprano, appears in operas, concerts, and recitals. She made her professional operatic debut in 1982 in Aix-en-Provence, soon moving on to numerous international engagements. She sings regularly for principal opera companies in the United Kingdom. Joan has appeared with such illustrious conductors as Zubin Mehta, Daniel Barenboim, and Sir Simon Rattle. She has made recordings of principal roles such as Susanna (*The Marriage of Figaro*), Zerlina (*Don Giovanni*), and Despina (*Così fan tutte*), along with numerous solo recordings covering the principal works in the recital repertoire. Joan received the Royal Philharmonic Society Award as Singer of the Year for 1997 and the 1997 Evening Standard Award for outstanding performance in opera for her performance as the governess in the Royal Opera House's production of *The Turn of the Screw*. She was awarded the Companion of the Order of the British Empire (CBE) in 2001.

First Steps to Freedom

LILIAS FOLAN

In *Yoga Sutra* 1:20, the definitive text on yoga, Sage Patanjali tells us that one of the things we need on our journey is *shraddha* (faith), a serene and unflappable confidence that even though we have not yet seen it and probably never will, the objective that we seek exists and can be attained. The path of yoga can be difficult to tread for, almost by definition, the ultimate end of spirit is unobservable. It is beyond. It is beyond description or viable step-by-step direction giving. Nevertheless, gurus, yoga teachers, and books on the subject exist, and they seem to give the guidance required. There must therefore be some pedagogy within yoga, some established art or method or science to being an imparter of this yogic wisdom.

But to think of *pedagogy* as "the correct use of teaching strategies" is to understand the word in a modern sense. It is actually derived from the ancient Greek *paidagogos*, a slave who imparted the techniques of the trade to others. However, those "others" were the children of slaves. No free person would take orders or instruction from a slave. The paidagogos simply made sure that all slaves under his care did everything according to the dictates of the master. Although the connotations of slavery play no part in the modern understanding of *pedagogy*, many educators still do not consider the word relevant to adult education. Some prefer to adopt the term *andragogy* in that context, because adults generally need to know why they are being asked to learn something; prefer to learn experientially rather than by rote; prefer specific applications and problem-solving to endless dry examples; and learn much better when the topic has some immediate value they can grasp. They are also much more self-directed and expect to take—and be given—greater responsibility within the educational process. Teachers in adult education settings can become much more like facilitators.

The issues raised by spiritual education are beautifully summarized in a famous story told by Swami Vivekananda (1863–1902):

There was once a minister to a great king. He fell into disgrace. The king, as a punishment, ordered him to be shut up in the top of a very high tower. This was done, and the minister was left there to perish. He had a faithful wife, however, who came to the tower at night and called to her husband at the top to know what she could do to help him. He told her to return to the tower the following night and bring with her a long rope, some stout twine, packthread, silken thread, a beetle, and a little honey. Wondering much, the good wife obeyed her husband and brought him the desired articles. The husband directed her to attach the silken thread firmly to the beetle, then to smear its horns with a drop of honey and to set it free on the wall of the tower, with its head pointing upward. She obeyed all these instructions, and the beetle started on its long journey. Smelling the honey ahead, it slowly crept onward in the hope of reaching the honey, until at last it reached the top of the tower, where the minister grasped the beetle and got possession of the silken thread. He told his wife to tie the other end to the packthread, and after he had drawn up the packthread, he repeated the process with the stout twine and lastly with the rope. Then the rest was easy. The minister descended from the tower by means of the rope and made his escape. In this body of ours the breath motion is the "silken thread"; by laying hold of and learning to control it, we grasp the packthread of the nerve currents, and from these, the stout twine of our thoughts, and lastly the rope of Prana, controlling which, we reach freedom.★

Swami Vivekananda's elegant story affirms the appropriateness of the ready confidence we can and should have in the aims and attainability of yoga's purpose, thus making our shraddha, or faith, appropriate. It also affirms the kind of learning and teaching—an andragogy rather than a pedagogy—that yoga inspires. The spirit cannot be seen. But like the honey dabbed on the horns of the beetle or the silken, near-invisible, and surely unreliable thread it carries, we can and will—with the certainty of serenity—be guided upward to it and the freedom it promises. The teacher is then our guide to and facilitator of that which is unseen. Sometimes, as Lilias Folan discovered, the pedagogy—the methodology, the set of instructions, the light on yoga—provided by the chosen

---

★ Swami Vivekananda, "The First Steps," in *Raja-Yoga* (New York: Ramakrishna-Vivekananda Center, 1956).

teacher is so fitting and complete that he or she readily facilitates the andragogy required, and we do not even need to meet or see that teacher for such guidance to occur.

B ack in the 1960s, the hatha yoga classes that I both took and taught were quite different than they are today. There might have been fifty students on an outdoor platform, and we were all doing the same yoga postures the same way. Ages twenty to eighty, all different sizes and shapes, many different fitness levels, yet we were not offered any variation in the way we did our postures. Few cautions were spoken. Everyone inhaled to the count of five and exhaled to the count of five. Each student tried to perform the postures perfectly, even if his or her body complained. There was not a sticky mat, belt, blanket, or block in sight.

During those years, I began to notice something very troubling. I was developing injuries where before there were none. My friends could do magnificent scorpion arm balances (vrschikasana) but in private told me how painful it was to sit straight in meditation. Almost everyone, including myself, had a callus or puffy bruise on the back of the neck from doing shoulderstands on a bare floor. How could yoga postures, so highly touted as vehicles of physical and mental health, cause such discomfort?

In light of these disturbing questions, I knew there had to be a better way. Some problems I could figure out for myself, but I could only go so far with my own limited experience and observations. Deep in my heart, I was seriously thinking of quitting my yoga practice.

Looking back on that time in the late 1970s, it is amazing to realize that the universe actually heard my plea for help. Like an echo from the Himalayas, a great teacher's voice came into my life—that of Mr. B. K. S. Iyengar. I would never study with him directly, but I learned from a few of his dedicated, close students at that time.

Bernard Rishi came to Cincinnati, Ohio, from Paris to give a workshop. Rishi was quick to give credit to his teacher, Mr. Iyengar. He listened quietly to my litany of physical discomforts and noticed my feelings of illogical shame that I was not able to solve these problems myself through my yoga practice. He pointed out that my body had been kind to me by giving me early signals to change my hatha yoga practice.

Out came the blankets, carefully folded under my shoulders for shoulderstand. Here were insights to body alignment, the use of props, and countless ways to help myself and my students avoid injury and enjoy the practice.

"Lilias," said Rishi, "you should go to India and greet the lion [the guru, Mr. Iyengar] in his lion's den." But it was not to be. Over the coming years, the brilliance of Mr. Iyengar's teachings would continue to echo in my direction through other teachers—Angela Farmer, Judith Hanson Lasater, and many more. Thank you, Namaste, and Pranams to you, Mr. Iyengar. I continue to be your long-distance student, and I am deeply grateful to you.

§

LILIAS FOLAN, known as the "First Lady of Yoga" since her groundbreaking 1972 yoga series *Lilias! Yoga and You,* is regarded as one of America's most knowledgeable and respected yoga teachers. Through her television shows, books, audiotapes, videos, workshops, and seminars, Folan has spent nearly three decades helping people learn about the benefits of yoga for the body, mind, and spirit. She first became involved with yoga at the age of thirty, when her doctor suggested trying the system of simple stretching and breathing techniques to help relieve a variety of ailments that included back pain, sleeping problems, and a general case of the "blahs." Finding that yoga renewed her vitality and energy, she continued her yoga practice in New York City, where she studied and taught with some of the finest teachers from Europe, India, and America.

Light on B. K. S. Iyengar

Maxine Tobias

A gem bestowed with good qualities ensures the good luck, prosperity and success of kings. Any with bad qualities will bring disaster and misfortune. Therefore the cognoscenti should assess their fortunes according to the state of these gems.
—Brihat Samhita of Varahamiriha, chapter 80, verses 1–3

A gem free from all defects and shining in its characteristic internal lustre should be regarded as the harbinger of good fortune. . . . Inward lustre, transparency, brilliancy of rays, sparkle, the lack of impurities, and good formation are the salient properties of good gems.
—Agni Purana, chapter 246, verses 7 and 13–14

On November 26, 1922, Howard Carter stood with Lord Carnarvon, Lord Carnarvon's daughter, and a few others in attendance. He stepped forward with his chisel and "with trembling hands" made the now-famous "tiny breach in the upper left hand corner" of the doorway that stood before him.* He then peered into the small hole he had made. He later wrote, "It was sometime before one could see. The hot air escaping caused the candle to flicker, but as soon as one's eyes became accustomed to the glimmer of light the interior of the chamber gradually loomed before one, with its strange and wonderful medley of extraordinary and beautiful objects heaped upon one another."† "I was struck dumb with amazement, and when asked 'Can you see anything?', it was all I could do to get out the words 'Yes, wonderful things.'"‡ Even as the pale candlelight flickered, Carter realized that he was looking at three-

---

* Howard Carter and A. C. Mace, *The Discovery of the Tomb of Tutankhamen* (New York: Dover, 1977).
† *Encyclopedia Britannica Online*, s.v. 2007, "Carter, Howard," http://www.britannica.com/eb/article-9020544.
‡ Carter and Mace, *The Discovery of the Tomb of Tutankhamen*.

dimensional objects in abundance. There appeared to be enormous gold bars stacked against the wall opposite him, along with ebony treasures. Transfixed and dumbfounded, he just continued to mutter, "Wonderful, marvelous, my God, wonderful." He had found something much more than a treasure for himself. He had fulfilled a dream. He had found a treasure for all humankind.

Carter's reaction was quite understandable. He and the Carnarvons were standing in front of the antechamber to Tutankhamen's burial chamber. They were to be the first people to set foot in it since it had been sealed three thousand years before. Three months later, on February 16, 1923, Carter opened the inner sealed doorway and found that it led to the burial chamber itself, where he got his first glimpse of Tutankhamen's sarcophagus: "The effect was bewildering, overwhelming."* "The golden sarcophagus is one of the greatest masterpieces of the goldsmiths' art of all time; it contains two hundred kilogrammes of gold, is one and a half meters high, and is encrusted with lapis lazuli, turquoise and cornelians."† Carter was enraptured. The deep significance of what he was looking at was not lost on him.

As human beings, we are prone to inner dialogues such as "If I had not been quite so prone to fear, I would have seen the truth of that situation more readily." Or "If I had looked a little more closely, I would have seen that that was a rope and not a snake." Patanjali tells us that the aim of yoga is to quiet the mind so that it no longer gives us this dangerous kind of flawed information about our selves, our capabilities, and the world around us. In *Yoga Sutra* I:41, he uses the word *kshina* to describe the gradual, yoga-induced wasting away of such proclivities. But what then steps forward to take their place?

A gem is often described as breathtaking in its beauty. When we hold it up to the light, it is so luminous and lustrous, such a purveyor of the light that falls upon it, that we are entranced not only by the gem itself, but by the whole scenario, as light and gem are mutually enhanced. When we take the gem out of the light, it immediately darkens, and we think more of its value and see its shape, structure, and so forth. Its ability to enrapture us with light is still there, but the rapture itself is gone.

Although most of the time we do not see it, the light of the spirit

---

* Carter and Mace, *The Discovery of the Tomb of Tutankhamen*, 95–96.
† A. Chalaby, *All of Egypt* (n.p.: Bonechi Guides, 1998).

shines constantly; it always has the ability to enrapture. A gem would surely help us see it. If we could only find one, then we could hold it up to the Light and be enraptured. Patanjali assures us that such a gem exists. But as we search for that gem, we should take heed of the warning given us in chapter 246, verse 8 of the *Agni Purana:* "A gem which is cracked, fissured, lacking in lustre, or that appears rough and sandy, should never be used." The *Garuda Purana* (chapter 70, verse 19) adds its voice by saying, "The person who, out of ignorance, wears a gem with many flaws will assuredly be tormented by grief, anxiety, sickness, death, a loss of wealth and other calamities." So how are we to avoid flawed gems and instead find only those gems that are even more delightful than those discovered by Howard Carter?

Flaws in gems are caused by *chitta vritti,* the mind's tendency to move, which it is yoga's mission to quell. *Yoga Sutra* 1:41 confirms this by saying that when the observer is so enraptured by the vision that even the sensation of seeing has gone, then it is the entirety of that person that becomes the precious gem. This is a gem that does nothing but glorify the Light seen, the person seeing, and itself. When we hold this gem and turn our attention to it, we find that it holds us instead. But where is that gem to be found?

As Maxine Tobias tells us, the best—and perhaps the only—way to find such a gem is to be shown it, be told about it, and see it in someone who has already found it.

A great teacher is like a precious jewel because we are illuminated by his or her presence. We all have enormous potential to develop as human beings, and a great teacher recognizes and helps that potential surface so that we shine brightly, too.

In the United Kingdom, I had searched far and wide for a yoga teacher, and I found Penny Nield-Smith, who was teaching Iyengar Yoga. I loved the structure and the liberation that I felt after a class with her. It was so different from the yoga I had been practicing. We were told that Guruji, although we did not refer to him by that title in those days, was coming to London to give classes and we could have as many as we could afford. I signed up with eager anticipation.

I remember the first glimpse I had of B. K. S. Iyengar in London in 1969. He entered the room, a small, quiet, unassuming man. He was dressed in a white dhoti, and I was already aware of something greater than I had imagined. I could smell the sandalwood oil emanating from his skin. From that very moment, I can say without any doubt that I was inspired by his presence alone. Then he changed into his green shorts for the class. What a transformation! Suddenly he was bigger, more physically there; energy was filling the room. From this small man had grown a giant of a teacher.

He organized those present into rows, with smaller people like me at the front and taller ones behind. It was all very precise and regimented. Then he said the name of the first pose in Sanskrit, which sounded so different from the way that I had heard it said before, but I understood and began to move. I wanted to give my all. He made you feel that way. We repeated the pose several times with a bit more instruction and, for some, the inevitable correction to their pose. What was it that made me want to do the pose with every fiber in my body? It was this great teacher bringing out my potential. I longed to be corrected by him and, like an overeager child, I tried far too hard in every movement and earned some correction. I can still remember every sensation of being adjusted in a pose by B. K. S. Iyengar, a privilege many students have never had.

Guruji came to London for a month every year, and each time was a revelation. Almost overnight, the students in the classes doubled, tripled, and soon we were making friends with people who had come from different countries and continents to be taught by him. His fame was growing. We were graded into A, B, and C classes and I was fortunate enough by now to be in the A stream. But it was terrifying! If we were in the top stream, then we had to *be* the top stream; there was no going back. We now had to practice, practice, practice to be ready for our teacher when he came back to us. I have been in classes where there were about fifty students, and Guruji dropped all of us back from standing into urdhva dhanurasana—not once, but over and over—and then he would throw our legs back into hand balance and down on two feet to the floor. His energy and strength were remarkable, because there were some big men in the class and we were all rather raw as students. I was seeing stars, but they were in heaven. He was like a lion—fierce, fearless, commanding, and exacting—but we still managed to laugh. He was putting us into kapotasana, and as he came to me, he tripped slightly. Recovering, he said to me, "You break my toe, I'll break your back!" And there I was in kapotasana seeing stars again. Everybody thought this hilarious but did not dare laugh out loud. I can remember coming from class and being able to see without my spectacles for about two hours.

In those days, we had lovely outings to parks for picnics, theater shows, and small gatherings to eat delicious food prepared by Silva Mehta, who cooked for B. K. S. (as we called him) when he was in London. Following the Hindu tradition, especially being of the Brahmin caste, he does not eat eggs or fermented foods. So there were the food police. I remember that once somebody who did not understand the seriousness of his dietary laws made him a cake but sloshed brandy into it. Alas, he could not eat it, but we all tucked in. Those outings were glorious, sunny, summer days, and we came home in a bus, having had the good fortune to be near Guruji and feel some of his love. Some of the teachers from that era have now passed away: Silva Mehta, who was one of the founding Iyengar Yoga teachers and who greatly influenced Iyengar's coming to England in the sixties; Bunny Read; Eileen Piercey, who did the wonderful illustrations in *Light on Yoga;* Penny Nield-Smith; and Clara Buck, to name but a few. Many of us who were "bright young things" in those days are now grandparents! I find that hard to believe and even harder to believe that Guruji will soon be ninety years old. His flame is still burning brightly, and we are still being illuminated by his presence.

Then there were the trips to Pune. It was like being in a large family. I remember in particular attending a "backbending" course given by Guruji for senior teachers in 1992, one that made us physically stronger and spiritually enriched. One morning, we were invited to watch Guruji go through his own backbending practice, which was truly a moving experience and one that shed light on the work that we were doing in the course. A great man, a great teacher, and a great artist. A Picasso in the yoga world, B. K. S. Iyengar must be ranked with other great thinkers and artists of the twentieth century—a man ahead of his time. He brought to the West the blueprint of yoga from which many styles have developed.

When we look at a great work of art, it has a universal quality that puts it in any time and surpasses its cultural limitations. In thirteenth-century England, man's spiritual aspirations found lofty expression in the building of Gothic cathedrals. Their vaulted ceilings served a spiritual purpose—to take the eyes and heart upward toward God. Guruji's back-bends expressed this spiritual quality: the height of the spine was breath-taking, and the arms and legs gave the pose support and energy that enabled him to remain in a perfect state of stillness for minutes. This was not a cosmetic performance, moving only the body; the spirit moved through it, an expression of the inner creative energy tempered by his intelligence and precision. This was so vital in his practice that I was moved to tears. A great teacher of yoga must be a great practitioner.

The opportunity to face this challenge and find this integrity in our own practice and self-development is one of the greatest gifts B. K. S. Iyengar gives us. When children are learning to walk, we do not stop them for fear of them falling over, but we remove the obstacles that get in their way or might harm them. We instill in our children love, kindness, fortitude, fidelity, and bravery so they will grow into humans with a conscience. We develop in our yoga just as children do, learning to be courageous, dedicated, and having moral strength. These qualities make us civilized. I believe that Guruji's teachings have furthered the course of humanity. I quote a few lines from Nelson Mandela, another man of great character, intelligence, and conscience, from his 1994 inaugural speech as president of South Africa:

> We are meant to shine, as children do.
> We were born to make manifest the glory of God that is within us.
> It is not just in some of us:
> It's in everyone, and as we let our own light shine,
> We unconsciously give other people permission to do the same.

—NELSON MANDELA

❦

MAXINE TOBIAS began teaching yoga in 1971 at the behest of B. K. S. Iyengar. For many years, she dedicated herself to teaching yoga in adult education for the Inner London Educational Authority. She served on the committee of the B. K. S. Iyengar Yoga Teacher's Association, edited the first Iyengar newsletter in the United Kingdom, and ran one of the first Iyengar teacher-training programs. She was accredited with an advanced-level certificate by B. K. S. Iyengar for her dedication and achievement in yoga. Tobias owns a studio in Chelsea, London, and is the author of several books, including *Stretch and Relax* and *Complete Stretching*. Her yoga expertise has led her to create a video, *Basic Yoga,* and to design the Chelsea Yoga Kit, a collection of yoga clothes.

The Dancer's Posture

Yana Lewis

According to the *Natya Shastra* and *Abhinaya Darpana,* treatises on dancing, dance was created by Brahma, the Creator, at the request of Indra
and the other gods, who desired some entertainment. Since the other
fourVedas were restricted to priests, Brahma went into a trance and drew
literature from the *Rig Veda,* song from the *Sama Veda, abhinaya* (expression) from the *Yajur Veda,* and *rasa* (aesthetic experience) from the
Atharva Veda. He combined these to create the *Natya Veda* as a fifthVeda
that was accessible to all. But since none of the gods could dance, Indra
was not able to use the *Natya Veda* to enlighten and entertain them.
Brahma therefore handed it on to his son, Bharata, who then handed it
on to his one hundred sons. Bharata staged his first play in the amphithe-
ater of the Himalayas with his hundred sons and the *apsaras* (celestial
dancers). Shiva was so taken by it that he sent his disciple Tandu to
Bharata to learn the elements of dance. Shiva ended up learning the *tan-
dava* (masculine form), while his consort, Parvati, learned the *lasya* (feminine form). Through Bharata, dance eventually came to earth.

Indian dance is a triple blend of *nritta* (rhythmic elements), *nritya* (a
combination of rhythm and expression), and *natya* (the dramatic element). It is usually necessary to be familiar with Indian legends in order
to comprehend natya (the dance dramas), because the vast majority of
dances take their themes from myth and legend. Nritta, being the entirely rhythmic component, is concerned exclusively with the movements of the body devoid of emotional content. Nritya, on the other
hand, uses the eyes, hands, and facial movements to convey that content.
It comprises abhinaya and depicts rasa and *bhava* (mood). A dance is
therefore made up of nritya combined with nritta in the service of a
natya.

Classical Indian dance is a combination of bhava, *raga* (melody), and
tala (rhythm). Each style of classical dance has its *gati* (stylized form or
gait). The *Natya Shastra* not only describes all the movements of the

*anga*s (major limbs)—the head, chest, sides, hips, hands, and feet—but also gives detailed descriptions of the *upanga*s (minor limbs). There are intricate movements of the eyebrows, eyeballs, eyelids, chin, and nose— sometimes described in excruciating detail, and all intended to create specific moods and effects. It takes a considerable amount of focus and concentration to keep a consistent rhythm while feet and body parts move and tilt in parallel and contrary directions, and hands and eyebrows follow their own precisely defined choreography—all the while allowing the mood and drama of the dance and the expressiveness of the dancer to be conveyed. Whether it searches for enlightenment and peace in dance or in asana, a dancer's body—such as Yana Lewis's—must obviously learn to align itself with precision, while at the same time being a vehicle for the expression of the universe.

Beloved Guruji,

I am deeply honored to be given this opportunity to thank you from my heart. Words cannot express the gratitude that I feel for your gift to all of us by sharing your immense knowledge and wisdom in the art of yoga. You have touched so many lives in so many different ways. You have given me so much. You have changed my life and given me a sense of belonging. You have given life to my life. You have given me the guidance to grow and the glimpse of harmony and oneness that I knew existed. You have given birth to the real me that was trapped inside for so many years, just waiting to grow. You nurtured that very essence, and it continues to grow new every day, and every day a step closer to *samadhi*.

Thank you from the depths of within. I write this as a practitioner of Iyengar Yoga for twenty years and a classical ballet dancer and teacher. My life's work is entirely in the field of dance. Iyengar Yoga has really shaped my teaching skills in classical ballet; enhanced my awareness of my own art; and given depth, musicality, and freedom for creativity in my field. I have also gained immensely from yoga on a personal level.

When I took my first yoga class, I was working as a professional ballet and jazz dancer. I had been in many companies and was appearing on television weekly. My job was very outward-oriented, performing and giving energy to the audience.

I never sat still as a child. In fact, I would spend much of my time in what I now know as sirsasana. My family used to tease me constantly that they saw more of my feet than my head. I studied dance and went to a full-time vocational ballet school at the age of twelve. My father would always say that I should do yoga, which I used to think was a joke, but as I reflect now, perhaps he had a greater insight into yoga than I realized. My father passed away when I was twenty-one, and I used to hear echoes of his advice about yoga.

One day I found myself in an Iyengar Yoga class. I spent the whole class thinking that I was a dancer and should be able to do this! When I tried these very strange positions people were calling asanas, I was like a child—shaky, wobbly, and feeling extremely awkward. My mind was so present; my ego was leaping up every few seconds; and my body, which I used on a daily basis and was so graceful and fluid, suddenly felt strange venturing into the unknown. I felt very much like a child learning to ride a bicycle. From that first class to now, it has been a very long road, with an abundance of learning, growing, feeling, awareness, and opening.

I was very curious after just one class and was drawn back to investigate further. I never left yoga from that day. Yoga has become a way of life for me. My life is so enriched on a daily basis. I thank Guruji for everything. The early days of yoga were very confrontational, dramatic, and life-changing. I gradually found myself becoming totally absorbed by it. I was very involved in Iyengar Yoga, as the details of the asanas intrigued me. The number of classes I attended started growing. My first impressions of Guruji came from my teacher in North London, Silvia Prescott, who passed on Guruji's teaching and words with intrinsic detail. Silvia would quote Guruji and recall his words and instructions in great detail. One in particular was about two rivers—one flowing up and one flowing down with energy—with relationship to the inner and outer leg, the spine, or the complete asana. I used the process and fields of direction and applied it to a dancer's class work. It gave a greater insight and technical advancement. In performance, it gives a more vibrant, dynamic quality.

Silvia knew my dancer's body, and I felt that in a class she would take it apart and put it back together for savasana. The effects it had on me internally were astounding. I was so peaceful, silent, and still and felt a deep sense of being connected to something universal. I felt centered and whole. For me, it was an incredible process of transformation that I felt so clearly and strongly.

I remember on a particular yoga weekend, where the focus for the first morning was on backbends, I thought I wouldn't survive the morning. I remember so clearly struggling as we were told to push up in urdhva dhanurasana. My dance teachers had told me that my shoulders were stiff. I never really fully understood why until this particular day, when all was revealed to me. My shoulders were so stiff that I could barely push up. I remember thinking, *Oh no, please don't say push up again and again*. The teacher came and tried to open them, but my body did not respond. I was just grateful for that brief moment of help! I had approached backbend before in classes but with a lot of preparations and props. This was just mat to wall and pushing up. The class was very full, and I was feeling like I just wanted to run away out the door and not return. I kept thinking, *Why are we not doing standing poses? I felt I was beginning to get a glimpse into those asanas. I was beginning to enjoy standing asanas.* I was immediately pulled back to the present and was told to push up into urdhva dhanurasana. I began to feel awkward, frustrated, and emotional. It seemed that every yoga class, or yoga day, or yoga intensive, the teacher just seemed to target what I clearly needed the most. I felt it was universal that I must be communicating in some way and being directed to all the classes that would do me good. I took a deep breath and knew I was not going to give up. I just channeled myself into yoga and tried to switch my mind off. I pushed up so many times that I lost count. We were given various instructions, but I could not follow any of them with any depth. I had little awareness at that time, especially when I was upside down.

I pushed on all morning, and by lunchtime I was in a quiet, sensitive space. A whole set of new doors had opened for me. I had to find my spine and my shoulders and open these areas. My lumbar region was always very flexible, but my thoracic was extremely stiff, and my shoulders had very little movement. I realized by reading *Light on Yoga* and *Light on the Yoga Sutras of Patanjali* that these were not just physical blocks, but emotional, spiritual blocks too. That very difficult backbend weekend helped me process so much new information and gave me a thirst to discover more about myself, the real me, the one beyond this body. The very reason that I had taken up yoga in the first place was my feeling of disconnection and knowing there was more to life than the surface level. I finally had taken a shift to a new dimension, the spiritual body.

During the first ten years of Iyengar Yoga, I realized just how much our beloved Guruji was giving to the West. He brought yoga to people like me with his intricate detail and understanding. It was tangible, and at that time in my life, that was a very important factor.

Dancers love to push themselves, so the discipline required for a regular yoga practice came very naturally to me. I would try to do all the asanas that I found very difficult on a daily basis. In the early days, it was virasana, so I would make myself sit in the asana to eat with blocks under my bottom, gradually reducing them over a period of few months. I would do adho mukha vrksasana at least ten times daily, as I could not stay in the pose at all. Forward bends came naturally, so I did not practice them so much. I used to practice everything I did not like or I felt awkward doing. I felt that way I would learn faster. I believed I was directing the pace of my yoga asanas, but now I know that the asanas themselves have to unfold, each with its own uniqueness from within me. I just cannot control it. I began my own daily practice as well as going to classes. It was not something I had planned. It just seemed to grow by itself and become a part of me, of my life.

I remember discovering so many new ways of looking at movement, alignment, and energy in my yoga classes that I would translate into my own practice for ballet. I discovered amazing new techniques to help dancers master difficulties in new, deeper ways, with more attention to the process of the movement than the result, as a dancer would normally see it. My teaching of classical ballet changed! I became very analytical yet creative with details, musicality, and energy flows. My choreographic ability improved, and it became so much easier to express myself fully through the music. I was enjoying and learning with my work as well as my yoga. There was a reason for everything, I was learning, and the speed seemed to increase. I had tapped into the vast reservoir of knowledge and was gaining so much joy in just absorbing what I could as I dived deeper and deeper into it.

I advise my students who wish to take up dance professionally to study yoga to prevent injuries due to the asymmetrical use of the body in performance. When I am doing remedial work with injured dancers or those with technical weakness, I often use yoga asanas.

The second decade of my yoga was very dramatic. It changed my life in many new and exciting ways. I had my own successful ballet school in North London for ten years and was still working as a dancer. The more I practiced yoga, the more I realized that my material possessions—a flat, a car, and so on—meant nothing to me. They did not feed my soul.

I was being drawn more and more toward India, and I wondered if it was the yoga or me. Or was the yoga so much a part of me now, that it was just my destiny? When Guruji's eightieth birthday celebrations were announced, I knew I had to attend—in India. I followed my intuition, as I felt I was being guided so strongly by it. I sold my house and gave away everything I owned. It was such a liberating experience, freedom from the clutter that I had collected over the years. It took approximately one and a half years to organize everything with business and home. What I was left with was a rucksack with a few clothes! I felt so free and eager to find out what was in store for me. I left the United Kingdom and arrived in India on November 3, 1998. I had planned to see a little of South India and then go to Pune for the celebrations of Guruji's birthday. I fell in love with India, the country, the vibration, the people, the culture, and the spirituality that is very present there. I could not leave, and I finally felt a sense of belonging. The simplicity, the harsh reality present on a daily basis; life is very real and uncomplicated away from the consumerism I find in the West. I have never left since that day except for vacation.

The celebration was so inspiring for me, to meet so many people from all walks of life coming to celebrate Guruji's birthday and learn more about yoga. For the first time, I felt I was among my kind of people. I have been to Pune several times since then. I have been privileged to be there when Guruji has taught. I have watched as Guruji made an unskillful trikonasana blossom like a flower opening. It was like poetry in motion to watch him teach. We can only practice and aspire to gain insight through Guruji's teachings.

My practice has evolved as I continue with it for two and a half to three hours daily. My stiff shoulders of the early classes have vanished completely, and I enjoy the freedom of a new thoracic spine for my dance as well as my yoga. In the early days, I used to stare at ekapada urdhva dhanurasana, rajakapotasana, kapotasana, and natarajasana in *Light on Yoga* and study the details. They used to be a target, a goal, and now they are a part of my daily practice. These asanas help to bring my body back to balance, harmony, and a sense of inner peace at the end of a long day of dance.

I live a beautiful, happy, holistic, and simple lifestyle with my wonderful Indian husband, whom I met in India and married in 2002. I look forward to the next decade of unfolding in yoga with an open heart and mind and all the enthusiasm I had in the early years. I owe it all to you, Guruji, and I thank you from the core of my heart.

YANA LEWIS is an international ballerina and choreographer from the United Kingdom. She holds an associate diploma from the Imperial Society of Teachers of Dancing; a certificate in anatomy and physiology from the Royal Society; and an arts educational diploma. She has performed leading roles in *Swan Lake*, *Sleeping Beauty*, *Coppelia*, and *Peter and the Wolf*, and has been a lead dancer in many television shows, music videos, and commercials. She has ballet schools in the United Kingdom and India, as well as her own dance company in India.

Yana is also the founder and managing trustee of the Lewis Foundation of Classical Ballet, a charitable trust to promote classical ballet in India and fund full-time vocational training for Indian dancers in Europe. The trust works with orphans and street children in India. Her deep interest in yoga took her to Pune, India, where she trained with B. K. S Iyengar, and has had an ongoing twenty-year practice. Her certificate in anatomy and physiology, combined with her deep understanding of movement and muscles, helps Yana bring fresh insights to yoga and dance. She combines yoga with Pilates to help injured dancers and improve muscle strength and flexibility, and she encourages her students to reach beyond their limitations to find new depths in their practice.

Being in the World

ANNETTE BENING

The drama of being in existence sometimes asks us to suppress or augment the various possibilities for action we have available within ourselves. We can consciously refer to a storehouse of subjective knowledge,
and we can respond unconsciously according to habit. In addition, we
have a storehouse of objective knowledge, which is our current stock of
information on the world. All of this is subject to change. Although these
internal and external kinds of knowledge influence each other, the link
is not always obvious, and we do not always bear their connections in
mind.

According to the view of yoga, we can only exist as individuals if we
have both the internal capacity to appreciate ourselves as doers and subjects, and the ability to perceive external objects. "I" must be able to do
something to "that." This can only happen if the "I" possesses *chitta*, or
pure consciousness. Chitta, therefore, has three important attributes:
ahamkara, or "I"-ness; *buddhi*, or intelligence; and *manas*, or mind.

Chitta has two facets. On the one hand, there is *vidya* (objective
knowledge), the knowledge that comes from learning and being edu-
cated in and by the outside world. It is gleaned by contact with objects
as they display their objectivity. On the other hand, there is *jnana* (subjective knowledge), an inner knowledge that can be gained only through
experiencing the inner world. It is a kind of "emotional intelligence,"
the nexus and recording of our many responses as we gradually stitch
them together into a coherent whole. We do this as we are buffeted
around by our reactions to the diversity of things we perceive. Thus we
attempt to navigate our way through fields of experience established by
such dualities as pleasure and pain, cold and heat, joy and sorrow, reality
and illusion, contentment and discontent, and so on. Such experiences
form our responses—as subjects—to objects and their objectivity.

As individuals, our struggle is to become actors in the drama of existence by enabling our selves to acquire and act out our jnana. We seek
to reconcile our subjective and objective stores of information. Our
characters and personalities then become what we choose to reveal and

conceal, to augment and suppress, to expose and impose at any given time. Yoga is the quest to bring the subjective and objective together, so both our existence and our awareness of existence stand in their own true light. This requires skill in the truth of being.

But there is another kind of quest for the truth of being, the one now addressed by Annette Bening. Although the craft of acting has many different approaches and philosophies, it can be seen as the attempt by an individual to portray a given character by adding to and subtracting from aspects of her own personality, so that she can—in truth and with complete believability—expose and convey whatever might be the "real" and "true" character hidden within. The actor tries to respond to the objective world not as she would in herself and as herself, but in ways that accord with whatever she is trying to emulate at the time. That is to say, the emotional intelligence of the actor must be deployed in such a way that something which lies entirely within stands revealed in its own true light.

Annette Bening was interviewed by Anne O'Brien in June 2006.

ANNE O'BRIEN: Annette, you have studied yoga for many years. When did you begin practicing Iyengar Yoga?

ANNETTE BENING: I began yoga when I was in acting school in San Francisco at the American Conservatory Theater (ACT). They brought in a yoga teacher, Bonita Bradley, an Iyengar Yoga teacher who had studied with Mr. Iyengar. She was my first teacher. We were also taking voice classes that seemed to be using yoga techniques as well. There was lots of concentration on opening the body, learning the physiology of breathing, the physiology of the ribs and the intercostal muscles, and just opening and stretching. Of course, voice production is air. It's just basically learning how to get lots of air and get rid of lots of air quickly, which produces volume. We were training to be in the theater, so they were trying to teach us how to find ways to produce a lot of volume and maintain a body that was not tense, a body that was relaxed, without unnecessary tension.

I responded to the yoga classes because there was so much stress being in acting school. It was an all-day program lasting three years. I found myself drawn to yoga right away because it was such a stress reliever. My first impression was that it affected my mind. That was the most pungent impression that I had to begin with: it calmed my mind. Over the years, reading and studying the whole philosophy behind yoga, I've learned that part of the whole aim is to address the mind. But of course when you're just starting out, you don't know that; you just experience it. I was very fortunate because that experience was palpable. It transcended the intellect. It transcended anything else. It was an experience of being able to really address my own mental activity.

AOB: Does that transcendent quality of yoga enter into other areas of your life?

AB: Sure. It's one of the basic principles, though it is not easy for me to articulate, which is why I like reading Iyengar's books. I feel like, "Oh, yeah, that's it!" I couldn't put it into words, but he sure could. I try to use the practice of maintaining an inner equanimity when working to my maximum in my professional life. Acting is a very physical activity. It's also psychological and mental and emotional and intellectual and all of those things, but it's certainly physical, especially working on the stage. So in a literal way, it's very applicable in that you want to find a way to use your body to its maximum and not have undue tension. From a psychological standpoint, it's the same. You want to find yourself on the edges of your capacity yet maintain some sort of inner calm. I guess *calm* is a good word, or at least the ability to direct oneself, rather than feeling a victim of whatever moment you're in, especially as an actor.

AOB: Many note that in Mr. Iyengar's presence, there's a feeling of light, a power that emanates from him and that is shed on those around him. Since you recently had the opportunity to share a stage with Mr. Iyengar to interview him, could you talk a little bit about your experience with this light and power that you might have felt?

AB: I found Mr. Iyengar to be very open, with a wonderful sense of humor, and he is more than happy to laugh at any moment about anything. In fact, my first question to him as I interviewed him was "How important is a sense of humor for a yoga practitioner?" With that, the one-thousand-plus audience cracked up, as did Mr. Iyengar. "If there is no sense of humor," he answered, "then life is not worth living."

I think that is an example to all of us about how to live life. The sharpness of his mind is so impressive. I have a lot of longevity in my family. One of my grandfathers lived to be one hundred. So when I look at Mr. Iyengar and other people who've achieved that age with such vitality, I think that gives me somewhere to strive. I think he's an incredibly accessible, open person. When he was here most recently, he was so obviously enjoying himself. He really seems to enjoy life. For someone with such discipline and who's so admired, that could be a burden—to deal with so many people wanting something from him. But he seems to have a kind of endless font inside of him that just comes out. It's like a fountain of energy and a fountain of joy. He was also very funny with me. I mean, some of the things I asked him about, he just enjoyed it so much and just laughed and giggled and made us all laugh. I think that lightness and that joy in life is what we're looking for when we're studying yoga. We're not looking to be in some room with our eyes closed, breathing; we want to be in the world. And I think he really stresses that in his books and in his practice—that this is a practice for those of us who are in the world and want to be involved in life and work and family and all of those things. The true test of all of this yoga is, how does it affect you when you are interacting in the world with everyone around you?

AOB: How does yoga affect you in your world? As we all go through life, our bodies change, perceptions change, roles in life change, and with luck, maturity comes. How has your practice changed as your life has evolved and continues to evolve, particularly thinking of your life as a well-known actress contrasted with balancing pregnancies, motherhood, and family life?

AB: It's the place I go to be able to absorb and quite frankly enjoy all of the things that I've got going on. I have four children. So it's a busy world, it's a busy life. I'm very grateful for that. And I work. Yoga is one of the constants. One of the things that is so beautiful about the Iyengar teachers and the teachers that I've had is they really teach you how to use the practice for what you need. Whether you're overly hyped-up and you need to calm yourself down, or whether you're feeling down and you need to find a way out of it. Or you just need to let go and do the restorative work. It becomes a tool to find a way to not feel like a victim of my own mental vicissitudes. This is something I strive for. I don't ever feel like I've gotten there completely, but it's a way to at least address a stressful, busy life and to be able to appreciate it and enjoy it. It's a big deal going through pregnancy, and going through it four times is pretty demanding! But having the yoga really helped, especially as I got bigger and bigger and couldn't move as much. It was a way, again, to take care of myself.

AOB: One of the things that you alluded to is that Mr. Iyengar is continually learning and curious. He uses the physical body as a window into that vast inquiry. He encourages his students to develop that same inquiry, to follow their own inward journey. Where is your curiosity taking you now?

AB: As we get older, we begin to shed skins, like a snake does, and there's a kind of . . . perhaps on a good day [chuckles] you lose some of the neuroses that you have when you're younger and you begin to really know yourself better. I guess one of the things that yoga gives us the opportunity to do is to face ourselves, which is not easy. It's not an easy task to face oneself honestly, but that's what we're doing when we go into a class or when we're practicing at home. As we get older and we face ourselves, hopefully, we're more familiar. We're more familiar with our own tendencies, mental and physical. Perhaps we can hone them a little bit and leave off the stuff that is counterproductive or just a waste of time. The process of studying is the same as the process of living. The way that you approach your practice is the way that you approach your kids and your work and the people around you. I feel so fortunate in my life. I feel like I've been given so much. I have such a wonderful family and do work that I enjoy. My practice gives me a chance to really feel grateful. It gives me the opportunity to really experience it. There's a kind of quality that I see in my teachers who are Iyengar practitioners; they are so in the moment. They are so present. And in that kind of learning mentality, there is a sense of "What are we doing right now? In this moment? With this pose or this series of poses? What are we getting at that perhaps we haven't gotten at before?" When I see people who are far more experienced and knowledgeable on the subject than I am approaching things with such a fresh perspective, it is inspiring to me. Then I feel like maybe I can bring that into my own life—not only my practice, but my life with my family and with my work. Life experience does teach you, but there's always something new, and there's always something new to study and to read. I certainly feel like that in my profession. It's like peeling away an onion: there's just more and more and more to discover.

AOB: And isn't it wonderful to be guided in that yogic discovery?

AB: Without question. I mean that's why Mr. Iyengar's teaching is so powerful. Since I've been the recipient of so much of his teachers' teaching, I can see how he has inspired them. So I think all great teachers have a love of passing things on, and he obviously is completely dedicated in that way. He is trying to give people a taste of what it's like to apply one's self and to care enough about one's self and one's own existence with discipline and energy. Because there are so many other things to do, you know? It's so much easier to just sit and do nothing. I think the beauty in his approach to life and teaching is his dedication to his students and his dedication to his teaching. That, in turn, is passed on to all of his students—their love of teaching, their desire to get something across and to share.

I would like to thank him for all of his incredible dedication to practice and to his students. We all appreciate so much his generosity in giving so much of himself to all of us. And we are awaiting his next visit to the United States!

§

ANNETTE BENING graduated from San Francisco State University and began her acting career with the American Conservatory Theater in San Francisco, eventually moving to New York, where she appeared on the stage. She has been featured in many theater productions and movies, including *The Grifters, Bugsy, American Beauty,* and *Being Julia,* receiving several Oscar nominations. She is married to actor Warren Beatty and has four children.

The Balance of the Self

ELISE BROWNING MILLER

There are two great systems of health and well-being based on the Sankhya philosophy: yoga and ayurveda. But although they both have the same foundation, their aims are somewhat different. The *Ashtangahridayam,* a medieval classic on ayurveda written by the Indian Buddhist practitioner Vagbhat, defines its aims by saying, *"Rogastu dosha vaisamyam, dosha samyam arogata,"* or "The imbalance of the *dosha*s (humors) is called disease, while the balance of the doshas is freedom from disease." Ayurveda therefore holds that diseases have two essential causes: imbalances of the body's energies, and karmic or psychological factors. Although the latter are felt to predominate over the former, both are present in most diseases. But whatever their precise relations, they ultimately result in a loss of the essential energetic balance of the body, which it is then the ayurvedic practitioner's duty to restore. Interestingly, however, the *Charaka Samhita,* the truly great classic of ayurveda, defines the aims a bit differently: *Vikaro dhatu vaisamyam samyam prakrtirucyate sukham samjnakam arogyam vikaro duhkhamevata,* or "Disease is any disturbance in the balance of the *dhatu*s (tissues). Health is their equilibrium state. Health and disease are each defined, respectively, as pleasure and pain."*

Having defined *yoga* in *Yoga Sutra* 1:2 as "the cessation of movements in the consciousness," Patanjali immediately tells us in the next verse what happens to the aspirant when that state is attained: *Tada drashtuh svarupe 'vasthanam,* or "Then the seer dwells in his own true splendor." Viewed in this light, any search for a more physical state of well-being—that is, having a more overtly medical approach—can be referred to as *svasthya* (health) in that it seeks for a sound mind-body complex. As defined by Patanjali, however, yoga's aim is somewhat different. It is to bring about *svarupavastha,* or the ability to abide in one's own true nature.

---

* *Charaka Samhita,* Sutrasthana 9.4.

Many people begin studying yoga, as Elise Browning Miller did, knowing that they are seeking some kind of "balance." They may even intuit that this balance is something far deeper than they originally suspected, even if an important component of their original search was for physical equilibrium. But the possibilities for any kind of balance ultimately depend on what is felt to exist. If the physical body is "real" in this sense and what we think it is, then we could say that any attempt for health or balance is a search to fulfill *roganirodha,* or the restraint of disease. Seeking to balance the doshas is certainly the aim of ayurveda. It is also the aim of any therapeutic modality seeking to produce a structural or physiological equilibrium. But since yoga is defined as "the cessation of movements in the consciousness," it clearly has a different overall ambition. Yoga tries to create *vrttinirodha,* or the restraint of the modifications of consciousness. That is to say, in yoga, the root cause of all imbalances or diseases is to be found in *chitta* ("pure consciousness") itself. Since the ultimate cause is in consciousness, then it must be addressed there. This invariably means that people start off believing they are aligning themselves with, resolving, and coming to a clearer understanding of one set of issues only to find that a very different set is involved.

A guided plan brought me to B. K. S. Iyengar. Originally, I came to Guruji to counter the physical effects of my severe scoliosis, as well as to learn proper alignment in the asanas. His impact, however, has been much deeper: he has truly been my guru. Through correcting my imbalances, Mr. Iyengar has taught me that if we quiet the mind and listen to our intelligence, we may be guided and provided for. He has helped me in my life and has given me the gift to reach my students.

Like many of my generation, after graduating from college, I longed for meaning in life that went beyond the "American dream" of getting a high-paying job, buying a nice house in the suburbs, and buying the latest fashion of clothes. So the search began.

In 1970, I joined the Peace Corps and was sent to Brazil to provide political consulting services. Realizing the futile nature of pushing U.S. policies on the Brazilian culture, I eventually withdrew from the Peace Corps but continued to live in Rio de Janeiro, teaching English. I had begun to comprehend the importance of ignoring the chattering of my mind and ego and of listening to my intelligence instead. While I was on the right track, I needed more guidance. So fate led me to yoga. One of my English students handed me *Autobiography of a Yogi* by Yogananda and ordered, "You must read this!" Inspired by the book, I started practicing yoga in Brazil and immediately discovered its therapeutic effects on my scoliosis.

Upon returning to the United States, I discovered the teachings of Swami Satchidananda. Although Swamiji led me in an essential journey, I needed more direction as to how to address my scoliosis with precision. After being introduced to Mr. Iyengar's style of yoga by Judith Hanson Lasater and consequently reading Guruji's book *Light on Yoga,* I was determined to meet him. It seemed that he could provide guidance in alleviating the physical ailments of my scoliosis, as well as teach me the proper alignment of the asanas. His book and reputation displayed an incredible technical knowledge of anatomy and proper alignments.

In 1974, I met Mr. Iyengar for the first time in San Francisco. I immediately noticed the difference in his style from that of the calm, peaceful Satchidananda. Mr. Iyengar had no pretenses. He was not dressed in orange robes but instead wore simple shorts that resembled boxer shorts. He certainly was not leading an OM SHANTI chant as Swami Satchidananda had often done. More striking, Guruji emanated fire. He was fired up to teach and adjust students with a *rajasic* nature that I had never before seen in a teacher. He had fire in his eyes, which were like the eyes of a hawk. He could see everything.

In addition to fire, Guruji possessed an incredible intuitive, as well as technical, knowledge of the body and the asanas, which his book and reputation had indicated. His hawk eyes immediately detected my scoliosis and gave me intense adjustments that made a lasting impression. I also felt for the first time that someone not only understood my imbalances but could guide *me* to find balance. At this point, I believed that his yoga was a science.

I felt so dedicated that I went back to my home in Oregon and began to practice three to four hours a day. Shortly after, I discovered that I was pregnant and practiced yoga throughout my pregnancy. Nine months later, I gave birth to a beautiful baby boy, who was delivered at home with no complications. I attribute the positive birthing experience to the Guruji-influenced yoga I did during my pregnancy.

In 1976, my husband and I moved to Palo Alto, California, and inspired from meeting Guruji, I attended the Iyengar Yoga Institute of San Francisco from 1976 to 1979. I made my first visit to Guruji in Pune, India, in 1978. Making the eighteen-hour trek, I had expectations of his attention, as well as being healed. Upon my arrival, however, Mr. Iyengar ignored me. Completely distraught, I realized that I could not rely on Iyengar to heal my ailments. Once he saw the shift, he focused his incredible energy on me and helped me tremendously with my scoliosis. Over the years, he has helped me counter the physical effects of my condition, while avoiding surgery, which Western physicians recommended. Additionally, he touched me in a way that displayed passion and care. I now realize that Guruji's seemingly harsh avoidance of me contained a purposeful lesson: I must learn the balance between seeking help and taking responsibility for my own growth.

Over the years of going to the Institute in Pune and attending conventions, B. K. S. Iyengar always had messages for me. As I have gone through many stages in life—marriage, raising a son, owning a yoga center, and teaching for thirty years—he has led me by teaching me to seek my inner intelligence through his teachings and through the example of his journey of life. His influence on my life has exceeded my original goal of learning alignment in the asanas. Mr. Iyengar is a guru in the true sense of the word, who brings one from darkness to light and who has inspired me in all areas of my life. I began to realize that Iyengar's yoga is definitely more than a science.

This inspiration-connection goes beyond having to be physically by his side or connected on a physical plane. Although I have not had the opportunity to go to the Institute every year, guidance comes from him in my practice. I realize that when one has a connection with Guruji, one does not always have to be in his physical presence or even hear his words. The heart speaks significantly louder if you are willing to be open to the teachings, quiet the mind, and listen from within. Although the delivery is not always how you expect it to be, it is no less significant.

When he has spoken to me or others with harsh words, it is not from anger but rather from impatience. His comments arise from his passion of wanting the Iyengar community to dedicate themselves, as he has, to this powerful system of yoga. Guruji has encouraged me to share this passion with my students. While he has never led me to believe that I must be like him, his inspiration has provided a fire within me to reach my students through my own intelligence. The root, however, is his intelligence. He has set an example for me to give completely to my students.

May we continue to pass Guruji's art and science on from generation to generation. Thank you for the light you have shared with us, Iyengar.

§

ELISE BROWNING MILLER is a senior certified Iyengar Yoga teacher and has been teaching since 1976. A founding director of the California Yoga Center in Mountain View, California, she teaches classes specializing in back and sports-related injuries. She is a faculty member at the Iyengar Yoga Institute of San Francisco and has published numerous articles on scoliosis.

For All We Know

BERYL BENDER BIRCH

The "story" that Western science offers for the mystery of existence is based on its acceptance of the subject–object division. According to that story, or metaphysics, complete knowledge of anything and everything studied, as an object, is possible. This approach has allowed the physical body—seen purely as a physical body—to be divided into the generally accepted structural and functional systems: urinary, skeletal, nervous, muscular, digestive, lymphatic, endocrine, respiratory, reproductive, cardiovascular, immunological, and integumentary. Unfortunately, this list tells us nothing about what it is like to be an owner. It does not tell us why we possess such systems. And it certainly does not provide any kind of "instruction manual" telling us the best and most propitious way to use all the attributes in our possession.

According to yoga's metaphysics, existence begins with *prakriti* (nature), originally in its *samayavastha* (balanced and unmanifest state). When *purusha* (the universal life principle) stirs it, it becomes *alinga parva* (the imperceptible, not-yet-differentiated universal and primordial substratum for existence). Its inherent *guna*s (qualities)—*sattva* (the illumined), *rajas* (the energetic), and *tamas* (the inert)—begin to vibrate. As the vibrations take hold, *mahat* (the cosmic intelligence) begins to manifest itself, and the possibility for differentiation begins to exist. The initial result is *linga matra parva,* which is an apprehensible, observable, and phenomenal but still-generalized state. Observers and objects have been created only in principle, the finer details still needing to be elucidated. Given that the three gunas remain essentially balanced, although vibrating, this is an *avishesha,* or nonparticulate condition of nature. It contains, first, *ahamkara* (the "I-sense"), which provides observers the ability to observe. Second, it contains *bhutadi ahamkara,* the potential for nature to be divided into the *bhutas* (gross elements) that will produce five perceptible things: earth, water, fire, air, and ether. Third, it contains *vaikharika ahamkara,* that part of nature that can modify and interact.

This part can both "do" things and allow things to be done. It leads to the five organs of action—walking, handling objects, excreting, procreating, and speaking—which allow the observers coming into being to interact with the objects being created. Fourth, the avishesha contains *taijas ahamkara,* that part of nature that can brighten and act on the mind. This provides us with the five senses of perception—smell, taste, sight, touch, and hearing—through which the objects created can be independently apprehended.

Once this entire process of evolution has been completed, *asamyavastha,* a definable and particularized condition, has been reached. This is what we see all around us. It is the *vishesha* (differentiated state). Its complete inventory of attributes comprises the five elements; the five organs of action; the five organs of perception; and last but not least, the mind, which allows them all to function together as inner, outer, and the gateway between. All this explains not only the objective "what," but also the subjective "who" and the actualizing "how." As to the "why," yoga recommends copious amounts of practice so that an answer can be seen.

Concerning that practice and the revelation of an answer, since everything in this world is systematically constructed from a primordial samayavastha, then it must be possible to sift and abstract that initial equilibrium out of everything we make contact with, because it is what is common to everything. All we have to do is suitably realign the complete inventory of things in our possession, and we will immediately have restored the cosmos to its original balanced state. Beryl Bender Birch now reflects on the process of discovering and experiencing that process of alignment and realignment.

It is the kind of day that you experience maybe a few times in your life—not often and never always. The air is crystal clear, a rare thing on the East Coast of the United States in the early twenty-first century. It is dry: not a harsh dry, but a clear Colorado mountain dry, a Himalayan dry, an easy-to-breathe dry, a dry that conducts prana like copper wire conducts electrical current, a dry that is free of water molecules hanging on to the dry emptiness and slowing down the process. A sweet, soft air that is just a little cooler than the skin.

And the sky, oh, the sky. Not a single cloud from horizon to horizon—just clear, dry blue. An incredible blue, an infinite blue that stretches out beyond the beyond—reaching out, ever expanding, creating blueness with every moment of its being. How do you speak of it? You don't; you can't. It's unspeakable. How do you give an experience of a blue sky to anyone who hasn't been there with you in that moment to see it with their own eyes? Describing blue, or any color really, has never been an easy thing to do. It isn't given to language. Blue is not even really something that is there. Modern physics tells us that the color itself, the "blueness," is created in the mind's eye. Ancient yoga philosophy tells us it is an arising of consciousness as we perceive it, as conditioned thought, as all things, all experiences, all situations, all thoughts, and all colors. Form arising out of the formless. The unmanifest becoming manifest. Purusha becoming prakriti. Blue is a particular vibration in the spectrum of light. It's a wave. It is hard to understand how we experience blue. How can it be that as I look at this blue sky in front of me now that the blue only exists in my mind? It isn't really blue in and of itself. It's only blue in my mind. Maybe there is no sky there at all.

Blue anything can be compared to other blue things, like the color of lapis lazuli from the mines of Afghanistan, or the blue of bluebells, or the blue of my dog Hopi's eyes. But does that help you to experience the blue, to know blue, to taste it and feel it? You, as you read this, can only go to your memory of blue, a stored image from a past experience of something blue, or you can look at something right now that you perceive as blue. You can't know this sky that I see right here, right now, because it exists only here and now—and the color only in my mind.

The Long Island Expressway isn't the kind of place one would expect to have an experience of *samadhi,* but then samadhi can sort of sneak up on you when you least expect it. I am feeling delicious—no stress, traffic moving freely. I had driven up-island earlier in the day to buy dog food. I have six racing Siberian huskies, and there is a small family business in Huntington, Long Island, about seventy-five miles from my home, that prepares an organic, freshly made dog food, then freezes it in two-pound containers and sells it to people like me. I pick up fifty pounds and begin my hour-and-a-half return journey home. I am feeling grateful, grateful for transportation, grateful for money to buy the gas to make the trip, grateful for my vehicle, grateful for no traffic, grateful for my dogs and the money to buy them organic food, and certainly, grateful for the sky.

The kind of grateful that comes up on you when things are going well and you are just so happy for no particular reason—the kind of gratitude that borders on just breaking into goose bumps.

Maybe part of the bliss has to do with the fact that I am listening to pop star Rod Stewart's CD *It Had to Be You*. Over the past few years, Stewart has recorded a couple of albums of tunes from the great American songbook of timeless standards, wonderful old love songs. And as I listen to his indelible voice singing fragrant old classics like "I'll Be Seeing You," "These Foolish Things Remind Me of You," "The Very Thought of You," and the Hoagy Carmichael classic "The Nearness of You," I am reminded of the great Persian mystic and Sufi poet of the fourteenth century, Hafiz. I think of his poems and his astonishing descriptions of his beloved. His poems are so grounded in the colors of earth and the senses. It's so easy to read his poems as poems for the secular world, the longing for "other," our loved one, thinking in our limited scope that he is talking about some woman, some lover, some special one. Yes, he is talking of a special one, the One. One Taste, the Boundless Beloved, Brahman.

I wonder how Hafiz would relate to contemporary poems and songs written to express the romantic pleas of the modern era, that of our love for some one person on whom we have pinned our expectations of happiness. Our joy, our bliss at the nearness of "you." Our aching for the girlfriend who left, or the boyfriend who didn't call, or the husband who is away on a trip.

The sun is shining. Rod is singing. I am driving my dog truck, only no dogs are traveling with me today. It's too hot. I start listening to the lyrics. All these old tunes, all composed by different writers, yet all longing for the same thing. Who were the writers of these songs talking to? They all seem to be talking to the same person, really. And although, for all I know, they weren't exactly written as lilting love songs to the divine, then again, perhaps they were.

These songs, the voice of Rod Stewart, begin to expand in my mind. The wonderful old tunes of my youth that brought longing for this boyfriend or that, for some future moment when everything would work out, for the finding of that like-minded energy that would complete my soul, I now begin to hear in a new way. I am listening with the ear of the seeker, the *sadhu,* the saint reaching out to the divine. Longing for sight of the Boundless One. Couldn't this be Krishna counseling Arjuna in the epic Indian classic, the *Bhagavad Gita*? "Look for me, Arjuna, look in the morning sun. I am there. You will be looking at the moon, but it will be Me you will see."

At this moment, this precise moment, as Rod is singing "tomorrow may never come," none other than perfectly now—no past, no future, no time—my eyes shift to the side of the road, and there is the body of a deer, crumpled, curled like an embryo, knocked to the ground by the modern age, precious and empty of life, dragged aside and dead. *We come and go like a ripple on a stream.* No longer a physical being—warm and breathing, heart beating, eyes gazing softly into the future. No longer filled with life and curiosity. In that moment, all the heavens opened and the light of the understanding was blinding. No words, no thoughts, just a boundless knowing. Infinite consciousness came flooding into the car, blinding the seers for miles around. Tears of joy and bliss ran down the road, and the deer ascended to the heavens in chariots of light. This is it. For the gazillionth time. None other than this. *Ishvara pranidhana,* surrender not to something out there. Not to form or name or image. Not to a thought or a picture. Not even to the guru. Surrender only to now. Not to anything of this world and yet to everything of this world. Surrender to this moment.

The light ahead on the road turned red, and I had to stop. I took a deep breath. What bliss. I reached out to catch hold of the moment, but it was gone. I was still grateful. I drove home, careful to keep an eye out for deer eating the new green grass growing along the side of the road.

When Kofi asked me to write a piece for this commemorative book on the lifework of Mr. B. K. S. Iyengar, I was so honored that I jumped at the chance. What an opportunity to pay tribute to one of the most respected teachers of yoga in the world and to a man who has affected every aspect of teaching yoga in the West. I had forgotten one very important piece of information—I had never met Mr. Iyengar! Not only that, I'd never even taken a class with him. How in the world could I have anything to contribute? What could I say that would be of interest? The work and teaching of Mr. Iyengar have been a pivotal influence in my life. Yes, it was true I had never met or studied with him, but perhaps I did have something to contribute. I might be typical of the many hundreds of thousands of yoga practitioners around the world who, like me, have never met him, but whose practice has been strongly affected by his teaching.

I had been a student of the eight-limbed path of ashtanga yoga since the early seventies. I had bought *Light on Yoga,* Iyengar's seminal work, in 1972, six years after its first publication. It was the first yoga book I bought. Back in the early seventies, there were not too many other choices. *Light on Yoga,* being the "bible" and consummate research source for almost any foray into yoga, is a complex text. As most serious practitioners of yoga know, the book not only describes the general philosophy of classical yoga as set down in the *Yoga Sutras* (the authoritative ancient text on the eight-limbed path), it also details the procedure for the practice of hundreds of asanas and outlines a number of potential asana sequence practices that one can take on to begin the study of yoga. So I sat down and looked through it. Whew, it was undoubtedly impressive, but it was a little overwhelming. The whole project seemed a little lengthy to me. I did not have that kind of time, I thought. There had to be a quicker/easier way to come to know God. I put the book up on the shelf. It looked good up there. I had *Light on Yoga* now; I could check that off the list of things to "get."

Patanjali, the author of the *Yoga Sutras,* does not say very much about asana. But he does make clear that the study of asana is meant to precede the study of more subtle aspects of the spiritual path of yoga, such as meditation, and that it is nearly impossible to train the mind for meditation without first training the body and mind in the practice of asana. So this study of asana is an important step.

This was a little disturbing for me to discover, because I had apparently done it all backward. I began the yoga path in 1971 with the study of meditation through biofeedback training and through the teachings of Munishree Chitrabhanu, a Jain monk, and Chögyam Trungpa Rinpoche, a Tibetan Buddhist monk. I took some asana classes here and there with Yogi Bhajan in the Kundalini tradition and Swami Vishnudevananda of the Sivananda Yoga organization. I even took enough classes to begin to realize the benefits of this "yoga stuff," and I began teaching the Sivananda style of asana in 1974 to skiers in Winter Park, Colorado. But compared to what was to come, I was still just dabbling around. I was serious about meditation but did not really "get" asana—all that was to change soon.

I decided to rethink the importance of this asana thing. One day in the mid-seventies, I signed up for a three-day workshop in Denver with Judith Hanson Lasater, another of Mr. Iyengar's "senior" students. It was hot, it was hard, it was precise, and it was technically difficult. I think on that day I understood the point of asana and realized, for the first time, the connection between entry-level asana and the more advanced "limbs" of the classical yoga path. On that day, I embarked on a lifelong journey in the yoga tradition of perhaps the most influential yoga teacher of this century, Sri Tirumalai Krishnamacharya. He was not only Iyengar's teacher, but also that of three other accomplished contemporary teachers: Indra Devi, K. Pattabhi Jois, and T. K. V. Desikachar (Krishnamacharya's son), all of whom have had a profound effect on the teaching of classical yoga and its powerful component of asana in the West.

I continued for the next six years or so to study and take workshops with some of Mr. Iyengar's top students, including Ramanand Patel, Aadil Palkhivala, and John Schumacher. I learned a great deal about the importance of the correct practice of asana from these teachers. And I began to read *Light on Yoga*. Then in 1980, I discovered a form of asana practice that its main proponent, Sri K. Pattabhi Jois, calls "Ashtanga."

My teacher was a man named Norman Allen, who had recently returned to New York after many years in India, where he had been the first Western student of Mr. Jois and the first to master the entire series of this demanding and difficult asana practice. After attending a yoga workshop given by Norman in 1980 in New York City, which included a short demonstration of the Ashtanga practice, I was completely captivated by its flowing strength and sequencing. The moment I saw it, I felt as if I had discovered an old friend and asked immediately to be taken on as a student.

The next day, filled with enthusiasm, I showed up at Norman's yoga *shala* with mat in hand. Norman welcomed me and said, "Oh, you are here. Welcome. Please sit." *Okay,* I thought. *I can do this.* I sat. There were two people in the middle of the room doing practice. After about twenty minutes, I got a little fidgety. Surely he was going to ask me to start any moment. I waited. Time passed. I cleared my throat. Norman didn't seem to notice me. An hour passed. Two hours. The two people who were practicing finished and left. Norman turned to me and said, "Oh, you are still here? Good. Yes, you come back tomorrow." That was it. I left.

I came back the next day, eager, with my mat under my arm once again. Surely today Norman would ask me to practice. "Oh, you are here again. Good. You sit. You watch." *Wait a minute,* I thought. *I sat yesterday. Wasn't that enough? He wants me to sit again? How long can this possibly go on?* I fidgeted, mostly thinking about how soon I could get started. An hour passed. Two. The two or three people practicing finished, took rest, and left.

"Yes, you, you are here? Good. You come back tomorrow." I came back tomorrow and the day after that and the day after that. Soon Norman didn't have to say anything. I knew the drill. I just came in and sat down, no longer with an impatient sigh, but with a developing interest in the practice and an emergent ability to actually *watch*. One day after a couple of weeks of this exercise, I arrived at the yoga shala and plunked myself down. On this day, I just finally surrendered. I gave up having any hope of ever learning or doing this practice. I did not even know what I was doing there any longer. At that moment, Norman walked over to me and said, "You, you do sun salutations."

"Oh, my God! Really?!" Well, needless to say, no one had to teach me sun salutations: I had been watching the damned things for nearly two weeks. I wasn't exactly sure of what the people I had been watching were doing with their breath, to make that funny sound, but I almost had it figured out. When I finished about three Surya Namaskar As and three Surya Namaskar Bs, Norman came over and suggested I do them again. He made some suggestions about my breathing and about my form and corrected a few mistakes. Then he went off to work with someone else who was just beginning. When I finished, he came back and said, "You lie down, you take rest. You come back tomorrow."

And so it went. I came to learn the practice of what Pattabhi Jois, Norman's teacher, called Ashtanga Yoga. One day at a time. Twenty-four days a month at 5:30 AM, twelve months a year. No practice on the full moon, the new moon, or Saturdays. Other than those six days a month, I was there every day, learning the practice posture by posture. This was the traditional way of teaching. Every day, you did what you did the day before, and maybe your teacher would give you a new posture or two when you were ready. Slowly you developed endurance and strength of body and mind. Not like today, where anyone can stumble into an "open" class at a gym or studio and nearly do themselves in trying to make it all the way through a Primary Series class, for example, with no training and no *watching*!

It was a wonderful time. I had just moved back to New York from Colorado. I was teaching a couple of yoga classes a week with one or two people in each class; so for all practical purposes, I had no money. I couldn't even afford to buy a subway token to go back and forth to the yoga shala, so I walked several miles a day to practice. The money I did manage to round up, I gave to Norman for my training. On one level, the practice was extremely difficult and challenging. My shoulders and rotator cuff muscles were as tight as the lid on the raspberry jam I tried to open this morning. They had been tight since my high school athletic days and were still tight. Every posture involving the shoulders—which, of course, is most of them—was difficult.

But then I think back to the ease with which I learned the practice and moved steadily through the sequences. How had that happened? Perhaps because of the intelligent and patient way I was taught the practice. But the other reason was that the postures were recognizable. Although there were some minor variations from the Iyengar tradition in a few postures, most were well-known to me, and I had blessedly learned the correct alignment for them. Although I couldn't always do them correctly, I knew to some degree how they were *supposed* to look. So I was trying to move in the right direction. For example, when Norman would assist me in marichyasana C, I remembered the posture from *Light on Yoga*. I remembered something Judith or Kofi or Aadil had said. I remember hearing, "As Mr. Iyengar says, 'Drag your organs through' before making the twist." I now use this quote when I teach. How in the world do I know what Mr. Iyengar says? The same way we know what Buddha or Einstein or Hafiz or Galileo said.

The alignment of every asana within every sequence I practice or teach is affected by the teachings of Mr. Iyengar. I have been teaching yoga since 1974 and training yoga teachers since 1985, and my abilities to think out of the box, to do original asana sequencing, to develop modifications within the Ashtanga system, and to work therapeutically with individuals have been augmented by my studies of Iyengar Yoga. With every breath I take through the incredibly brilliant methodology of the eight-limbed path of classical yoga, there is not a moment that passes that my *abhyasa* (practice) is not influenced either directly or indirectly by the dedication and hard work of this man from Pune. The contribution his work has made to the general understanding in all yoga schools of how postures are to be practiced, both safely and therapeutically, is immeasurable. It is impossible to comprehend the scope of his teaching and wisdom.

I am out driving on the Long Island Expressway again today. The fog is rolling in off the ocean, and the air is heavy and wet. Rod Stewart is not singing, and no CD is playing. There is a little traffic. I don't see any deer on the side of the road. I wonder about the unique sets of circumstances that bring us to yoga. Where did the journey start? How many lifetimes ago? Can you remember the first glimmer of wakefulness? Who called to you? Who set you on your journey? Do you know? Maybe it was that first yoga class you took, when Mr. Iyengar (or your teacher) said to you, "Hey, you over there! Hello! Yo, you there! Pay attention! Bring your big toes together. Internally rotate the femur bones. Lift the sternum. Tuck the tailbone. Level the chin. Let the scapulae slide down your back."

Pay attention? Pay attention to what? you wondered.

"Be mindful of your alignment," Mr. Iyengar prompted.

You surrender to the idea that you could use a little restructuring. It *might* help. And then that radiant moment arrives when you turn your attention to the physical structure of self. When you first realize that you can have some effect, some control, over how you stack up, how you go through the world, how purusha particularizes in you. That you can actually sit back and observe yourself. That *who you truly are* and the *form* of your body are not stuck together with insoluble superglue. That who you are can stand back and take an objective look at yourself. How amazing. This is a big jump in perception.

Slowly this leads to the discovery, perhaps a little farther down the road, that the same thing is true for your thoughts. One day, while attempting to find the correct alignment of trikonasana, your mind spins through and ticks off the directives: *Keep my quadriceps lifted, my spine extended, my arches lifted and my feet anchored, my breath even, and my gaze steady.* Then out of nowhere, imperceptibly, for a second or two it all comes together. You relax, and your attention is steadfast. You are *there,* actually, more correctly, you are *here.* Boom. Just like that. Bliss. Then, blam, a thought interrupts: *Gee, I wonder if my teacher is seeing how good I am in this posture at this moment?* You shifted slightly, the breath wavered. And a bell rang, and you noticed! You noticed your distraction. You *actually noticed* that your attention wavered. You came off the breath and on to the movie of hope that your teacher was watching you. And in that instant you actually separated from conditioned thought and noticed your new position, The Witness. In that moment, perhaps for the first time, you recognized that the true self is separate from your thoughts. And your journey has begun.

Abhyasa means "effort toward steadiness of mind." If you aren't making an effort to "pay attention" in your asana practice, well, it just isn't *practice.* Your practice teaches you to focus, to pay attention, or as I like to say, it teaches you to get your attention in present time. It is that struggle to stay firmly rooted in the present that enables you, for a moment, an instant, to have a true *experience* of yoga, the result of the quieting of the mind. The mind "quiets" because it is busy directing its attention to something. The mind becomes, through your efforts and training, very interested in your point of focus, and distractions—both outer and inner—fall away. You start with asana on the physical plane and work from there. Slowly over the years, your sense of awareness grows, and you begin to disconnect from conditioned thought—for even just a moment. In that instant, the *vrittis* are still. You breathe. You find stillness in the posture for a moment. Slowly, the obstacles diminish. You practice for a long time, without a break, with earnestness. Ever seeing the bigger picture. Ever becoming more wakeful. Not finished. Not perfect. Not realized. Just working to be here. Just this.

As I look back on my journey and that of so many others who began yoga in the late sixties and early seventies in this country, and as I imagine the voyage of those who are just starting today, I am reminded again and again of the importance of the tangible methodology of the eight-limbed path, this set of instructions, created thousands of years ago in the *Yoga Sutras* and carried impeccably forward over the generations to this day, to Krishnamacharya and through him to Mr. Iyengar. I am taken with the applicability of the ancient *Yoga Sutras* for the modern world and simultaneously with the incredible evolution of this system called yoga. Its ability to be fixed and flexible, unchanging yet impermanent, dual and nondual, all at the same time, is a mystery understood only by those who *know* yoga. Mr. Iyengar, through his tireless personal abhayasa (practice), his endless experimentation and *viveka* (discernment), and his constant *svadhyaya* (self-study), has walked this path and knows this journey. He has made the trip himself, realizing slow, steady evolution—from his very first day of asana practice to the experience of yoga itself.

Thank you, Mr. Iyengar, for all you do in this world. *Soham.*

§

BERYL BENDER BIRCH has been a student of yoga since 1971 and is the author of the best-selling books *Power Yoga* and *Beyond Power Yoga,* poetic and philosophical tours of the eight limbs. She is the founder/director of The Hard & The Soft Ashtanga Yoga Institute in East Hampton, New York. She now travels and teaches yoga all over the world, guiding and inspiring students of all levels with her down-to-earth style. Her school has been training yoga teachers in the nondual methodology of classical yoga since 1980.

The Light of Yoga

ALI MACGRAW

According to yoga, the cause of all life's troubles is *avidya* (ignorance) of our true nature. Removing that ignorance is yoga's primary objective. Its cosmology makes it very clear that the universe knew exactly what it was doing when it first created the world, and that it knows exactly what it is doing as it is creating this world right now. It is only we, its end products, who do forget or have forgotten. The fact that the universe can be brought into being is personified by Brahma, the Creator. Brahma therefore represents that faculty of ourselves, in this present universe, that produced and produces this world. But the knowledge he needs to do this is vested in his consort, the goddess Sarasvati, who is the goddess of learning. By tradition, Sarasvati has four arms representing *manas* (mind); *buddhi* (intelligence); *ahamkara* (ego, or "I"-sense); and *chitta* (pure consciousness). She therefore represents the part of us that knows but also seeks *vidya* (truth).

Once created, the universe must be maintained. This is given over to Vishnu. His ability to find all the resources necessary to achieve his goal is assigned to his consort Lakshmi, the goddess of wealth.

The universe will eventually come to an end. The transformation of all things back to their original condition is undertaken by Shiva, whose name means "beneficent one." All materiality along with the potential for destructibility is the property of his consort, Parvati (also known as Annapurna, which means "giver of food"). It is she who gives the senses of perception the "food" they need to perceive objects, all of which Shiva can then remove and destroy.

The three goddesses—Sarasvati, Lakshmi, and Parvati—represent aspects of us that gradually awaken as we embark on the practice of yoga. In *Yoga Sutra* II:2, Sage Patanjali tells us that yoga can remove all the afflictions of life. As those afflictions are removed, a deep *santosha* (contentment) comes as a prerequisite for *samadhi* (enlightenment). That contentment is a gift from these three divine ladies who also reside within us.

Unfortunately, and as Ali MacGraw describes, our modern world makes it difficult to appreciate such things. It almost seems to be the duty of our hurly-burly society, with all its advertisements and imperatives, to bombard us with a string of wants and desires, all of which foster a discontent that we must then seek to satisfy through the goods and activities society proffers. But new cravings simply step forward to take the place of old ones. We proceed to identify ourselves with those lusts and cravings and are lost.

Patanjali tells us however, that this ignorance can be destroyed. The net result is a truer and deeper contentment or serenity (santosha). That serenity comes because we make a firm, almost moral decision to live and think in a particular way. We place our faith in our selves—and in our three goddesses. We sense that these personalized gifts from Sarasvati, Lakshmi, and Parvati are within us and that they cannot be lost even when we find ourselves surrounded by chaos, disharmony, and crises of all kinds. As Ali MacGraw describes here, the purpose of the eight limbs of yoga—as of the three goddesses—is to give us a way to realize our full potential as human beings and thus seek liberation.

M y first exposure to yoga? I can remember my mother—nearly seventy years old at the time—walking shyly through our living room in a black leotard. She told me that she had just joined a yoga class in our rural neighborhood and that everyone else in the class was in their thirties. This was in the 1970s, and I did not pay that much attention; I was used to her unusual interests and did not realize that this one went beyond esoteric exercise. I admired both of my parents very much; they were what today would be called bohemians, artists, or individuals. So much of what they did and talked about and read seemed so exotic, even peculiar, to me then. I was not ready to investigate my mother's yoga or my father's many books by Krishnamurti—not yet.

It was not until I was living in Los Angeles, years and lifetimes later, that I happened upon yoga for myself. I was at a gathering of women where I noticed that an old friend whom I had known and admired for years (and through more than one of life's dramas) seemed to have an altogether different energy about her. When I asked her what was going on in her life, she answered that she had been practicing yoga for a while and that it had changed her life. I could see that. There was a stillness and a focus about her that was completely new: she seemed entirely present. She invited me to join her in a class that very day, and I have been practicing ever since. Yoga has utterly changed my life, and today, although I have been practicing for more than fifteen years, I write this as a virtual beginner.

Each day I bring my old/new body to the mat and wait to see what will be revealed by the asana. I have learned that, for me, it changes every single day. For someone who lived her life in an almost manic state of attempted overachievement and goals, this new acceptance of "What is today?" is brand-new; it has taken me a long time. I see how I sped through my life from the very beginning—through schools and college and assorted "shiny" jobs with a focus that was so result driven that I barely experienced the minutiae of the present as I strove for the illusion of "perfect." When I was going to school, no one ever told us that living life was about the ongoing micromoments of our everyday lives; we were all geared up to try to excel, to be perfect. As the years have flown by, I have learned—largely through the tools of yoga—that this old behavior very often produces anxiety, self-involvement, a sense of separation, and even sadness. Where is the joy in all that constant judgment of performance? Could the journey become the destination? And when was there ever a mention of humility, of the real connection with all of life? How was it possible, with the old behaviors, to feel the thrill of being a part of a much bigger whole (instead of the overrated "star" piece)? And how was it possible to dare to free-fall into the even bigger mystery of life?

Today I know that I know nothing. I have started my daily yoga practice all over again, partly because of a shoulder injury, and partly because I have at last encountered the yoga teachings of B. K. S. Iyengar. Over the years, I have studied with various gifted teachers, have learned from all of them, and have tried to incorporate their best teachings into my own private practice. I am grateful to so many of them for the ways they have changed my life.

But it was only when I had the honor of participating in a Los Angeles celebration of the life and work of Mr. Iyengar and to be in his presence that I felt, for the first time, the ecstatic light that is in yoga. I honor and respect the daily discipline, the ongoing *practice* of yoga. I have stopped beating myself up for not being able to "do" certain aspects or asanas. My meditation practice is still uneven; there are many days when I am disappointed by my lack of focus. But I am learning a bit of patience, and this has taken an incredibly long time. I am beginning to understand the concept of not comparing myself to others, which is a real stumbling block to happiness. I have begun to accept the limitations of aging (that most negative of events in our youth-obsessed American society). I feel less separate from people and from the whole of creation. I feel the possibility of faith and joy.

I am indebted to Sri B. K. S. Iyengar and all of the men and women he has guided and taught over the ninety years of his own journey. I am deeply humbled to be invited to write this for him. Thank you.

ALI MACGRAW is an alumna of Wellesley College. She began working in 1960 as a photographic assistant at *Harper's Bazaar;* she then worked as an assistant to the legendary fashion maven, Diana Vreeland, at *Vogue;* as a fashion model; and as a photographer's stylist. She gained notice for her acting in *Goodbye, Columbus,* but real stardom came in 1970 with *Love Story,* for which she was nominated for the Academy Award for Best Actress. MacGraw's keen eye and sense of style were celebrated on the cover of *Time.* She wrote a well-received autobiography, *Moving Pictures.* In 1991, *People* magazine chose her as one of the 50 Most Beautiful People in the World. She has resided in New Mexico for many years and in 2006 made her Broadway debut (at age sixty-eight) as a dysfunctional matriarch in the drama *Festen (The Celebration).* Ali has practiced yoga for many years and produced a well-loved video with Erich Schiffmann.

APPENDIX

The Yogacharya Festival in Honor of B. K. S. Iyengar

The following two contributions were written especially for the catalog of the Yogacharya Festival, a gathering in 2007 to celebrate B. K. S. Iyengar's life's work and teaching.

FROM JOYCE STUART

The inspiration I received from attending a 1967 yoga course in London has never waned in the forty years since. My contact with the great master B. K. S. Iyengar has been maintained and has allowed his "light" to penetrate more deeply. As my personal studies and practice have continued, I have developed a greater awareness and widened my channel of knowledge.

As teachers, we start by working with basically healthy people to enable them to remain that way and gradually develop an understanding of the methods necessary to treat certain ailments. Having observed and occasionally assisted in the medical classes in Pune, our eyes are opened to the necessity of helping people who require more personal attention. Our confidence in our abilities to aid those in need develops, but we always acknowledge the source that makes it possible for us to give that aid. Our reward is the deepening of a personal knowledge that will always be open to a higher authority.

A study of the *Yoga Sutras* of Patanjali gives us a greater understanding of the philosophy on which the great soul, known affectionately to us as "Guruji," bases his system of yoga. The union of body, mind, and spirit that emanates from him is its essence and is based on his personal experience. This is perhaps one of the most telling facets of Guruji's awareness. He never teaches anything he has not already experienced and thereafter checked with the source sutras.

In his role of "darkness dispeller" may the Lord grant B. K. S. Iyengar many more years of abundant life to enable his students around the globe to be led from "darkness to light." May the purity of his teachings be maintained worldwide on this auspicious occasion.

From Baron Baptiste

Dear Mr. Iyengar,

You are a source of profound knowledge, and you have been a light in my life and my teaching.

We all have our share of difficulties and challenges, and we all look for sources of inspiration to carry us through. In my case, much inspiration as a teacher and person has come from you.

My first introduction to you and your work came to me through my parents at the age of sixteen, when you were visiting San Francisco in the early 1980s. At that early age, you helped to spark a flame in me that to this day has not died. More recently, I had the opportunity to spend several days with you at Estes Park in Colorado, which was a confirmation that even today you remain a man of remarkable strength, insight, and common sense, who always seems to know what to do in every situation. It is very helpful to me that I have found someone in you who is stronger than I am, but human too.

You are an inspiration to me in the following ways: You have beliefs and the courage to communicate them. You see things for yourself from your inner light. You set an example. You stand up to bullies or those who would attempt to malign your name or words. You deal with first things first. Loyalty is a vital virtue to be developed in those you surround yourself with.

Also, I have learned from you that throughout your teachings you seek to demonstrate the effectiveness of the lessons you have learned with hard evidence. You seem to believe and therefore demonstrate *proof more than theories, results more than rhetoric.* You did what you had to do, and you saw it through without exception, rather than following the crowd.

As a younger man, I am learning that being grateful for what I have, and for those who inspire me, is often my greatest balm. Mr. Iyengar, to you I am grateful for staying the course, for staying true to yourself and your god, and for never losing belief in your own voice and inner sense in a world that would have us conform.

That is how you live, and your belief in yourself is a great inspiration to me.

Salutations,

BARON BAPTISTE
OCTOBER 2, 2006

Acknowledgments

First and foremost, I would like to thank my Beloved Guruji, Yogacharya Sri B. K. S. Iyengar, for his lifelong inspiration and guidance. I would also like to thank all the contributors to this commemorative volume for the selfless and enthusiastic way in which they responded to my request to offer one chapter each in honor of him, and as a way of assisting him in his work to help the citizens of his home village, Bellur, Karnataka State, India.

I acknowledge the most kind assistance of Philippe Harari and Judith Jones in helping me piece together the early history of Iyengar Yoga in the U. K. I also acknowledge the kindness, dedication, enthusiasm, and assistance given to me well beyond the call of duty by Jonathan Green, Emily Bower, Sara Bercholz, and all the other employees of Shambhala Publications who kindly agreed to help this book see the light of day. I give my sincere thanks to my literary agent, Jeanne Fredericks, who had enough faith to convert the germ of my idea into publishable form.

And finally, there are not enough words to thank Anne O'Brien, who oversaw this project from the time that I first approached her, close to its inception, right through to its completion. She came up with several ideas for its improvement, prepared the book proposal, gathered the materials together, liaised with selected contributors, conducted and edited all the interviews, and performed so many other services with a constant and unfailing enthusiasm, that if I were to list them all they would probably double the length of this book.

Index of Contributors